EDITION

T0210288

Mosby's
Exam Review
for COMPUTED
TOMOGRAPHY

Daniel N. DeMaio, MEd, RT(R)(CT)
Chair
Department of Health Sciences and Nursing
Director
Radiologic Technology Program
University of Hartford
West Hartford, Connecticut

ELSEVIER

ELSEVIER

3251 Riverport Lane
St. Louis, Missouri 63043

MOSBY'S EXAM REVIEW FOR COMPUTED TOMOGRAPHY, THIRD EDITION

ISBN: 978-0-323-41633-7

Notices

Knowledge and best practice in this field are constantly changing. As new research and experience broaden our understanding, changes in research methods, professional practices, or medical treatment may become necessary.

Practitioners and researchers must always rely on their own experience and knowledge in evaluating and using any information, methods, compounds, or experiments described herein. In using such information or methods they should be mindful of their own safety and the safety of others, including parties for whom they have a professional responsibility.

With respect to any drug or pharmaceutical products identified, readers are advised to check the most current information provided (i) on procedures featured or (ii) by the manufacturer of each product to be administered, to verify the recommended dose or formula, the method and duration of administration, and contraindications. It is the responsibility of practitioners, relying on their own experience and knowledge of their patients, to make diagnoses, to determine dosages and the best treatment for each individual patient, and to take all appropriate safety precautions.

To the fullest extent of the law, neither the Publisher nor the authors, contributors, or editors, assume any liability for any injury and/or damage to persons or property as a matter of products liability, negligence or otherwise, or from any use or operation of any methods, products, instructions, or ideas contained in the material herein.

Library of Congress Cataloging-in-Publication Data

Names: DeMaio, Daniel N., author.
Title: Mosby's exam review for computed tomography / Daniel N. DeMaio.
Other titles: Exam review for computed tomography
Description: Third edition. | St. Louis, Missouri : Elsevier, [2018] |
   Includes bibliographical references and index.
Identifiers: LCCN 2017035969 | ISBN 9780323416337 (paperback)
Subjects: | MESH: Tomography, X-Ray Computed | Examination Questions
Classification: LCC RC78.7.T6 | NLM WN 18.2 | DDC 616.07/57076–dc23 LC record available at https://lccn.loc.gov/2017035969

Senior Content Strategist: Sonya Seigafuse
Senior Content Development Manager: Ellen Wurm-Cutter
Content Development Specialist: Sarah Vora/ Charlene Ketchum
Publishing Services Manager: Deepthi Unni
Project Manager: Janish Ashwin Paul
Designer: Ryan Cook

Working together
to grow libraries in
developing countries

www.elsevier.com • www.bookaid.org

Printed in India
Last digit is the print number: 9 8 7

For my family – Christine, Ryan, and Emily.

CONTENT AND ORGANIZATION

Mosby's Exam Review for Computed Tomography is designed to prepare the radiologic technologist for successful completion of the American Registry of Radiologic Technologists (ARRT) Advanced Certification Examination for Computed Tomography. This review text will also help prepare the nuclear medicine technologist for the Computed Tomography certification examination offered by the Nuclear Medicine Technology Certification Board (NMTCB). Because many general radiographers and nuclear medicine technologists are now cross-training in computed tomography and are performing computed tomography as part of their daily practice, this text will be a valuable resource for preparing for the applicable CT certification examination.

This text first offers a thorough review in an outline format of the content areas on the ARRT Computed Tomography Examination: Patient Care, Safety, Image Production, and Procedures. The review is followed by three 165-question mock examinations and answer keys.

FEATURES

Simulated Examinations

The format of the questions is similar to the ARRT examination. Answers and rationales are provided for each question.

Evolve Resources

One of the most valuable features of this review resource is the accompanying Evolve site, **http://evolve.elsevier. com/DeMaio/CT**. The Evolve site contains questions that can be randomly accessed to compile an unlimited number of variations of mock examinations. Examinations on the Evolve site may be taken in quiz mode with immediate feedback or in a timed mode to simulate the actual examination experience.

Daniel N. DeMaio

Sincere thanks to the superb staff of Elsevier, including Sonya Seigafuse, Sarah Vora, and Janish Paul. Working with editor Charlene Ketchum was an absolute pleasure, and I am very appreciative of her guidance and support throughout this project.

I am truly grateful to Mr. Steven Ahrenstein. Not only did he provide me with some excellent images for this revised edition, but he was also my first CT teacher and helped instill within me a love for this imaging modality that I still carry to this day.

To my friends and colleagues at the University of Hartford, thanks for all that you do in support of me, our programs, and our students. I could not ask for a better group of professionals to work with.

To my students, past and present, it remains a distinct honor for me to be a part of your education in the radiologic sciences. I have the best job in the world, and so much of that is because of you.

To my wife and best friend Christine, our son Ryan, and our daughter Emily, you make me the proudest husband and father on the planet. I love you all more than I'll ever be able to describe with words on a page.

Daniel N. DeMaio

CONTENTS

PART 1

CHAPTER OUTLINE

AMERICAN REGISTRY OF RADIOLOGIC TECHNOLOGISTS POSTPRIMARY CERTIFICATION IN COMPUTED TOMOGRAPHY

Technologists who wish to enter the postprimary pathway to certification in computed tomography (CT) must hold a registration in one of the following supporting categories:
- Radiography
- Nuclear Medicine Technology
- Radiation Therapy

To attain eligibility for American Registry of Radiologic Technologists (ARRT) certification in CT, technologists must complete a minimum of 16 hours of structured education credits in topics that reflect the certification examination content. In addition, candidates for CT certification are required to document performance of core clinical procedures to establish eligibility. Specific educational and clinical requirements and documentation procedures may be obtained from the ARRT.

The ARRT postprimary examination in CT was first offered in March 1995. It was designed to give the technologist an opportunity to become certified in the specific modality of CT. The CT registry is a 165-question, multiple-choice examination covering four major subject areas in the following manner:
- Patient Care: 22 questions
- Safety: 20 questions
- Image Production: 55 questions
- Procedures: 68 questions

The latest content specifications for the ARRT examination in CT are provided in the box at the end of this chapter. The approximate number of test questions for each major topic is provided in parentheses. The computer-based CT certification examination is currently given at specific test centers located throughout the United States. Please contact the ARRT (www.ARRT.org) for additional information regarding application procedures, deadlines, testing center locations, and so on.

NUCLEAR MEDICINE TECHNOLOGY CERTIFICATION BOARD POSTPRIMARY CERTIFICATION IN COMPUTED TOMOGRAPHY

Nuclear medicine technologists certified by the Nuclear Medicine Technology Certification Board (NMTCB), the Canadian Association of Medical Radiation Technologists (CAMRT), or the ARRT may be eligible to sit for the new CT certification examination offered by the NMTCB. First offered in 2014, this 200-question multiple-choice examination covers much of the information included on the ARRT certification examination in CT. However, the NMTCB/CT certification examination also includes information pertaining to the hybrid imaging studies that combine CT with molecular imaging techniques such as positron emission tomography (PET) and single-photon emission computed tomography (SPECT).

To attain eligibility for NMTCB certification in CT, technologists must complete a minimum of 35 contact hours of instruction in the following topics:
- Contrast administration
- Cross-sectional anatomy
- X-ray physics
- CT radiation safety

In addition, appropriately credentialed nuclear medicine technologists must complete a minimum of 500 clinical hours in CT, PET/CT, and/or SPECT/CT. Specific educational and clinical requirements and documentation procedures/forms may be obtained from the NMTCB.

USING THIS REVIEW BOOK

The first edition of this book, titled *Registry Review in Computed Tomography,* was developed shortly after I had successfully completed the CT registry examination in March 1995. A second edition published in 2011 was vastly updated and expanded. This third edition incorporates much of the information included in the second edition, but has been completely revised and updated to include the latest information on this dynamic imaging modality. This review text is essentially designed for two different groups of examination applicants. For the established CT technologist, the review outline and examination questions help bridge the gap between clinical experience and cognitive knowledge. Those of you who are experienced in CT will already be familiar with much of the subject matter covered. This review book allows you to answer questions concerning the principles and procedures that you put into practice each day. Used in conjunction with some additional reference materials, this book should adequately prepare you for the CT certification examination.

Keep in mind that the ARRT and NMTCB CT certification examinations are "advanced-level" examinations. Some of the subject matter may go beyond the standard responsibilities of the staff CT technologist. Practical experience in CT does not eliminate the need for study and preparation in order to achieve success on this examination.

Many examinees may be looking to use an advanced-level certification examination as a vehicle toward developing a career in CT. This second group of test applicants may have little experience in CT beyond the ARRT or NMTCB clinical requirements. If you are among this group, you have a significantly larger amount of work ahead of you. It would certainly be advisable to use several of the textbooks listed as references in the bibliography during the initial stages of preparation. It is extremely important to review the physical principles of CT imaging along with the many clinical applications, such as patient care, scanning protocols, cross-sectional anatomy, and the identification of pathology on the CT image. *Mosby's Exam Review for Computed Tomography* will then serve as an invaluable tool to test your newly acquired knowledge and practice "registry-type" questions.

Please remember that the best way to reap benefits from review books such as this one is to concentrate on the material you are unfamiliar with: the questions that you *incorrectly* answer. It is not sufficient to simply grade each examination and calculate your score to determine whether or not you passed the examination. Take the time to carefully review each chapter. If you find that you are in need of further explanation, turn to the bibliography for additional study materials. Attempt the practice examinations with the mind-set that they are "dry runs" for the real thing. After grading a practice examination, concentrate on the questions that you answered incorrectly. Look up each correct answer, read the brief explanation given, and then further review the topic in the review chapter and/or bibliography provided. You have much more to learn from the mistakes that you make, and when properly used, this book will give you the information you need.

TEXT FORMAT

Part I of *Mosby's Exam Review for Computed Tomography* contains a review in outline form of the four content areas covered on the ARRT certification examination in CT. In addition, information specific to the NMTCB certification examination in CT is included in the outline.

Part II contains three examinations and the answers for each examination. A brief explanation accompanies each correct answer, and more detailed information about the question's subject may be found in the review chapters.

Many of the questions in each examination pertain to an included CT image. Be sure to use all of the information provided by the image when attempting to correctly answer these questions. Each examination contains 165 multiple-choice questions. The topics for questions follow the latest content specifications of the ARRT and NMTCB advanced-level examination in CT. Each practice examination is weighted by subject area in a similar manner to the ARRT certification examination."

STUDY HABITS AND TEST-TAKING TECHNIQUES

Each of you preparing to take an advanced-level certification examination in CT is a registered and/or licensed medical imaging technologist. Most of you have already successfully completed a similar certification examination in an imaging discipline. You undoubtedly know how to take standardized examinations, and your previous results support this assumption. However, it may have been some time since you participated in a standardized examination, so here are some points to assist you in your preparation.

1. Do Not Wait Until the Last Minute to Prepare!

Although easier said than done, beginning to study early definitely improves your potential for success. The review chapters are just that—a review! They provide succinct outlines of the pertinent material and will serve as an excellent resource. But you may also find yourself in need of additional, more in-depth information. There is a multitude of excellent resources in both print and online form. Start with a general text in the physical principles of CT and progress through the many clinical applications. Also, a large proportion of the examination pertains to cross-sectional anatomy. Do not rely only on your practical experience in this area. Take care to review the CT images in this text. You may want to refer to the cross-sectional anatomy books listed in the bibliography for additional review. For some people, this book may be sufficient as the sole preparatory tool for the CT examination. However, it is not a "quick fix" and will not make up for lack of adequate experience, research, and study.

2. Practice Your Time Management Skills

Time management is equally important during preparation and while you are taking the actual examination. The ARRT allows you 3.5 hours to complete 165 questions. This should be more than sufficient if you take care to keep track of your progress during the examination. You will be provided with a countdown timer during the computerized examination and should follow the standard rule of not spending too much time on any one question.

3. Zero In on the Correct Answer

Success on standardized examinations relies on your ability not only to choose the correct answer, but also to identify the incorrect ones. The process of elimination is your most valued asset when you encounter a multiple-choice question. Carefully examine each answer, and eliminate those that are obviously incorrect. This step often narrows the possible choices and improves your chances when guessing becomes a necessity.

4. Have Confidence!

You are in the midst of a successful career in medical imaging. Your interest in the field and your dedication to continued learning have brought you here to this advanced-level examination. Have confidence in your ability, and put some faith in your preparation and experience: you know the material, so relax, and simply tap into this knowledge.

AMERICAN REGISTRY OF RADIOLOGIC TECHNOLOGISTS COMPUTED TOMOGRAPHY CERTIFICATION EXAMINATION: CONTENT SPECIFICATIONS

Patient Care (22)
1. Patient interactions and management (22)
   A. Patient assessment and preparation
      1. Clinical history
      2. Scheduling and screening
      3. Education
      4. Consent
      5. Immobilization
      6. Monitoring
         a. Level of consciousness
         b. Vital signs
         c. Heart rhythm and cardiac cycle
         d. Oximetry
      7. Management of accessory medical devices
         a. Oxygen delivery systems
         b. Chest tubes
         c. In-dwelling catheters
      8. Lab values
         a. Renal function (e.g., BUN, eGFR, creatinine)
         b. Other (e.g., D-dimer, LFT, INR)
      9. Medications and dosage
         a. Current
         b. Preprocedure medications (e.g., steroid, antianxiety)
         c. Postprocedure instructions (e.g., diabetic patient)
   B. Contrast administration
      1. Contrast media
         a. Ionic, nonionic
         b. Osmolarity
         c. Barium sulfate
         d. Water soluble (iodinated)
         e. Air
         f. Water
         g. Other
      2. Special contrast considerations
         a. Contraindications
         b. Indications
         c. Pregnancy
         d. Lactation
         e. Dialysis patients
      3. Administration route and dose calculations
         a. IV
         b. Oral
         c. Rectal
         d. Intrathecal
         e. Catheters (e.g., peripheral line, central line, PICC line)
         f. Other (e.g., stoma, intraarticular)
      4. Venipuncture
         a. Site selection
         b. Aseptic and sterile technique
         c. Documentation (e.g., site, amount, gauge, concentration, rate, and number of attempts)
      5. Injection techniques
         a. Safety
         b. Manual
         c. Power injector options
            1. Single or dual head
            2. Single phase
            3. Multiphase
            4. Flow rate
            5. Timing bolus
            6. Bolus tracking

Continued

AMERICAN REGISTRY OF RADIOLOGIC TECHNOLOGISTS COMPUTED TOMOGRAPHY CERTIFICATION EXAMINATION: CONTENT SPECIFICATIONS—cont'd

6. Postprocedure care
   a. Treatment of contrast extravasation
   b. Documentation
7. Adverse reactions
   a. Recognition and assessment
   b. Treatment
   c. Documentation

Safety (20)
1. Radiation safety and dose
   A. Radiation physics
      1. Radiation interaction with matter
      2. Acquisition (geometry)
      3. Physical principles (attenuation)
   B. Radiation protection
      1. Minimizing patient exposure
         a. kVp
         b. mAs
         c. Pitch
         d. Collimation/beam width
         e. Multidetector configuration
         f. Gating
      2. Personnel protection
         a. Controlled access
         b. Education
      3. Shielding
         a. Traditional (e.g., lead apron)
         b. Nontraditional (e.g., bismuth)
      4. Dose measurement
         a. CT dose index (CTDI)
         b. Dose length product (DLP)
         c. Documentation
      5. Patient dose reduction and optimization
         a. Pediatric
         b. Adult
         c. Dose modulation techniques (e.g., SMART mA, auto mA, CARE dose, and SURE exposure)
         d. Iterative reconstruction
         e. Dose notification
         f. Dose alert

Image Production (55)
1. Image formation (30)
   A. CT system principles, operation, and components
      1. Tube
         a. X-ray production
         b. Warm-up procedures
      2. Collimation/beam width
      3. Generator
      4. Detectors
         a. Detector configuration
         b. Detector collimation
      5. Data acquisition system (DAS)
      6. Computer and array processor
   B. Imaging parameters and data acquisition
      1. Parameters
         a. kVp
         b. mAs
         c. Pitch
         d. Acquisition thickness

e. x, y, z planes
f. Scan field of view
2. Acquisition
   a. Axial/sequential
   b. Helical/spiral
   c. Volumetric
C. Image processing
   1. Reconstruction
      a. Filtered back projection reconstruction
      b. Iterative reconstruction
      c. Interpolation
      d. Reconstruction algorithm
      e. Raw data vs. image data
      f. Prospective/retrospective reconstruction
      g. Reconstruction thickness
      h. Reconstruction interval
   2. Postprocessing
      a. Multi-planar reformation (MPR)
      b. 3-D rendering (MIP, SSD, VR)
      c. Quantitative analysis (e.g., distance, diameter, calcium scoring, ejection fraction)
2. Image evaluation and archiving (25)
   A. Image display
      1. Pixel, voxel
      2. Matrix
      3. Image magnification
      4. Display field of view (DFOV)
      5. Window level, window width
      6. Cine
      7. Geometric distance or region of interest (ROI) (e.g., mean, standard deviation [SD])
   B. Image quality
      1. Spatial resolution
      2. Contrast resolution
      3. Temporal resolution
      4. Noise and uniformity
      5. Quality assurance and accreditation
      6. CT number (Hounsfield units)
      7. Linearity
   C. Artifact recognition and reduction
      1. Beam hardening or cupping
      2. Partial volume averaging
      3. Motion
      4. Metallic
      5. Edge gradient
      6. Patient positioning (out-of-field)
      7. Equipment induced
         a. Rings
         b. Streaks
         c. Tube arcing
         d. Cone beam
         e. Capping
   D. Informatics
      1. Hard/electronic copy (e.g., DICOM file format)
      2. Archive
      3. PACS and electronic medical record (EMR)
      4. Security and confidentiality
      5. Networking

PROCEDURES (68)

Type of Study

1. Head, spine, and musculoskeletal (24)
   A. Head
      1. Temporal bones/internal auditory canal (IAC)
      2. Pituitary fossa
      3. Orbits
      4. Sinuses
      5. Maxillofacial and/or mandible
      6. Temporomandibular joint (TMJ)
      7. Base of skull
      8. Brain
      9. Cranium
      10. Brain perfusion
   B. Spine
      1. Cervical
      2. Thoracic
      3. Lumbar
      4. Sacrum/coccyx
      5. Post myelography
      6. Discography
   C. Musculoskeletal
      1. Upper extremity
      2. Lower extremity
      3. Bony pelvis and/or hips
      4. Shoulder and/or scapula
      5. Sternum and/or ribs
      6. Arthrography
2. Neck and chest
   A. Neck
      1. Larynx
      2. Soft tissue, neck
   B. Chest
      1. Mediastinum
      2. Lung
      3. Heart
      4. Airway
      5. Low-dose screening
3. Abdomen and pelvis
   A. Abdomen
      1. Liver
      2. Biliary
      3. Spleen
      4. Pancreas
      5. Adrenals
      6. Kidneys and/or ureters
      7. GI tract
   B. Pelvis
      1. Bladder
      2. Colorectal
      3. Reproductive organs

Focus of Questions

Questions about each of the studies listed on the left may focus on any of the following relevant factors:

Anatomy
- Imaging planes
- Pathological considerations/recognition
- Protocol considerations
- Patient considerations (e.g., pediatric, geriatric, bariatric)
- Postprocessing presentations
- Landmarks

Contrast media
- Indications
- Scan/prep delay
- Effect on images

Additional procedures
- Vascular (CTA, CTV) (e.g., PE, dissection, runoff, venogram)
- Biopsies
- Drainages
- Aspirations

Source: The American Registry of Radiologic Technologists at www.arrt.org.

Review of Patient Care in Computed Tomography

CHAPTER OUTLINE

PATIENT ASSESSMENT AND PREPARATION

A. Clinical History

1. Obtaining an accurate and pertinent patient history is one of the most important responsibilities of the computed tomography (CT) technologist.
2. Proper documentation of the patient's recent procedures, surgeries, symptoms, possible trauma, and specific areas of pain or discomfort can greatly assist the interpreting physician in the diagnostic process.
3. General practices necessary to obtain a good patient history include the following:
   a. Nonleading or open-ended questions that allow the patient to provide the history in his or her own words.
   b. Keen listening and encouragement to maximize the information provided by the patient.
   c. Focused questioning for additional information.
   d. Repeating and summarizing the information provided by the patient to check for accuracy.

B. Scheduling and Screening

1. Communication is the key to any successful patient interaction.

2. It should begin during the scheduling/screening process to identify concerns regarding examination tolerance, potential contrast agent contraindications, and so on.
3. CT examinations of the trunk (chest, abdomen, pelvis) should be scheduled before an imaging procedure that requires high-density oral contrast (barium) or only after sufficient time to allow for bowel clearance. High-density or metallic items, such as jewelry, hair fasteners, and electronic devices, should be removed when necessary and appropriate.
4. Care must be taken to ensure patient comfort on the CT table. This comfort will result in less patient motion and lead to higher-quality CT examinations.

C. Education

1. It is typically the responsibility of the technologist to fully explain the CT procedure to the patient and/or their authorized representative.
2. Clear and thorough explanation by the technologist at the point of care helps make certain that the patient follows the instructions necessary for optimum examination quality.
3. Review breathing instructions when necessary, and include an opportunity for the patient to practice to ensure understanding and compliance.

4. During the CT procedure, the technologist should remain in constant communication with the patient and/or their authorized representative to ensure patient comfort and cooperation.

5. Particularly during contrast studies, the patient should be instructed to empty the bladder before the start of the examination to reduce the possibility of discomfort or interruption.

6. Before contrast agent administration, discuss potential physical effects, such as warm sensation and metallic taste so that the patient is not surprised and upset during data acquisition.

7. Upon examination completion, the CT technologist must provide postprocedural instructions that are appropriate to the age and level of understanding of the patient and/or their authorized representative.

8. The CT technologist should communicate with other authorized service providers to coordinate all necessary follow-up care.

D. Consent

1. The patient is required to provide informed consent before the start of any invasive procedure.

2. Patient consent may be deemed "informed" only when the procedure, including its risks, benefits, and alternatives, are clearly explained in a language the patient fully comprehends.

3. Any patient questions must be adequately answered by qualified personnel before the procedure is begun.

4. The patient or a competent, legal representative must sign a form documenting informed consent for the procedure.

5. A parent or legal guardian must sign the informed consent form for a minor.

6. *Implied consent* occurs when a patient is in need of immediate medical services but is unconscious or is physically unable to consent to treatment. In this case, services are rendered with the assumption that the patient would consent if able.

E. Immobilization

1. As with any imaging procedure, patient motion during the CT examination can cause substantial image degradation.

2. CT scan manufacturers routinely include a variety of cushions, straps, and other safety devices that may be carefully used to help the patient hold still during data acquisition. These items are typically nonabrasive and can be utilized in place of medical tape.

3. The *breath-hold* is another form of patient immobilization required during many CT examinations. Carefully instruct the patient to suspend respiration at the end of inhalation or exhalation, providing a visual example when necessary. Cessation of breathing works to reduce motion and is particularly important during CT imaging of the chest and abdomen.

F. Monitoring

1. A patient who is awake, alert, and responsive is considered to exhibit a normal level of consciousness.

2. There are varying abnormal levels of consciousness:
   a. Patients who are alert and conscious have the ability to fully respond to all stimuli, including the ability to fully answer questions.
   b. In a *lethargic* state, the patient appears drowsy but can be aroused.
   c. The *obtunded* patient is in a more depressed level of consciousness and may not easily be aroused from a state of confusion.
   d. *Stupor* describes a state of near unresponsiveness (semicomatose).
   e. When in a *coma*, the patient is completely unresponsive to stimuli.

3. Vital sign assessment is the measurement of basic body functions to monitor critical information regarding the patient's physical condition.

4. Vital signs are temperature, pulse, blood pressure, and respirations:
   a. Normal body temperature is 97.7° to 99.5°F (36.5° to 37.5°C).
   b. Pulse rate for adults ranges from 60 to 100 beats per minute (bpm). Pulse rate for children ranges from 70 to 120 bpm.
   c. *Systolic blood pressure* indicates the pressure within arteries during cardiac contraction and should be less than 120 mm Hg. *Diastolic pressure* is measured during relaxation of the heart and should be less than 80 mm Hg.
   d. Normal respiration rate for an adult is 12 to 20 breaths per minute and that for a child is 20 to 30 breaths per minute.

5. A *pulse oximeter* is an electronic device used to measure pulse and respiratory status. Placed on a patient's finger, toe, or earlobe, the pulse oximeter measures blood oxygen levels, which are normally between 95% and 100%.

6. The *cardiac cycle* refers to the series of blood flow–related events that occur from the beginning of one heartbeat to that of the next.

7. It is the frequency of the cardiac cycle that determines the patient's heart rate.

8. As related to the cardiac cycle, *diastole* refers to relaxation of heart muscle and *systole* refers to contraction of the heart muscle.

9. An electrocardiogram (ECG) is a graphic representation of the electrical activity of the heart. It is used particularly during cardiac CT procedures to evaluate the heart rhythm and cycle (Fig. 2.1).

10. The cardiac cycle can be divided into the following three distinct stages:
    a. Atrial systole:
       • Contraction of the left and right atria.
       • Corresponds to the onset of the P wave of the ECG.

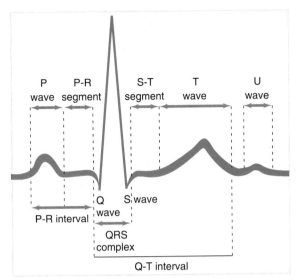

FIG. 2.1 Normal ECG waveform. *(From Ehrlich RA, Daley JA:* Patient care in radiography, *ed 7, St Louis, 2009, Mosby.)*

  b. Ventricular systole:
  - Contraction of the left and right ventricles.
  - Beginning of the QRS complex on the ECG.
  c. Complete cardiac diastole:
  - Period of relaxation after heart contraction.
  - Consists of ventricular diastole and atrial diastole.
  - Corresponds to the T wave of the ECG.
11. Cardiac CT images are typically reconstructed from data acquired during the diastolic phase.
12. Patients with slower heart rates exhibit longer diastolic phases, which yield higher-quality cardiac CT examinations.
13. β-Adrenergic receptor blocking agents (β-blockers) may be used to reduce a patient's heart rate. Sixty-five bpm is the preferred rate for optimal imaging on most multidetector CT (MDCT) systems.
14. Newer systems at the 64-slice level and beyond are capable of acquiring adequate cardiac CT images at higher heart rates. This capability may preclude the need for pharmaceutical intervention as clinically indicated.
15. If not contraindicated, sublingual nitroglycerine may be administered just before the cardiac MSCT study to cause dilation of the coronary vessels, improving their visualization.
16. Please consult the physician and/or department protocol for further information regarding administration of pharmaceuticals for cardiac CT procedures.

G. Management of Accessory Medical Devices

1. Oxygen delivery systems
  a. *Hypoxemia* refers to a condition whereby the patient suffers from a low concentration of oxygen in the blood. The term *hypoxia* describes insufficient oxygenation of tissue at the cellular level.
  b. Hypoxia can lead to general physiologic concerns, including headache, dizziness, and nausea, leading to more serious complications such as *ataxia* (loss of muscular coordination), tachycardia, and *pulmonary hypertension* (increased blood pressure in the pulmonary vasculature). Left untreated, hypoxia can result in *cyanosis* (blue coloration of the skin), low blood pressure, and death.
  c. Localized hypoxia can result in tissue effect such as pain, cyanosis, and eventual gangrene.
  d. Oxygen is considered a drug, and it is typically administered under the order of a physician.
  e. A device is typically used to deliver oxygen in units of liters per minute (LPM) or in a specific concentration (percentage, %).
  f. Most importantly, the CT technologists must never completely remove an oxygen delivery device from the patient without permission from a supervising nurse, respiratory care professional, or independent licensed practitioner (physician, physician's assistant, advanced-practice registered nurse).
  g. Oxygen is typically stored in either gas or liquid form.
  i. Oxygen gas may be supplied in metal tanks that accompany the patient or through an oxygen supply system that is integrated within the facility and accessed via a wall-mounted port within the treatment or scan room.
  ii. In liquid form, oxygen may be supplied in a concentrated and more convenient manner in small, portable tanks.
  h. An *oxygen flow meter* is a valve used to control the rate of oxygen gas delivery in LPM. It may be mounted on a wall outlet or attached to a portable cylinder and will be green in color. There are several options for oxygen delivery:
  i. Nasal cannula, a two-pronged tube inserted into the nose for delivery of oxygen. Typically used to deliver 1 to 5 LPM of oxygen.
  ii. Mask, a simple oxygen mask covers the patient's nose and mouth to deliver oxygen flow rates of 6 LPM or higher.
  - A *nonrebreathing* mask includes an attached reservoir that fills with oxygen and provides a higher percentage of delivery. A nonrebreathing mask includes a one-way valve that prevents the patient from exhaling into the reservoir.
  iii. Ventilator, patients with an insufficient airway or the inability to maintain adequate oxygenation may require intubation with an endotracheal tube and mechanical ventilation.
  - A mechanical ventilator maintains the appropriate volume of delivered oxygen at a controlled pressure and delivery rate.
  - Oxygen and carbon dioxide are exchanged through an artificial airway consisting of either an *endotracheal tube* that has been inserted

into the patient's trachea through the mouth or nose or a *tracheostomy tube* that has been inserted into the trachea through a surgical opening (*tracheotomy*).

- The CT technologist must take great precautions not to disrupt the artificial airway of the ventilated patient. The CT technologist should enlist the assistance of appropriate health care personnel (physician, nurse, respiratory care specialist) when moving and/or positioning the ventilated patient.
- If disruption to the maintained airway occurs, the ventilator may sound an auditory alarm. This alarm should not be silenced by the CT technologist, and an appropriate health care professional (physician, nurse, respiratory care specialist) should be immediately notified.

2. A thoracostomy tube (chest tube) may be in place to drain fluid from the intrapleural space of the ill or injured CT patient.

   a. Chest tubes are commonly used to reestablish and maintain proper intrapleural pressure in patients who have a fluid collection in the lungs (pleural effusion, hemothorax) or a pneumothorax (abnormal collection of air in the pleural space).

   b. The CT technologist must take great caution not to displace or dislodge a chest tube during the transport and positioning of the patient.

3. An in-dwelling catheter is one that remains in place to provide a physiologic function within the patient.

   a. The bladder is a common location for an indwelling catheter, which is used to collect urine into a drainage bag.

   b. Urinary catheterization is the process by which a catheter has been placed into the bladder.

      i. A *Foley* catheter includes a balloon that is inflated after insertion to keep it in place (in-dwelling), whereas a *straight-type* catheter may be used for temporary drainage purposes.

   c. When imaging a patient with an in-dwelling catheter, the CT technologist must take care to ensure that the urine drainage bag be kept below the patient's bladder at all times to prevent the backflow (reflux) of urine.

H. Lab Values

1. A number of lab values are important for the CT technologist to recognize and understand, particularly as they relate to the patient's capacity to undergo iodinated contrast agent administration (Table 2.1).

2. Blood urea nitrogen (BUN) and creatinine level are lab values used to indicate renal function. These values may be examined individually or in ratio form, as follows:

   a. Normal BUN values in adults range from 7 to 25 mg/dL. Range may vary depending on lab testing

TABLE 2.1	Normal Assessment Signs and Lab Values in the Adult Patient
Temperature	97.7° to 99.5°F (36.5° to 37.5°C)
Pulse	60–100 beats per minute
Blood pressure	Systolic—less than 120 mm Hg
	Diastolic—less than 80 mm Hg
Respiration rate	12–20 breaths per minute
Pulse oximetry	95%–100%
Blood urea nitrogen (BUN)	7–25 mg/dL
Creatinine (Cr)	0.5–1.5 mg/dL
BUN/Cr ratio	6–22:1
Glomerular filtration rate (GFR)	70 ± 14 mL/min/m^2 for men
	60 ± 10 mL/min/m^2 for women
Prothrombin time (PT)	12–15 seconds
Partial thromboplastin time (PTT)	25–35 seconds
International normalized ratio (INR)	0.8–1.2
Platelet count	140,000–440,000 µL of blood

TABLE 2.2	Stages of Chronic Kidney Disease (Adapted From the National Kidney Foundation)	
Stage	Description	GFR
1	Kidney damage with normal function.	>90
2	Mild loss of kidney function.	89–60
3a	Mild-to-moderate loss of kidney function.	59–44
3b	Moderate-to-severe loss of kidney function.	44–30
4	Severe loss of kidney function.	29–15
5	Kidney failure.	<15

GFR, Glomerular filtration rate.

reference. By itself, BUN is not a sufficient indicator of renal insufficiency.

   b. Normal creatinine levels range from 0.5 to 1.5 mg/dL. Range may also vary with lab reference. An elevated creatinine value (>1.5 mg/dL) may not always indicate renal function compromise because this value can vary widely with different populations. Recent changes in a patient's creatinine level are thought to be more informative as a renal function indicator.

   c. The BUN/creatinine ratio may also be used to evaluate renal function. A normal BUN/creatinine ratio is approximately 6:1 to 22:1, and this reference is lab specific.

3. Glomerular filtration rate (GFR) is a more accurate measure of renal function. Estimated GFR (eGFR) is an approximation of creatinine clearance or the rate by which creatinine is filtered from the blood stream. eGFR is calculated using the patient's measured serum creatinine level and takes into account the patient's age, sex, and race. An eGFR measurement greater than 90 to 120 mL/min indicates normal kidney function (Table 2.2). Decreasing kidney function is indicated by a decreasing eGFR measurement.

TABLE 2.3	Normal Liver Function Test Values for an Adult Male	
Test	**Normal Value Range**	**Condition**
Alanine transaminase (ALT)	7–55 units per liter (U/L)	Elevated ALT may be indicative of hepatitis, cirrhosis, blocked bile ducts, or liver malignancy.
Aspartate transaminase (AST)	8–48 units per liter (U/L)	Elevated AST may be indicative of hepatitis, cirrhosis, blocked bile ducts, or liver malignancy.
Alkaline phosphate (ALP)	45–115 units per liter (U/L)	Elevated ALP may be indicative of hepatitis, cirrhosis, blocked bile ducts, or liver malignancy.
Bilirubin	0.1–1.2 milligrams per deciliter (mg/dL)	Increased bilirubin causes jaundice (yellowed pigmentation of the skin, orbits, and other mucous membranes).
Albumin	3.5–5.0 grams per deciliter (g/dL)	Elevated albumin may be indicative of chronic liver disease such as cirrhosis.
Total protein (TP)	6.3–7.9 grams per deciliter (g/dL)	Liver disease may be indicated by a low TP measurement.
Gamma-glutamyltransferase (GGT)	9–48 units per liter (U/L)	Used to determine the cause of elevated ALP that can occur in certain liver diseases.
ʟ-Lactate dehydrogenase (LD)	122–222 units per liter (U/L)	Elevated LD may be indicative of liver disease such as hepatitis.

4. Prothrombin time (PT) is a measure of blood coagulation. The normal range for PT is approximately 12 to 15 seconds.

5. PT is measured in the lab after the addition of a protein called *tissue factor* to a patient's blood sample.

6. Because of the inherent differences in manufactured batches of tissue factor, the international normalized ratio (INR) is calculated to standardize PT results. The INR compares a patient's PT with a control sample for a more accurate result.

7. The normal range for INR is 0.8 to 1.2.

8. Partial thromboplastin time (PTT) is an additional lab value used to detect abnormalities in blood clotting. Normal range for clotting time is generally 25 to 35 seconds.

9. Platelet count is also used to assess the patient's clotting ability. Normal platelet count is 140,000 to 440,000 per mm^3 (or μL) of blood.

10. ᴅ-Dimer testing is utilized for the diagnosis of deep vein thrombosis and pulmonary embolism. Although nonspecific, the presence of elevated amounts of ᴅ-dimer in the bloodstream may indicate recently degraded blood clots. If the ᴅ-dimer value is elevated, additional testing such as CT angiography of the pulmonary arteries may be indicated.

11. A liver function test (LFT) is used to screen for damage to the patient's liver and consists of a panel of blood tests that measure the levels of various enzymes and proteins in circulating blood.

12. Table 2.3 provides a range of normal LFT values for an adult male.

I. Medications and Dosage

1. The CT technologist plays a role in preventing an *adverse drug event (ADE)* in the patient.

2. During the various transitions of care for a patient during their admission to a hospital or other health care encounter, clinician-ordered changes in their prescribed medications may occur.

3. Maintaining an up-to-date and accurate record of all current patient medications is necessary to eliminate errors and potential ADEs.

4. *Medication reconciliation* refers to the process of reviewing the patient's medication record at all points of care, including admission, transfer of service (i.e., imaging procedures), and discharge.

5. The medication record should include all details about the medication(s) a patient is currently taking, including the name, dosage, frequency, and route of administration.

6. Coumadin is a proprietary name for the generic drug warfarin, an anticoagulant. This drug is used to prevent the formation of blood clots in veins and arteries and may reduce the incidence of heart attack and stroke. Patients undergoing therapy with warfarin or any other anticoagulant are prone to excessive bleeding caused by trauma, including intravenous (IV) access for contrast agent administration. The CT professional must take special precautions when providing care to the patient undergoing anticoagulant therapy. Adequate pressure must be applied to the site after IV removal to avoid excessive bleeding and bruising.

7. Metformin, also commonly referred to by the brand name glucophage, is a drug used to treat type 2 diabetes. Patients with acute injury to the kidney(s) or with severe chronic kidney disease may be instructed not to take a metformin product before the administration of iodinated contrast media (ICM) and for up to 2 days after a contrast-enhanced CT examination. There is a small risk of renal impairment from iodinated contrast agents, and reduced renal function can cause the potentially harmful retention of metformin within the body. The patient should consult the referring physician for instructions before resuming metformin treatment. A blood test to check renal function may be required.

8. Although CT is typically less anxiety provoking because of *claustrophobia* (fear of enclosed spaces) than other

medical imaging procedures such as magnetic resonance imaging, patients may be prescribed an antianxiety medication to take before their CT examination.

a. *Anxiolytic* medications may be prescribed to reduce patient anxiety during a CT examination.

i. Benzodiazepines are a class of anxiolytic drugs that include diazepam (Valium), alprazolam (Xanax), clonazepam (Klonopin), and lorazepam (Ativan).

ii. Selective serotonin reuptake inhibitors such as paroxetine (Paxil), sertraline (Zoloft), fluoxetine (Prozac), and escitalopram (Lexapro) may also be prescribed.

b. The CT technologist should carefully monitor patients who are known to have taken an anxiolytic medication before their procedure.

CONTRAST ADMINISTRATION

A. Contrast Media

1. Contrast media are used during many CT procedures in an effort to increase the contrast between, and subsequent visibility of, the multitude of anatomic structures and pathologic conditions whose radiographic densities are too similar to be adequately separated.

2. The contrast agents utilized during CT procedures can be broken down into two basic types: positive and negative.

3. The positive contrast agents belong to a class of substances known as *radiopaque contrast media* (RCM).

4. The RCM typically used for CT examinations are iodine and barium.

5. The degree of radiopacity exhibited by an iodinated contrast agent is directly proportional to the agent's concentration of iodine.

6. The degree of radiopacity exhibited by a barium contrast agent is directly proportional to the agent's concentration of barium.

7. Iodinated RCM are water-soluble compounds that may be administered:

a. Generally into the bloodstream intravenously.

b. Directly into a targeted vein or artery for localized enhancement.

c. Directly into the intrathecal space during CT myelography.

d. Into the joint space during CT arthrography.

e. Orally to opacify the gastrointestinal (GI) tract.

8. Suspensions of barium sulfate are commonly employed as positive contrast agents for opacification of the GI tract.

B. Types

1. Intravascular Radiopaque Contrast Media

a. Initial opacification of blood vessels allows for their anatomic visualization and differentiation from surrounding structures. Contrast enhancement of vasculature greatly aids in the diagnosis of many disorders, including aneurysm, thrombus, and stenosis.

b. Over time the contrast agent is distributed from the vasculature into the extravascular space. This interstitial redistribution of contrast agent can result in differentiation of normal from abnormal soft tissue on the basis of enhancement patterns.

c. As the kidneys excrete the contrast agent, opacification of the renal collecting system occurs. This process improves visualization of the renal pelvis, ureters, and bladder.

d. *Osmolality* is an important characteristic of an iodinated radiopaque contrast agent. It describes the agent's propensity to cause fluid from outside the blood vessel (extravascular space) to move into the bloodstream (intravascular space).

e. Iodinated RCM can be generally divided into the following categories:

• *Ionic contrast media* are salts consisting of sodium and/or meglumine. Each molecule of ionic contrast agent consists of three iodine atoms. When injected into the bloodstream, each molecule dissociates into two charged particles, or ions. The production of osmotic ions is indicative of high-osmolar contrast media (HOCM). Examples of HOCM are iothalamate meglumine (Conray) and diatrizoate sodium (Hypaque).

• *Nonionic contrast media* are nonsalt chemical compounds that also contain three atoms of iodine per molecule. They do not dissociate in solution. These substances are commonly referred to as *low-osmolar contrast media (LOCM)*. Examples of LOCM are iohexol (Omnipaque), iopamidol (Isovue), and ioversol (Optiray).

f. The osmolality of an iodinated radiopaque contrast medium greatly affects its potential for adverse effects in the patient.

g. Nonionic low-osmolar contrast agents are less likely to produce adverse side effects and/or reactions than ionic high-osmolar RCM.

h. Iso-osmolar contrast media (IOCM) have the same osmolality as blood and therefore may offer improved patient comfort and a reduced potential for untoward side effects.

i. Iodixanol (Visipaque) is an example of an IOCM.

2. Enteral Radiopaque Contrast Media

a. Enteral RCM are administered orally and/or rectally to opacify the GI tract.

b. Generally an enteral agent is either a water-soluble iodinated solution or a suspension of barium sulfate.

c. Barium sulfate suspensions are readily used as oral and rectal contrast agents for opacification of the GI tract.

d. Barium sulfate is an inert compound with excellent attenuation properties.

e. Routine transit time for barium sulfate through the GI tract is typically between 30 and 90 minutes.

f. Water-soluble oral contrast media can also be either high-osmolar or low-osmolar iodinated solutions.

g. High-osmolar contrast agents, such as diatrizoate meglumine and diatrizoate sodium, have traditionally been used as oral/rectal CT contrast media.

h. Newer low-osmolar contrasts such as iohexol may also be used as oral/rectal contrast media for CT.

i. Routine transit time for water-soluble iodinated contrast agents through the GI tract is typically between 30 and 90 minutes.

j. The important considerations in the choice between a water-soluble iodine oral contrast agent and barium sulfate are as follows:
   • Barium sulfate may be not be utilized in cases of suspected perforation because it may be toxic to the peritoneum.
   • Barium sulfate is contraindicated in patients who are to undergo surgery or other invasive procedures of the abdomen and/or pelvis.
   • Barium sulfate can be potentially harmful if aspirated.
   • Water-soluble oral contrast agents, particularly of the low-osmolar type, are usually more palatable and result in less GI distress.
   • Water-soluble oral contrast agents may be contraindicated in patients with known iodine allergy.

k. The contrast agent used for rectal CT may be administered via enema to opacify the distal large colon and rectum.

3. Negative Contrast Agents

a. Air, gases, and water may be used as negative contrast agents during CT examination.

b. Water may be used as an oral contrast agent to fill the GI tract. Advantages include:
   • Increased palatability and improved patient comfort.
   • Better demonstration of the enhancing bowel wall.
   • Does not interfere with three-dimensional (3-D) applications.

c. Effervescent granules used to treat gas and acid indigestion may also be administered as negative oral contrast agents. When swallowed, these granules add negative contrast in the form of gas to the stomach and proximal small bowel, allowing for better visualization of these structures.

d. Water-soluble iodinated solutions may be mixed with carbonated beverages to add negative contrast to the GI tract, improving the demonstration of subtle disease.

e. Air acts as a contrast agent during CT imaging of the chest much like it does on a chest radiograph. Image acquisition at the end of full inspiration improves image quality during a CT examination of the chest.

f. Air may also be administered via enema to insufflate the large bowel to improve image quality during CT colonography.

g. CT colonography may also involve insufflation of the large intestine with CO_2. Distention of the large intestine

with room air or CO_2 is necessary for optimal visualization of the bowel wall.

4. Neutral Contrast Agents

a. Neutral oral contrast agents may be administered to opacify the small bowel during procedures such as CT enteroclysis and CT enterography.

b. Neutral contrast media distend the GI tract while still allowing for clear visualization of the bowel wall.

c. Very low-density (0.1%) barium sulfate solutions such as VoLumen may be administered for detailed CT examination of the small bowel.

C. Special Contrast Considerations

1. In general, for patients who are to undergo administration of iodinated contrast agent, attention should be paid to the four Hs as outlined by the American College of Radiology (ACR):
   a. *History:* The CT professional should obtain a thorough patient history. Details regarding the patient's allergic and contrast agent history must be reviewed.
   b. *Hydration:* Particularly with patients who may be renally compromised, adequate hydration must be ensured before, during, and after the examination.
   c. *Have equipment and expertise ready:* A detailed plan to treat contrast agent reactions should be in place and should be practiced regularly.
   d. *Heads up!* Constant assessment of the patient's condition is vital for early identification and proper treatment of an adverse reaction.

2. Patients with increased risk of adverse reaction to iodinated contrast agents may be required to undergo a premedication regimen.

3. Each CT department should have a specific regimen for pretreatment of patients who are at increased risk for adverse reaction to iodinated contrast agents. The regimen typically consists of a combination of an antihistamine such as diphenhydramine HCl (Benadryl) and a corticosteroid (prednisone or methylprednisone) taken at timed intervals beginning as early as 12 to 24 hours before contrast agent injection.

4. Please consult the radiologist, ordering physician, and/or department protocol for a specific contrast premedication protocol.

5. The term *breakthrough reaction* refers to a repeat adverse reaction to iodinated contrast material in the patient who has undergone a pretreatment regimen. Patients who develop a breakthrough reaction are at greater risk for moderate or severe allergic reactions during subsequent administration of iodinated contrast material.

6. Physiologic and pathologic processes that may increase the risk of adverse reaction or other untoward outcome from iodinated contrast include:

a. Asthma.

b. Environmental and/or food allergies.

c. Renal disease.

d. Multiple myeloma.

e. Diabetes mellitus.

f. Pheochromocytoma.

g. Sickle cell disease.

h. Hyperthyroidism.

i. Significant cardiac disease.

j. Anxiety.

7. Contraindications to IV iodinated contrast agents include:

   a. Allergy to iodine.

   b. Prior severe allergic reaction to an iodinated contrast agent.

   c. Renal insufficiency/failure.

8. Patients who are in chronic renal failure and undergoing dialysis may be candidates for IV contrast agent administration at the discretion of the radiologist and referring physician.

9. Although ICM are known to cross the placental barrier, pregnancy is not a direct contraindication to their administration. However, caution must be used in determining the potential benefit of contrast agent administration in the pregnant patient because the risk of adverse reaction in the fetus is unknown.

10. Nursing mothers may be injected with iodinated contrast agents as clinically warranted. Caution again must be exercised because many such agents are excreted in breast milk. Nursing mothers are typically instructed to pump and discard breast milk for 24 hours after administration of a contrast agent to effectively eliminate risk to the infant.

D. Administrative Route and Dose Calculations

1. The IV administration of a contrast agent typically consists of an IV bolus injection through an 18- to 23-gauge angiocatheter or butterfly needle.

2. An *angiocatheter* is an IV catheter placed within a vein and used to administer fluids, medication, and/or contrast media.

3. It consists of a small plastic catheter surrounding a solid needle that acts as a stylet to allow the catheter to be placed within a vein. Once the angiocatheter is inside the vessel, the needle is retracted and the catheter is advanced into the vein.

4. The angiocatheter may be connected to a contrast agent syringe or an automated contrast agent delivery system. Connective tubing may be attached to facilitate the administration of fluids and/or medications.

5. Most current angiocatheters contain a built-in safety shield or retraction mechanism that guards against accidental sharps exposure.

6. *Needleless* IV access systems feature a reusable port device that allows the blunt plastic cannulas of syringes and connective tubing to be attached without needles. Needleless systems improve occupational safety by reducing the risk of accidental needlesticks.

7. A *butterfly needle* consists of a hollow needle surrounded by plastic flaps, or "wings." The wings are grasped and lightly pinched together to facilitate insertion of the needle into a vein. The needle is attached to a short length of connective tubing. Once the needle is inserted into a vein, the plastic wings are secured with tape, and the tubing is attached to a syringe or IV drip.

8. Intravascular RCM are generally administered in doses ranging from 50 to 150 mL. Specific dose depends on the patient's age, weight, and renal function and on the clinical indication for the CT procedure as directed by a radiologist.

9. The serum iodine concentration is a measure of the amount of iodine within the bloodstream. The range of serum iodine concentration for adequate opacification during CT examination is 2 to 8 mg/mL.

10. An IV contrast agent may also be administered through a central venous catheter if it is of adequate type, material, and diameter. The manufacturer of the venous catheter should be consulted for specific tolerances before contrast agent administration.

11. Common types of central venous catheters are subclavian lines, implanted access ports, and peripherally inserted central catheters (PICC lines).

12. Flow rates for injections through central venous catheters such as PICC lines are typically reduced to well below 2 mL/sec. Please refer to the manufacturer and the department's specific protocol before using a central venous catheter for contrast agent administration.

13. Patency of central venous catheters should be tested for venous backflow and may require a test injection of saline for complete assurance.

14. The total volume of oral contrast agent administered for a CT examination should be adjusted according to the extent of bowel opacification required clinically, that is, proximal small bowel, distal small bowel, proximal large bowel, and so on.

15. An example of oral contrast agent protocol for CT examinations limited to the abdomen is as follows:

    a. 300 mL of oral contrast agent 30 minutes before scan.

    b. 150 mL of oral contrast agent immediately before scan.

16. For CT examinations of the entire abdomen and pelvis, substantial opacification of the stomach, small bowel, and proximal large bowel is typically required. An example protocol is:

    a. 450 mL of oral contrast agent 60 to 90 minutes before scan.

    b. 300 mL of oral contrast agent 30 minutes before scan.

    c. 150 mL of oral contrast agent immediately before scan.

17. If complete distention of the stomach is clinically necessary, the last dose of oral contrast agent may be accompanied by a dose of effervescent granules.

18. For studies of the distal large bowel, including the sigmoid colon and/or rectum, an oral contrast agent may need to be administered 4 to 6 hours before scan time to ensure sufficient opacification.

19. When this delay is not clinically appropriate, an oral contrast agent may be administered rectally through an enema.

20. A 150- to 300-mL CT contrast agent enema is usually sufficient to adequately opacify the rectum, sigmoid, and distal large bowel.

21. A small amount of air (negative contrast) may also be administered rectally to improve bowel distention when clinically indicated.

22. *Intrathecal* administration of an iodinated contrast agent is the injection of the agent directly into the space surrounding the spinal cord.

23. Intrathecal injections are performed during CT myelography for evaluation of the spinal cord and nerve roots.

24. *Intraarticular* administration of a contrast agent is the injection of the agent directly into a joint space.

25. Intraarticular injections are performed during CT arthrography of joints, including the shoulder, wrist, and knee.

E. Venipuncture

1. The injection of a medication or contrast agent directly into the bloodstream is a type of parenteral administration.

2. Iodinated contrast agents are typically administered intravenously during CT examinations.

3. Sites commonly used for IV administration of radiopaque contrast agents include (Fig. 2.2):
   a. The anterior recess of the elbow, or antecubital space.
   b. The radial aspect of the wrist.
   c. The anterior surface of the forearm.
   d. The posterior portion of the hand.

4. IV administration requires strict adherence to standard precautions and aseptic technique.

5. *Aseptic technique* refers to the practices and procedures that a practitioner employs to reduce the risk of infection during the IV administration of contrast media.

6. Components of aseptic technique include:
   a. Thorough hand washing between patients.
   b. Wearing of disposable gloves.
   c. Cleaning of the site of venipuncture in a circular motion with an alcohol swab, moving from the center to the outside.
   d. Application of gentle pressure with an alcohol swab to the venipuncture site after removal of the needle/catheter.

7. *Sterile technique* refers to the practices and procedures used to maintain a sterile, microorganism-free

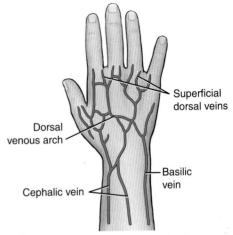

FIG. 2.2 Upper extremity veins commonly used for venipuncture. *(From Jensen SC, Peppers MP: Pharmacology and drug administration for imaging technologists, ed 2, St Louis, 2005, Mosby.)*

environment during invasive CT procedures such as biopsy, aspiration, and CT arthrogram.

8. Sterile technique involves establishing a field around the area of interest that is free of all microorganisms. The procedure is performed within this sterile field with the use of sterile equipment and supplies.

F. Injection Techniques

1. There are generally two approaches to IV administration of iodinated contrast agents, as follows:
   a. *Drip infusion,* whereby the volume of contrast agent is administered at a slow rate over a long period. Because this method results in a slow rise in blood iodine concentration, it is no longer typically used in most CT procedures.
   b. *Bolus injection,* whereby the iodinated contrast agent is "pushed" into the bloodstream at a rapid rate over a short period. This results in a sharp peak of iodine concentration in the blood, yielding a more pronounced pattern of contrast enhancement.

2. Bolus administration may be accomplished by hand, meaning that the volume of contrast agent is manually injected into the bloodstream.

3. Automatic power injectors are commonly used for IV administration of contrast agents during CT examinations.

4. Power injectors are capable of consistently injecting large volumes of contrast agent at flow rates up to 5 to 6 mL/sec. Flow rate is determined by several factors, including clinical area of interest, contrast volume, venous access, patient condition, and pressure capacity of the IV materials utilized.

5. A flow rate less than 1.5 mL/sec is typically recommended for catheters placed in a peripheral (e.g., hand or wrist) venipuncture location.

6. IV administration of contrast agent by power injector should be performed through flexible plastic angiocatheters rather than standard metal needles.

7. Twenty-two–gauge angiocatheters are sufficient for flow rates up to 3 mL/sec. Twenty-gauge or larger angiocatheters should be utilized whenever flow rates exceed 3 mL/sec.

8. Care must be taken to remove air from the injector syringe and connective tubing to eliminate the risk of air embolism.

9. Proper "bleeding" of the tubing eliminates air, and the injector syringe should remain in a downward position before administration of the contrast agent.

10. Once the total volume of contrast agent has been administered, scanning proceeds at set intervals based on the anatomic area of interest and the rate at which enhancement occurs.

11. Many CT systems have bolus tracking software to assist the technologist in acquiring CT images during periods of peak contrast enhancement.

12. During *single-phase imaging,* CT image acquisition occurs at a single specific time during or after the injection of the contrast agent. Images are acquired in this fashion during a single period of contrast enhancement.

13. *Multiphase imaging* involves the acquisition of multiple series of CT images over timed intervals. CT images may be acquired before, during, and after the administration of iodinated contrast agent. The periods of delay between subsequent acquisitions are determined by the clinical indication.

14. Automatic power injectors offer several advantages over manual injection of iodinated contrast during CT examination, including:
    a. Consistent, reproducible flow rates.
    b. Precise volume/dosage control.
    c. Higher injection rates for optimal contrast enhancement.
    d. Automatic delays for proper enhancement patterns and multiphase imaging.

15. The ability to administer normal saline as a flushing agent is an additional advantage of automatic power injectors in CT. Flushing the tubing with a volume of saline (30 to 50 mL) immediately after the contrast agent bolus allows for a reduction of contrast agent dose and helps eliminate the streaking artifact that often results from a high concentration of iodine in the mediastinal vasculature.

16. A saline test flush may also be appropriate to test the patency of the venipuncture site in an effort to avoid contrast media extravasation.

17. Dual-head power injectors can accommodate both the dose of iodinated contrast agent and the volume of saline flush in a convenient and accurate manner.

18. The major disadvantage of the use of a CT power injector is the increased risk of *extravasation,* or infiltration of the contrast agent outside the blood vessel. Extravasation of contrast agent into the surrounding tissue is extremely painful and a potentially serious consequence.

19. The technologist must take care to ensure the patency of the venous access before power injection. Before the injection is initialized, the technologist should check venous backflow by drawing back manually on the injector and observing blood flow into the connective tubing.

20. If venous backflow is not obtained, the catheter may need repositioning and should be checked with a test injection of saline before contrast administration.

21. The technologist must closely observe the contrast agent administration with initial palpation of the IV site. Power injection must be stopped immediately if extravasation occurs.

22. In the event of extravasation, the needle/catheter should be removed, and pressure applied with a warm, moist compress.

23. Extravasation events should be thoroughly documented in the patient's medical record with immediate notification to the referring physician and/or other appropriate health care provider.

G. Postprocedure Care

1. Appropriate postprocedure care must be coordinated by the CT technologist for patients who have undergone an invasive CT examination or one that involved the administration of oral and/or IV contrast.
2. The patient should be provided with detailed instructions on how to identify any untoward late effects of contrast administration, such as bleeding (hemorrhage), infection, or discomfort related to invasive procedures, or any additional concern related to the CT procedure.
3. Referral to the appropriate health care provider (physician, nurse, etc.) must be coordinated by the CT technologist before release of the patient from the current procedure.

H. Adverse Reactions

1. The frequency of adverse reaction to ICM is low, and most adverse side effects require only monitoring of the patient with efforts to decrease their anxiety and increase their comfort.
2. The use of nonionic or LOCM significantly reduces the incidence of adverse reactions in comparison with the use of ionic or HOCM.
3. Although the likelihood of severe adverse reaction to LOCM is low, the exact incidence is not known.
4. A severe, life-threatening reaction to iodinated contrast is most likely to occur within the first 20 minutes after administration.
5. Adverse reactions to iodinated contrast are classified as either:
   a. Allergic-like: Similar to other allergic reactions to food or medicine, with a mechanism of adverse response that is not fully understood.
   b. Physiologic: Effects of ICM that include cardiac arrhythmia, seizure, and pulmonary edema, likely related to the general toxicity of the contrast agent.
6. The majority of both allergic-like and physiologic adverse reactions to iodinated contrast agents can be characterized as mild and non–life-threatening.
7. Mild reactions to ICM include:
   a. Allergic-like:
   - Mild urticaria (hives).
   - Mild cutaneous edema (swelling).
   - Nasal stuffiness/sneezing.
   - Scratchy/itchy throat.
   b. Physiologic:
   - Nausea/vomiting.
   - Pronounced sensation of warmth and/or flushing.
   - Sweats/chills.

- Anxiety.
- Altered taste.
- Mild hypertension.
- Transient vasovagal reaction.

8. Mild reactions to iodinated contrast agents typically require no treatment. The patient should be positively reassured and closely observed until the symptoms dissipate.
9. Moderate reactions are also usually non–life-threatening. However, they may progress rapidly, so treatment may be necessary.
10. Moderate reactions to iodinated contrast include:
    a. Allergic-like:
    - Moderate-to-severe urticaria.
    - Diffuse erythema.
    - Facial edema.
    - Tightening throat, hoarse voice.
    - Wheezing.
    b. Physiologic:
    - Moderate-to-severe nausea and vomiting.
    - Vasovagal response requiring treatment.
    - Tachycardia from hypotension.
    - Chest pain.
11. Treatment for moderate adverse reactions to iodinated contrast includes:
    a. Bronchodilator inhaler and/or oxygen therapy for bronchospasm (wheezing).
    b. Diphenhydramine (Benadryl) for urticaria.
    c. Elevation of legs and IV fluids for hypotension.
12. Severe reactions to iodinated contrast agents are those that are potentially life-threatening and require immediate treatment.
13. Severe adverse reactions are rare.
14. They may begin with mild symptoms, such as anxiety and respiratory distress, and then progress rapidly.
15. Severe reactions to iodinated contrast include:
    a. Allergic-like:
    - Facial, laryngeal, and/or pulmonary edema.
    - Anaphylactic shock.
    - Severe erythema.
    - Profound hypotension.
    - Severe wheezing and/or bronchospasm.
    b. Physiologic:
    - Cardiac arrhythmia.
    - Seizure.
    - Severe hypertension.
    - Cardiopulmonary arrest.
    - Death.
16. Box 2.1 summarizes the treatment for severe adverse reactions to iodinated contrast agents in adults, as recommended by the ACR.
17. Delayed reactions to contrast agent administration can occur in a small percentage of patients.
18. Common delayed reactions include:
    a. Urticaria (hives).
    b. Pruritus (itchiness).
    c. Nausea/vomiting.

BOX 2.1 MANAGEMENT OF ACUTE REACTIONS IN ADULTS

Urticaria

1. Discontinue injection if not completed; maintain IV access and monitor vital signs.
2. No treatment needed in most cases.
3. Dependent upon severity, administer: diphenhydramine (Benadryl) PO/IM/IV 25 to 50 mg or fexofenadine (Allegra) 180 mg PO.

Facial or Laryngeal Edema

1. Give O_2 6 to 10 liters/min (via mask).
2. Give epinephrine IV 1 mL of 1:10,000 dilution (0.1 mg) slowly; repeat as needed up to 10 mL (1 mg); or, IM 0.3 mL of 1:1,000 dilution (0.3 mg). Repeat as needed up to a maximum of 1 mL (1 mg) total.

   If not responsive to therapy or if there is obvious acute laryngeal edema, seek appropriate assistance (e.g., cardiopulmonary arrest response team).

Bronchospasm

1. Give O_2 6 to 10 liters/min (via mask). Monitor ECG, O_2 saturation (pulse oximeter), and blood pressure.
2. Give beta-agonist inhaler such as albuterol (Proventil or Ventolin) 2 to 3 puffs; repeat as necessary up to three times. If unresponsive to inhalers, IM or IV epinephrine.
3. Give epinephrine IM 0.3 mL of 1:1,000 dilution (0.3 mg). Repeat as needed up to a maximum of 1 mL (1 mg) total; or, IV 1 mL of 1:10,000 dilution (0.1 mg) slowly; repeat as needed up to 10 mL (1 mg) total.

   Call for assistance (e.g., cardiopulmonary arrest response team, 911) for severe bronchospasm.

Hypotension with Tachycardia (pulse >100 bpm) – Anaphylactoid Reaction

1. Legs elevated 60 degrees or more (preferred) or Trendelenburg position.
2. Monitor ECG, pulse oximeter, blood pressure.
3. Give O_2 6 to 10 liters/min (via mask).
4. Rapid IV administration of large volumes of Ringer's lactate or normal saline (10 to 20 mL/kg, max of 500 to 1000 mL).

   If poorly responsive: epinephrine (1:10,000 dilution) 0.01 mg/kg; maximum single dose of 1.0 mL (0.1 mg). Repeat as needed up to a maximum of 1 mg. If still poorly responsive, seek appropriate assistance (e.g., cardiopulmonary arrest response team).

Hypotension with Bradycardia (pulse <60 bpm) – Vasovagal Reaction

1. Secure airway: give O_2 6 to 10 liters/min (via mask).
2. Monitor vital signs.
3. Legs elevated 60 degrees or more (preferred) or Trendelenburg position.
4. Secure IV access: rapid administration of Ringer's lactate or normal saline.
5. Give atropine 0.6 to 1 mg IV slowly into IV fluids. Repeat as necessary up to 3 mg total.
6. Repeat atropine up to a total dose of 0.04 mg/kg (2 to 3 mg) in adult.
7. Consider call for assistance (e.g., cardiopulmonary arrest response team, 911).

Hypertension, Severe

1. Give O_2 6 to 10 liters/min (via mask).
2. Monitor electrocardiogram, pulse oximeter, blood pressure.
3. Administer 20 mg labetalol IV slowly; may double dose every 10 minutes to 80 mg at 30 minutes, as necessary.
4. May consider nitroglycerine 0.4-mg tablet, sublingual repeated every 5 to 10 minutes, as necessary.
5. Call for appropriate assistance (e.g., cardiopulmonary arrest response team).

Seizures or Convulsions

1. Carefully monitor patient, turned on side to avoid aspiration.
2. Give O_2 6 to 10 liters/min (via mask).
3. As needed, administer 2 to 4 mg IV lorazepam slowly; may repeat to maximum of 4 mg.
4. Consider using cardiopulmonary arrest response team for intubation if needed.

Pulmonary Edema

1. Give O_2 6 to 10 liters/min (via mask).
2. Elevate torso.
3. Administer diuretics: furosemide (Lasix) 20 to 40 mg IV, slowly.
4. Call for appropriate assistance (e.g., cardiopulmonary arrest response team).

IM, Intramuscular; *IV,* intravenous; *SC,* subcutaneous; *PO,* orally.
From American College of Radiology: *Manual on contrast media, Version 10.2.* Reston, VA, 2016, American College of Radiology.

   d. Drowsiness.
   e. Headache.
   f. Fever/chills.
19. Cutaneous reactions are the most common and can occur within 3 hours to 7 days after administration of a contrast agent.
20. Delayed reactions to a contrast agent must be well documented, followed closely, and treated appropriately as needed.
21. Contrast-induced nephrotoxicity (CIN) is a potentially serious delayed effect of contrast agent administration.
22. It is a considerable decline in renal function that can occur after a patient receives an IV contrast agent.

23. CIN has varied definitions, but is usually signified by a marked increase in serum creatinine level over a baseline measurement obtained before contrast agent administration.
24. The causative relationship between contrast agent administration and CIN is not completely understood, but may be related to renal vasoconstriction and/or the toxicity of the contrast medium itself.
25. The overall risk of CIN is directly related to the patient's preexisting renal function and hydration level.
26. Other risk factors for CIN include:
   a. Diabetes.
   b. Myeloma.

   c. Advanced age.

   d. Cardiovascular disease.

27. Adequate hydration of the patient is the best method of CIN prevention.

28. In the patient with normal renal function, the risk for development of CIN is extremely low.

29. A baseline serum creatinine measurement should be obtained in all patients who are determined to be at risk for CIN.

30. If the patient is deemed renally impaired, alternative imaging options that do not involve contrast agent administration may be indicated.

31. Patients with non–insulin-dependent diabetes who are taking an oral biguanide (metformin) drug may also have a higher risk of CIN-related effects.

32. Patients receiving metformin drug therapy are at increased risk for lactic acidosis, a condition that may be exacerbated by renal insufficiency.

33. If the patient's renal function is adversely affected by administration of a contrast agent, there is a potential increase in incidence of lactic acidosis in the metformin-treated patient.

34. Patients who have associated risk factors for renal insufficiency and are currently taking a metformin drug are typically instructed not to take the metformin after the contrast study.

35. A lab test of renal function may be necessary before the patient resumes metformin therapy.

36. Please refer to the department protocol and/or the appropriate physician guidelines when administering contrast agents to patients receiving metformin drugs.

37. All information regarding patient care, including the procedure(s) performed, contrast/medication administered, untoward event(s), and final outcomes, must be documented by the practitioner.

38. Documentation within the patient's medical record must be clear, concise, and recorded in a timely manner.

Review of Safety in Computed Tomography

CHAPTER OUTLINE

RADIATION SAFETY AND DOSE

A. Radiation Physics

1. The primary physical issue of CT imaging is the measurement of the attenuation exhibited by a volume of tissue. In its most basic form, the reconstructed CT image is a two-dimensional map of the measured attenuation values.
2. Attenuation itself is defined as the reduction of intensity of a radiation beam as it passes through a substance.
3. During transmission through an object, radiation quanta may be absorbed due to the photoelectric effect. *Photoelectric absorption* occurs when the energy of an incoming (incident) x-ray photon is completely absorbed through the ionization of an inner-shell electron of the target atom (Fig. 3.1).
4. X-ray photons within the primary CT beam may also undergo the interaction known as *Compton scattering*. When incident x-ray photons interact with a target atom's outer-shell electron, a transfer of energy may occur which ejects the outer-shell electron (ionization), resulting in a loss of energy for the incident x-ray photon and a subsequent change in direction (Fig. 3.2).
5. Overall, attenuation of the CT x-ray beam depends on the beam quality (photon energy) and the atomic density of the imaged tissue. After passing through the patient, the transmitted radiation is incident upon an array of CT detectors.
6. The individual technical configuration of a CT system determines several characteristics that may affect patient dose:
   a. Source–detector distance: As the distance from the x-ray tube to the detectors decreases, dose increases.
   - The *focus-to-isocenter distance* describes the distance from the x-ray source (CT tube) to the center of the gantry opening, where the patient should be positioned.
   - The *focus-to-detector distance* describes the distance between the x-ray source (CT tube) and the detector array.
   - A structural increase by the CT manufacturer of either distance will result in a decrease in patient dose, based upon the inverse square law.
   b. Filtration within the CT x-ray tube varies between approximately 6 and 9 mm aluminum (Al) or equivalent material. Filtration acts to remove the unwanted, "low-quality" portion of the x-ray beam that adds to the patient radiation dose while failing to yield useful acquisition data. Beam-shaping or bowtie filters are also added to the x-ray tube to compensate for the noncylindrical nature of most body shapes. Additional filtration material along the periphery of the x-ray beam absorbs radiation where it is not necessary, thereby reducing the overall patient dose.
   - Positioning the patient in the center of the gantry (isocenter) is critical when a bowtie filter is employed. Positioning the patient off-center relative to the gantry and the bowtie filter can result in unwanted variations in patient exposure and dose.
   c. Detector efficiency plays an important role in patient radiation dose and can be described in several ways:
   - The *inherent absorption efficiency* of each detector element describes the ability of the detector to capture transmitted x-ray quanta and produce the appropriate response. Inefficiency here can

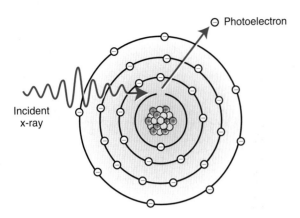

FIG. 3.1 Photoelectric absorption occurs when an incident x-ray photon interacts with an inner-shell target electron, resulting in a total loss of x-ray energy. During this ionization process, a photoelectron is ejected from the target atom. *(From Bushong SC:* Radiologic Science for Technologists: Physics, Biology, and Protection, *11th ed., St Louis, 2016, Mosby.)*

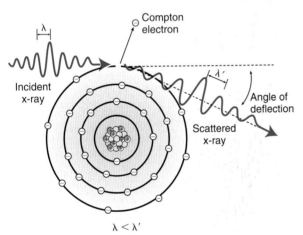

FIG. 3.2 Compton scatter occurs when an incident x-ray photon interacts with an outer-shell electron of a target atom. The photon loses some energy in this ionization interaction and undergoes a resultant change in direction. *(From Bushong SC:* Radiologic Science for Technologists: Physics, Biology, and Protection, *11th ed., St Louis, 2016, Mosby.)*

result in the loss of data and a subsequent compensatory increase in patient dose.

- The *geometric efficiency* of a detector array describes the spatial arrangement of detector elements, including the amount of interspace material required between adjacent elements. The interspace material absorbs transmitted radiation but yields no response. This results in a loss of acquisition data (signal) and requires an increase in radiation dose to compensate. This is of particular importance in MDCT, in which the complex arrangement of multiple rows of detectors requires increased interspace material, resulting in a reduction in geometric efficiency.

d. To expose the widened detector array equally, MDCT utilizes a cone-shaped beam instead of the fan-shaped beam traditionally used by single-slice CT (SSCT) systems. All detectors of the array must be exposed to x-radiation of equal intensity. The beam must be expanded even further to avoid exposing the detectors to undesirable "penumbra." This process is referred to as *overbeaming*. CT image data are acquired from only a portion of the exposed detector array. This results in a radiation dose to the patient that does not contribute to the formation of the CT image. Some CT manufacturers employ focal spot tracking systems to finely control the position of the x-ray beam on the detectors, reducing overbeaming and subsequent radiation exposure.

e. Overranging occurs when radiation dose is applied before and after the acquisition volume to ensure sufficient data collection for the interpolation algorithms inherent in spiral CT. Up to a half-rotation both before and after the spiral scan are common and add to the patient radiation dose.

f. Noise reduction algorithms, or adaptive filters, are employed during the reconstruction process to reduce displayed noise within the CT image. Reduction of displayed noise allows for lower mAs (milliampere-seconds) settings during data acquisition.

7. Use of an MDCT rather than an SSCT system is associated with several technical pitfalls, with the potential to increase the patient radiation dose. Dose can be considerably higher with MDCT because of:

a. Decrease in the focus-to-detector distance.

b. Use of a cone beam instead of a fan beam that is tightly collimated along the z-axis.

c. Increases in the number of phases of acquisition enabled by decreased scan times.

d. Use of thinner section widths for improvement of 3-D and multiplanar reformation images.

B. Radiation Protection

1. Radiation protection in CT should follow the ALARA (*as low as reasonably achievable*) concept.

2. Radiation protection of the CT patient should also encompass three general principles:

a. Strict clinical indication.

b. Protocol optimization.

c. Shielding.

3. Limiting CT examination to strict indications is the best way to reduce radiation exposure.

4. Scan lengths should be limited to the clinically indicated region(s).

5. Multiple-phase acquisitions should be held at a minimum.

6. An optimized protocol is one that acquires CT images with acceptable levels of noise at the lowest possible dose, while still delivering images of diagnostic quality.

7. Scanning parameters should be optimized in an effort to minimize patient radiation dose. Adjustments should

consider the examination indication, region(s) of interest, and patient's age and body habitus.

8. *Protocol optimization* is the process of adjusting parameters such as mA/kVp, slice thickness, and pitch for the purpose of reducing patient radiation dose while maintaining adequate image quality.

9. There is a directly proportional relationship between the milliampere (mA) setting, scan time, and patient radiation dose. For example, if the mAs value is doubled, the patient radiation dose is doubled.

10. There is a direct and exponential relationship between the kilovoltage-peak (kVp) setting and patient radiation dose. A decrease in kVp with no compensatory change in other technical factors (mA, scan time, pitch, etc.) will result in a significant decrease in the quantity of x-radiation produced by the CT tube and a subsequent decrease in patient exposure and dose

11. In certain applications, such as pediatric scanning and CT angiography, reduced kVp settings may be used without a loss in image quality, resulting in a dose reduction.

12. During CT data acquisition, the section of the patient exposed to radiation may be referred to as the *dose profile*. As measured at the isocenter of the gantry, the longitudinal (z-axis) dimension of the dose profile is directly controlled by collimation of the x-ray beam.

13. When only a single slice is scanned, an increase in collimation (thinner section width) will result in a decrease in patient radiation dose. However, CT examinations rarely consist of a single slice.

14. Within the context of the standard CT examination, collimation may indirectly affect patient radiation dose. Increases in collimation (i.e., thinner slices) yield images with more noise. Although usually unnecessary, it is common practice for the user and/or system to compensate for the resultant noise generated by thin sections with an increase in mA, thereby increasing patient dose.

15. During multidetector CT (MDCT), wider collimation results in improved dose efficiency because less overbeaming occurs. Narrow beam widths (i.e., thin slices) increase overbeaming and reduce dose efficiency.

16. Although selected reconstruction algorithm (*kernel*) and window width and level settings are not primary controllers of patient radiation dose, they can play an indirect role. Noise levels in the CT image are a function of dose—decreased dose typically yields an increase in image noise. Displayed noise can be reduced with the utilization of an appropriate reconstruction algorithm, or kernel. Also, displaying the reconstructed image with the correct window settings can help reduce the low image qualities inherent with noise. Both of these solutions are alternatives to increasing the patient dose.

17. Image noise is directly related to patient size. As a patient size decreases, noise decreases. Protocol optimization should include size-based dose (mAs) adjustments. For example, optimal scans in children can be acquired with a substantially lower radiation dose than scans in larger patients.

18. The clinical indication for a CT study should also be considered in the attempt to reduce patient radiation dose. For example, during renal stone survey scans of the abdomen and pelvis, more noise can be tolerated because of the high inherent contrast of the pathology in question.

19. During SSCT, pitch values greater than 1 allow for the acquisition of a given scan volume in a shorter time, resulting in a reduction in patient radiation dose.

20. However, an increase in pitch during MDCT results in a marked increase in image noise. It is typically compensated for by an increase in mA, yielding little net improvement in patient radiation dose.

21. The modern CT scanner comes equipped with a form of automatic exposure control (AEC) to manage patient radiation dose on the basis of the size, density, and overall attenuation of the part being examined. Automatic tube current modulation (ATCM) can occur as either:

    a. Angular (x- and y-axis) tube current modulation, whereby the mA setting is adjusted according to the difference in thickness of the part as the tube rotates. For example, during imaging of the oval torso, mA can be reduced as the beam passes from anterior to posterior. Less attenuation occurs in the anteroposterior (AP) path than in the lateral path through the patient.

    b. Longitudinal (z-axis) tube current modulation, which allows for the adjustment of the mA setting as the scan proceeds along the z-axis of the patient. Differences in attenuation as the body thickness and tissue density change from the chest to the abdomen and so on are met with appropriate adjustments in mA, resulting in an overall reduction in radiation dose.

22. Radiation dose reduction is maximized in CT scanners that employ both the angular and longitudinal current modulation techniques.

23. During MDCT cardiac studies, prospective gating can be used to reduce the patient radiation dose. ECG-triggered tube current modulation allows for pulses of x-ray energy rather than continuous exposure to be used.

24. Tube current is reduced during the cardiac phase not utilized for image reconstruction.

25. The potential radiation dose savings gained with ECG-triggered tube current modulation depend on the patient's heart rate. As heart rate increases, the radiation dose savings decrease.

26. Automated tube voltage selection (Auto kV) may also be available on certain CT systems to automatically adjust tube kilovoltage according to varying patient attenuation during CT acquisition.

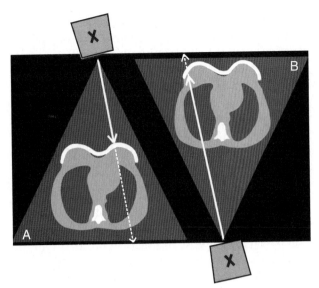

FIG. 3.3 Typical placement of bismuth shielding during a chest CT. (A) With the x-ray tube in the AP position, dose to radiosensitive breast tissue is reduced. (B) During PA exposure, transmitted radiation (data, signal) is lost, resulting in image noise and/or artifact.

27. Out-of-plane lead (or equivalent) contact shielding can be utilized during CT to reduce scatter radiation dose to sensitive tissues that lie outside of the scan acquisition range.
28. Shielding of radiosensitive tissues, such as the breasts and gonads, may be particularly important.
29. To maximize dose reduction, lead shielding must be applied both above and below the patient to account for the rotational nature of the exposure in CT.
30. When employing ATCM, the CT technologist must ensure that the shielding material remains outside of the anticipated acquisition range to avoid an inadvertent increase in radiation exposure to the patient.
31. In-plane bismuth shielding of particularly radiosensitive areas, such as the orbits, thyroid, and breast tissue, can substantially reduce the effective radiation dose.
32. Rubber impregnated with bismuth serves as a selective shield, reducing dose to sensitive tissue areas on which the shielding has been placed.
33. A disadvantage of bismuth shielding is the streaking artifact that may occur on the image.
34. A thin foam spacer may be placed between the patient surface and the bismuth shielding material to reduce the scatter artifact. Fig. 3.3 illustrates the typical placement of bismuth shielding to reduce breast tissue exposure during a CT of the chest.
35. The American Association of Physicists in Medicine (AAPM) recommends against the use of bismuth shielding in favor of more comprehensive dose reduction techniques.
36. Scatter radiation does occur in the immediate area surrounding the CT scanner.
37. Room shielding requirements must be evaluated by a qualified radiologic health physicist.

38. Consideration for shielding requirements should account for examination workload; scanner position; and construction of doors, windows, and so on.
39. The CT technologist is responsible for controlling access to the scan room, ensuring that only the patient remain in the room during radiation exposure.
40. When it is clinically necessary to have the patient accompanied by a guardian or family member during a CT procedure, or when essential health personnel must remain in the room during scanning, the guardian/family member or health personnel must wear appropriate lead shielding.
41. The CT technologist must make every effort to remain educated on the latest developments in dose reduction during CT.
42. Remaining current on best practices in protocol optimization, technological advances and dose reduction techniques enables the CT technologist to keep patient radiation dose to a minimum.

C. Dose Measurement

1. *Slice sensitivity profile* (SSP) may be used to describe the reconstructed CT section.
2. However, the section of tissue exposed to ionizing radiation, or *dose profile*, is greater in width than the SSP. The accurate calculation of CT patient radiation dose must take this fact into account.
3. *Exposure* is the term used to describe the ability of x-rays to ionize a volume of air. It is measured in roentgens (R).
4. *Absorbed dose* describes the amount of x-ray energy absorbed in a unit of mass. It is measured in grays (Gy).
5. *Kerma* may also be used to describe absorbed dose. *Air kerma* describes the amount of radiation absorbed in a quantity of air.
6. *Effective dose (EfD)* accounts for the type of tissue that the radiation is deposited in. Different tissues are assigned weighting factors based on their individual radiosensitivity. Effective dose approximates the relative risk from exposure to ionizing radiation. It is measured in sieverts (Sv).
7. EfD is an estimation of the whole-body dose equivalent that results from the partial body exposure the patient receives during a CT procedure. EfD may be used to estimate the risk of a given CT procedure when compared with epidemiological data.
8. The CT dose index (CTDI) is an approximate measure of the dose received in a single CT section or slice.
9. CTDI is calculated for the central slice in a series that is surrounded by seven slices on each side.
10. CTDI is measured by performing scans of both head- and body-sized CT phantoms using specific technical parameters. A radiation dosimeter, such as an ionization chamber is placed within each phantom during the scans.

11. The exposure measured by the dosimeter is used to calculate the CTDI for each acquisition.
12. Exposure from the scan is measured by the dosimeter, and the CTDI is calculated from those measurements.
13. $CTDI_{100}$ is a fixed measurement taken with a 100-mm-long pencil ionization chamber and makes no reference to a specific number of slices.
14. Because of absorption, dose varies within the CT image across the acquired field of view. $CTDI_w$ is an internationally accepted weighted dose index. It is calculated by summing two-thirds of the exposure recorded at the periphery of the field with one-third of the centrally recorded dose. This weighting yields a more accurate dose approximation.
15. $CTDI_w$ is calculated from measurements made with TLDs positioned at the center and periphery of the phantom to account for the variance in dose distribution.
16. The $CTDI_w$ is measured utilizing a conventional step-and-shoot mode of axial CT scanning and does not account for the effects of helical scanning on patient radiation dose.
17. $CTDI_{vol}$ is used to approximate the radiation dose for each section obtained during a helical scan.
18. It corresponds to the axially acquired $CTDI_w$ divided by the helical pitch, as follows:

$$CTDI_{vol} = \frac{CTDI_w}{pitch}$$

19. As the pitch increases, the dose per section ($CTDI_{vol}$) decreases.
20. $CTDI_w$ approximates dose along the x- and y-axes of the acquired CT image. $CTDI_{vol}$ also includes the dose along the z-axis of the scan acquisition; it is given in units of milligrays (mGy).
21. $CTDI_{vol}$ is similar in principle to an older term used for conventional step-and-shoot scanning, *multiple scan average dose* (MSAD).
22. MSAD is a calculation of the average cumulative dose to each slice within the center of a scan consisting of multiple slices.
23. The MSAD is higher than the dose from an acquisition of a single slice because of the contribution of scatter radiation.
24. The doses at the beginning and end slices in a series are slightly less due to the lack of dose from their outer sides.
25. MSAD may be calculated for axial scanning as follows:

$$MSAD = \frac{T}{I} \times CTDI$$

where *T* is slice thickness and *I* is increment or image spacing.
26. MSAD accounts for the effects of image spacing, or *bed index*, on the patient dose during axial scanning.
27. During axial scanning, overlapping scans increase the patient radiation dose, whereas gaps between slices decrease it.

28. MSAD increases when slice thickness is greater than image spacing—overlapping scans.
29. MSAD decreases when slice thickness is less than the bed index—noncontiguous scans.
30. When slice thickness equals the bed index, MSAD is equal to CTDI.
31. During spiral or helical scanning, MSAD is controlled by pitch, as follows:

$$MSAD = \frac{CTDI}{pitch}$$

where *pitch* is the amount of table travel per tube rotation divided by the collimation.
32. MSAD is most accurate at the center of a scan series. At either end of an acquisition, MSAD tends to overestimate patient radiation dose.
33. Both $CTDI_{vol}$ and MSAD are used to approximate average radiation dose within a scan volume. Total scan length along the z-axis is not considered. Therefore neither provides an estimate of the total dose along a given scan volume.
34. *Dose length product* (DLP) is an internationally accepted measure of CT patient dose defined as:

$$DLP = MSAD \times slice\ width\ (cm) \times No.\ of\ slices\ in\ scan\ volume$$

where *slice* again equals the prepatient collimator setting and *not* the reconstructed slice thickness.
35. The DLP can also be illustrated as the product of $CTDI_{vol}$ and scan length and is given in units of milligray-centimeters (mGy-cm), as follows:

$$DLP = CTDI_{vol} \times scan\ length$$

36. When evaluating patient radiation dose from an MDCT study, one must bear in mind that $CTDI_{vol}$ is still controlled by the prepatient collimator setting, regardless of the number of reconstructed slices.
37. Because direct measurement of effective dose from CT is not possible, estimations must be made on the basis of exposure to a phantom. Once the air kerma or absorbed dose in a phantom is measured, an estimate of effective dose can be calculated.
38. $CTDI_{vol}$ and DLP are displayed on many CT scanners to help the technologist achieve protocol optimization.
39. It is important to remember that $CTDI_{vol}$ and DLP do not account for patient size and so overestimate the radiation dose to the larger patient and underestimate the dose to the smaller patient.
40. $CTDI_{vol}$ and DLP may also be expressed by the newer terms *computed tomography air kerma index* (C_a) and *air kerma length product* (P_{kl}), respectively.
41. The Digital Imaging and Communications in Medicine (DICOM) standard includes a defined Radiation Dose Structured Report (RDSR) that serves as a standardized method of archiving the patient exposure information for each CT acquisition.
42. The RDSR includes information related to the tube's radiation output during CT data acquisition, including

tube current and voltage, scan time, acquisition length, pitch, collimation width, etc.

43. The RDSR documents the exposure data from all acquired CT images, including those acquired but not permanently archived due to low quality or other issues.

44. Current industry standards require that a CT system automatically transmit the RDSR to the patient's electronic medical record for permanent archival.

45. Modern CT systems may also employ an automated alert system called *dose check* that indicates when the anticipated dose for a given acquisition exceeds the recommended maximum. A dose check system typically consists of two levels of notification or alert:

    a. *Dose notification* describes an automated software feature that informs the technologist when the prescribed technical settings for an individual CT acquisition may result in a $CTDI_{vol}$ or DLP that is higher than a preset recommended value.

       i. Prior to initiating the acquisition, the CT technologist must confirm that the settings are correct and appropriate.

       ii. The CT system automatically records identifying information about the acquisition, including date/time, specific dose values, and any comments entered by the technologist.

    b. *Dose alert* describes an automated software feature that alerts the technologist whenever the prescribed acquisitions for an entire CT examination may result in a $CTDI_{vol}$ or DLP that is higher than a preset recommended value.

       i. If the anticipated $CTDI_{vol}$ or DLP for the prescribed CT examination consisting of multiple acquisitions is higher than a preset recommended value, the dose alert system will require the technologist to either:

          1. adjust the technical settings to reduce patient dose;

          2. or, confirm the settings and indicate a personal identifier (name initials) to proceed.

       ii. While the individual acquisitions may not trigger a dose notification, the anticipated cumulative dose index for the prescribed CT examination might cause a dose alert that would prevent additional scanning until the technical parameters are reviewed and adjusted by the CT technologist.

46. These dose notification systems are designed to ensure safe radiation exposure to the patient, prior to each CT acquisition.

47. Current industry standards require that CT systems employ dose reduction techniques and innovations to reduce patient dose to a minimum. These requirements include:

    a. Automated CT dose check

    b. Adult and pediatric reference protocols

    c. DICOM Radiation Dose Structured Reporting

    d. Automatic Exposure Control (AEC)

D. Patient Dose Reduction and Optimization

1. A dose gradient exists across the field of view of the CT image.

2. Doses at the periphery can be markedly greater than that at the center of the image, along the x- and y-axes.

3. The magnitude of this gradient is size dependent. The difference in absorbed dose is greater in larger patients.

4. Smaller adults and pediatric patients exhibit little to no radial dose gradient.

5. For smaller patients, the entrance radiation and exit radiation are equal in intensity, resulting in a more uniform distribution of dose.

6. When all other technical factors remain constant, absorbed dose is greater in the smaller patient.

7. This difference in dose distribution illustrates the importance of dose reduction for the smaller (i.e., pediatric) patient.

8. Recommendations for the reduction of pediatric dose include:

   a. Eliminate CT scans for inappropriate indication.

   b. Reduce multiphase scanning (precontrast, delays, and so on).

   c. Reduce mA.

   d. Reduce kVp

   e. Increase pitch.

9. Regardless of age, the CT protocol should be optimized on the basis of the individual patient's size and/or weight.

10. Patient size–based protocols should be developed for each specific CT system to include adjustments in mA, kVp, and pitch.

11. The *Image Gently* campaign was developed by the Alliance for Radiation Safety in Pediatric Imaging and sponsored by the Society for Pediatric Radiology. The widely recognized campaign offers guidelines to help reduce pediatric radiation exposure from CT imaging. Like the dose reduction techniques listed here, the *Image Gently* guidelines suggest that:

    a. mA and kVp should be "child-sized."

    b. One single-acquisition phase is often enough.

    c. Only the indicated area should be scanned.

12. *Iterative reconstruction* techniques may be used by a CT system to reduce patient dose. As compared with the standard filtered back-projection method of CT image reconstruction, iterative reconstruction can reduce image noise associated with the low-dose techniques employed to reduce patient exposure.

13. The use of iterative reconstruction algorithms can result in significant dose savings to the CT patient. This reconstruction method is discussed further in Chapter 5.

Review of Imaging Procedures in Computed Tomography

CHAPTER OUTLINE

HEAD

Technical Considerations

A. Brain

1. Axial plane computed tomography (CT) images are acquired parallel to the infraorbital-meatal line (IOML) on the sagittal localizer (scout, topogram) image. Acquisition may be performed at an angle 15 degrees above the IOML, parallel to the skull base, to reduce orbital dose and minimize beam-hardening artifact (Figs. 4.1 to 4.5).

2. The axial (sequential) mode of data acquisition may be used for improved z-axis resolution. Thin sections (2 to 5 mm) are acquired from the skull base through the posterior fossa, then 5- to 10-mm sections through the vertex. Thinner sections through the posterior fossa reduce the beam-hardening artifact caused by the petrous pyramids.

3. The excellent z-axis resolution of thin-section volumetric multidetector CT (MDCT) studies allows for high-quality helical examinations of the brain. Helical (volumetric) acquisition may also be preferred whenever multiplanar reformation (MPR) or

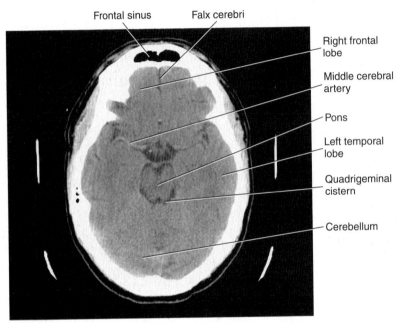

FIG. 4.1 Brain—axial image.

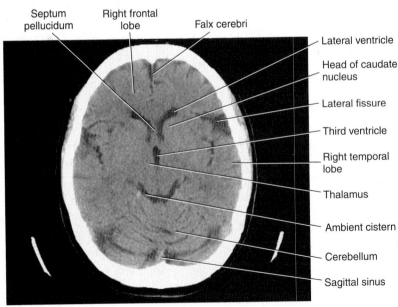

FIG. 4.2 Brain—axial image.

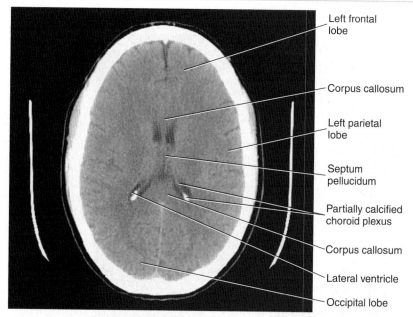

FIG. 4.3 Brain—axial image.

Left frontal lobe
Corpus callosum
Left parietal lobe
Septum pellucidum
Partially calcified choroid plexus
Corpus callosum
Lateral ventricle
Occipital lobe

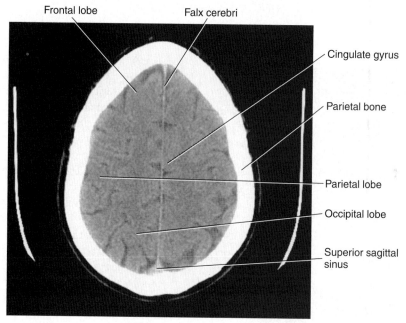

FIG. 4.4 Brain—axial image.

Frontal lobe
Falx cerebri
Cingulate gyrus
Parietal bone
Parietal lobe
Occipital lobe
Superior sagittal sinus

three-dimensional (3-D) imaging is anticipated or when examination speed is a critical issue.

4. Thin (~0.6 mm) detector configuration may be used for data acquisition, with thicker reconstruction settings used per department protocol.

5. A standard or soft tissue reconstruction algorithm (filter, kernel) is used.

6. Additional image reconstruction with a high spatial frequency (bone) algorithm may be used to maximize bony detail for suspected fractures or other skeletal anomalies.

7. Sample window level (WL) and window width (WW) settings for optimal image display of various structures or irregularities are as follows:

a. Gray/white matter: WL 35, WW 100.

b. Bone: WL 400, WW 3000.

c. Hemorrhage/hematoma: WL 75, WW 150.

d. Acute ischemia: WL 35, WW 25 (variable, high-contrast windowing improves the CT visualization of acute stroke).

8. Noncontrast CT examinations of the brain are routinely indicated for trauma to diagnose intracranial hemorrhage or hematoma. Administration of contrast media (CM) in the trauma patient is initially contra-indicated because contrast enhancement may mask subtle signs of hemorrhage (Fig. 4.6).

9. Unenhanced CT of the brain is also typically the first component of a comprehensive protocol for the

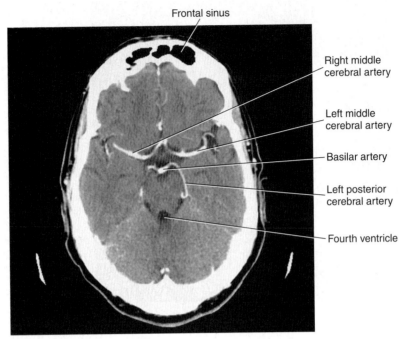

Frontal sinus

Right middle
cerebral artery

Left middle
cerebral artery

Basilar artery

Left posterior
cerebral artery

Fourth ventricle

FIG. 4.5 Brain—axial image.

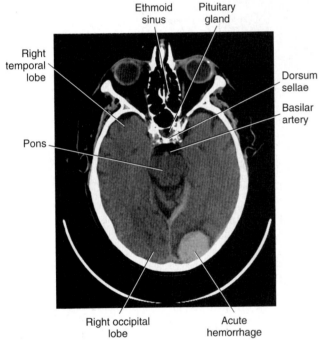

Ethmoid sinus   Pituitary gland

Right temporal lobe

Dorsum sellae

Basilar artery

Pons

Right occipital lobe   Acute hemorrhage

FIG. 4.6 Brain—axial image of acute intracranial hemorrhage (ICH) in left occipital lobe. *(Adapted from Fig. 31.4 in* Vascular Medicine: A Companion to Braunwald's Heart Disease, *2013.)*

evaluation of acute stroke. Hemorrhage must be first excluded on the noncontrast images obtained before thrombolytic therapy.

10. Other indications include:
  a. Congenital abnormalities.
  b. Hydrocephalus (abnormal accumulation of cerebrospinal fluid [CSF] on the ventricles).
  c. Mass or tumor.

d. Primary neoplasms of the brain, including meningioma, schwannoma, and gliomas such as astrocytoma.
  e. Metastatic lesions, which are commonly from lung, breast, renal, or gastrointestinal (GI) cancer.
  f. Infectious fluid collections or abscess.
  g. Bony abnormalities.
  h. Endocrine pathology.
11. Unless contraindicated, intravenous (IV) administration of an iodinated contrast agent is essential in cases of arteriovenous malformation, suspected neoplasm, or attention to the pituitary gland.
12. Coronal plane, thin-section (1 to 3 mm) helical imaging may be performed through the pituitary gland.
13. CT studies of the temporal bones and internal auditory canal require a high-resolution imaging technique, which consists of the following:
  a. Thin slices.
  b. Small targeted display field of view (DFOV).
  c. High-resolution reconstruction algorithm.
14. Thin sections (0.6 to 2 mm) are obtained in both the axial and coronal planes (Figs. 4.7 to 4.10). Multidetector CT (MDCT) axial acquisitions allow for isotropic MPR, which can eliminate the added patient radiation dose from direct coronal acquisition.
15. Targeted thin-section (0.6 to 2 mm) reconstructions should be performed bilaterally utilizing a small DFOV or increased zoom factor to maximize resolution of the small bony components of the inner ear.
16. CT images of the temporal bones are reconstructed with a high spatial frequency (bone) algorithm.
17. The patient must be instructed to hold completely still, because even the slightest motion may cause severe image degradation.

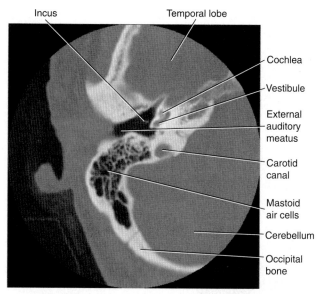

FIG. 4.7 Internal auditory canal (IAC)—axial image.

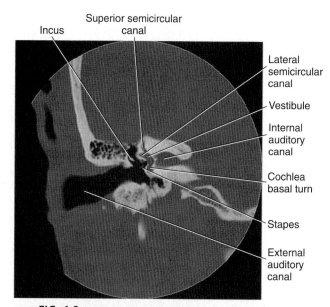

FIG. 4.9 Internal auditory canal (IAC)—coronal image.

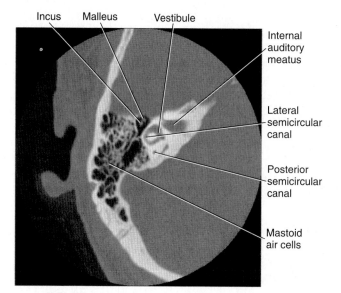

FIG. 4.8 Internal auditory canal (IAC)—axial image.

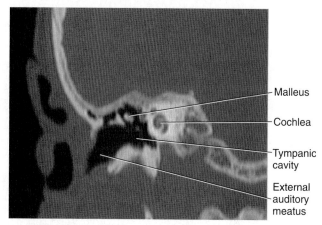

FIG. 4.10 Internal auditory canal (IAC)—coronal image.

18. CT examinations of the temporal bones are typically performed without contrast enhancement, although IV CM may be indicated in cases of suspected soft tissue neoplasm, vascular anomalies, and so on.

B. Orbits

1. For imaging of the orbits, axial plane, thin-section (1 to 3 mm) images are acquired parallel to the IOML (Fig. 4.11).
2. Direct thin-section (1 to 3 mm) coronal images may be acquired perpendicular to the axial plane (Fig. 4.12). The acquisition angle may be adjusted slightly to avoid streaking from metal dental apparatus.
3. MDCT axial acquisitions allow for isotropic MPR, which can eliminate the added patient radiation dose from direct coronal acquisition.

4. Oblique sagittal and/or oblique coronal MPR images through the optic nerve may be included (Fig. 4.13).
5. A standard or soft tissue reconstruction algorithm is used.
6. Additional image reconstruction with a high spatial frequency (bone) algorithm may be used for trauma indications.
7. Sample WL and WW settings for optimal image display are:
   a. Soft tissue: WL 40, WW 400.
   b. Bone: WL 400, WW 3000.
8. Protocol optimization is vital to limit unnecessary exposure of the highly radiosensitive eye lenses.
9. IV administration of an iodinated contrast agent is indicated for evaluation of vascular abnormalities, inflammation, suspected neoplasm, and so on.

C. Sinuses and Facial Bones

1. CT examinations of the sinuses should include axial images parallel to the hard palate (Figs. 4.14 and 4.15).

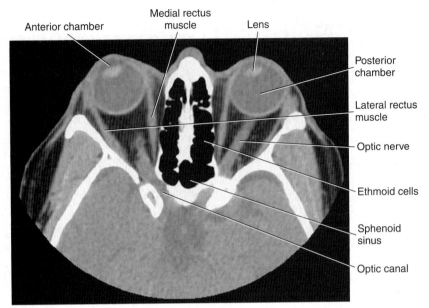

FIG. 4.11 Orbits—axial image.

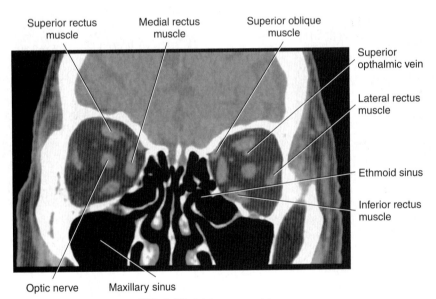

FIG. 4.12 Orbits—coronal image.

2. Acquisition should extend inferiorly and anteriorly to include the maxillary and ethmoid sinuses, superiorly to include the frontal sinus, and posteriorly to include the sphenoid sinus.

3. Direct coronal imaging perpendicular to the axial plane may be obtained with the patient in the prone position. The supine position with the head dropped back may also be used.

4. MDCT axial acquisitions allow for isotropic MPR, which can eliminate the added patient radiation dose from direct coronal acquisition. However, the additional coronal position may be valuable in demonstrating changing air–fluid levels and other sinus-related disease.

5. Coronal plane imaging best visualizes the osteomeatal complex, a common site for sinus inflammation (Figs. 4.16 and 4.17). Sagittal MPR images are also useful for demonstrating the osteomeatal complex.

6. Low-dose survey CT scans consisting of limited coronal acquisition through the sinuses are common.

7. Examination of the facial bones should also include axial and coronal images. Scan coverage should be adjusted to the area(s) of interest.

8. Both standard algorithm and bone algorithm reconstructions are necessary to optimally display soft tissue and bony structures.

9. Sample WL and WW settings for optimal image display are:

a. Soft tissue: WL 40, WW 400.

b. Bone: WL 400, WW 3000.

10. CT examinations of the temporomandibular joints (TMJ) also include axial and coronal thin sections (1 to 3 mm).

11. Images may be acquired in both the open-mouth and closed-mouth positions, as clinically indicated.

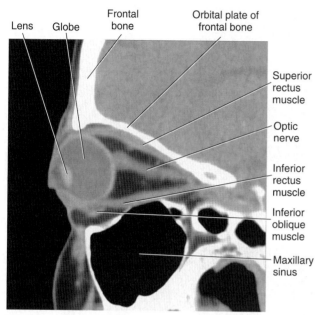

FIG. 4.13 Orbit—multiplanar reformation (MPR) image in the sagittal plane.

12. Examinations of the sinuses and facial bones are usually performed without IV contrast media, except in cases of suspected neoplasm.

Contrast Media

1. The administration of IV iodinated CM during CT examinations of the head has multiple indications, including:

a. Neoplasm.

b. Inflammatory processes.

c. Vascular abnormalities.

2. Administration of an iodinated contrast agent raises the attenuation values of normal brain gray matter, thereby increasing contrast and CT visualization.

3. A contrast agent enhances an intracranial neoplasm that has disrupted the normal blood–brain barrier.

4. Total volumes of nonionic contrast agents typically range between 75 and 150 mL, according to study type, patient weight, renal function, and so on.

5. Injection rates vary from less than 1 mL/sec during general examinations of the brain to upwards of 4 mL/sec during angiographic or perfusion studies.

6. Scan timing for general contrast-enhanced studies of the brain is not as critical as in other applications. In fact, delays of up to 5 minutes may be utilized to maximize sensitivity of the CT scan to detect neoplasm.

7. Contrast-enhanced CT studies of the temporal bones, pituitary, and facial bones follow department-specific protocols with regard to volumes, flow rates, and scan delays.

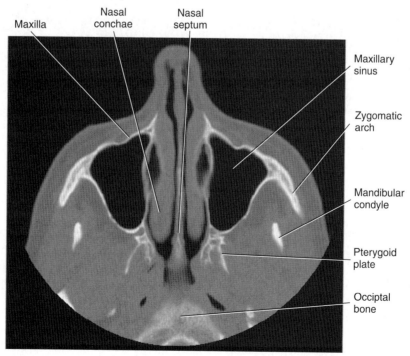

FIG. 4.14 Sinus—axial image.

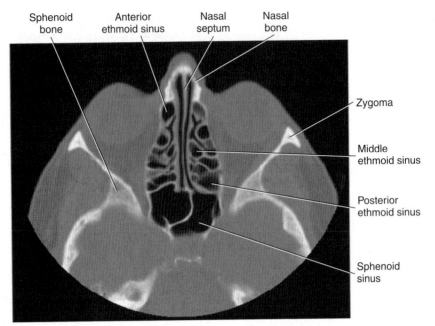

FIG. 4.15 Sinus—axial image.

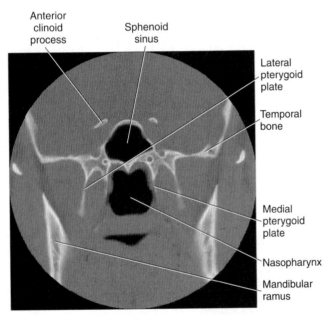

FIG. 4.16 Sinus—coronal image.

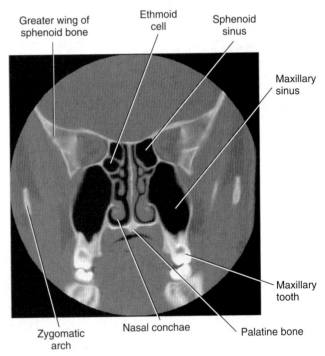

FIG. 4.17 Sinus—coronal image.

8. An example general protocol is as follows: 100 mL of a nonionic contrast agent, 1 to 3 mL/sec injection rate, 60-second scan delay.

Special Procedures

A. Brain CT Angiography

1. Brain CT angiography (CTA) consists of advanced multidimensional CT imaging of the cranial blood vessels (circle of Willis), which have been opacified by an intravenously administered iodinated contrast agent (Fig. 4.18).

2. The vascular components of the circle of Willis are as follows:
   a. Right and left anterior cerebral arteries.
   b. Anterior communicating artery.
   c. Right and left internal carotid arteries.
   d. Right and left posterior cerebral arteries.
   e. Right and left posterior communicating arteries.

3. Although they do not form part of the circle of Willis, the basilar artery and middle cerebral arteries are also of importance during CTA imaging of the brain and its blood supply.

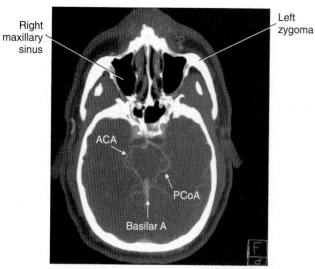

Right maxillary sinus

Left zygoma

ACA

PCoA

Basilar A

FIG. 4.18 Computed tomography angiography (CTA) of the head. ACA – anterior cerebral artery, basilar A – basilar artery, PCoA – posterior communicating artery. *(From Nguyen L, Cook SC: Coarctation of the aorta.* Cardiol Clin *2015;33[4]:521–530.)*

4. CTA of the brain is used to identify and evaluate cerebral aneurysm, intracranial thrombosis, traumatic cerebrovascular injury, arteriovenous malformation, and stenosis.

5. Thin-section (0.5 to 1.5 mm) helical acquisition is performed in the caudocranial direction from the level of the second cervical vertebra (C2) to at least 1 cm above the dorsum sella. CT systems with sufficient technical capabilities (16-slice or greater) may extend the acquisition through the vertex.

6. Before contrast agent administration, a survey scan of the brain is performed to evaluate anatomy and to identify underlying pathology.

7. The CTA spiral acquisition is then made during a rapid bolus infusion of iodinated contrast agent at a rate of 3 to 4 mL/sec.

8. Proper timing of the acquisition with regard to the contrast agent bolus is critical and may be accomplished by:
   a. Use of an empiric delay of 12 to 20 seconds.
   b. Performing a bolus-timing sequence, whereby multiple scans through the cranial vessels are acquired during a test bolus. The proper delay can be determined by visually identifying the time at which peak vessel enhancement occurs.
   c. Use of automated triggering or bolus-tracking software that monitors vessel opacification during contrast agent administration. The scan automatically begins once a predetermined Hounsfield unit (HU) value of attenuation within the target vessel(s) is reached.

9. Thin sections are reconstructed with a minimum 50% overlap to maximize the quality of MPR and 3-D images.

10. The axial "source" images are reformatted into various coronal, sagittal, and oblique planes.

11. 3-D techniques such as maximum intensity projection (MIP), surface rendering, and volume rendering are employed (Fig. 4.19).

12. Protocols for brain CTA depend strictly on the technical capabilities of the CT system employed. Example technical parameters for a CTA of the brain (COW) using a 64-slice system are:
    a. Performance of a standard noncontrast axial brain sequence first.
    b. 50 to 75 mL of a nonionic contrast agent at 4 mL/sec (15- to 20-second scan delay).
    c. Helical CTA acquisition with 0.625-mm collimation.
    d. 80 to 120 kVp/300 mA/0.4 sec.
    e. Overlapping 0.75-mm source images reformatted into coronal and sagittal MPR, MIP, and volume-rendered 3-D images.

13. CT angiography in the emergency setting is often deployed as part of a comprehensive acute stroke imaging protocol.

14. For evaluation of acute stroke, both the intracranial and extracranial vessels are included in the CTA acquisition, which extends from the aortic arch through the circle of Willis.

15. CT angiography source images (CTA SIs) can be utilized to produce subtraction maps, which may provide valuable information about acute brain infarct. The maps are obtained by subtracting the unenhanced CT brain images from the contrast-enhanced CTA source images.

16. CT venography (CTV) of the brain is a variation of the CTA technique. The CTA protocols can be modified with respect to bolus timing to evaluate venous structures.

B. CT Perfusion of the Brain

1. The comprehensive MDCT management of acute stroke consists of:
   a. Precontrast head CT.
   b. CTA of the brain and carotid arteries.
   c. CT perfusion (CTP) imaging.

2. *Cerebral perfusion* refers to the level of blood flow throughout brain tissue.

3. CT perfusion evaluates cerebral perfusion by monitoring the initial passing of iodinated CM through the vasculature of the brain.

4. The factors used to describe cerebral perfusion are as follows:
   a. *Cerebral blood volume (CBV):* The quantity of blood (in mL) contained within a 100-g volume of brain tissue. Normal range is 4 to 5 mL/100 g.
   b. *Cerebral blood flow (CBF):* The quantity of blood (mL) that moves through 100 g of brain tissue each minute. Normal range in gray matter is 50 to 60 mL/100 g/min.
   c. *Mean transit time (MTT):* The average transit time, in seconds, for blood to pass through a given region of brain tissue. MTT varies according to the

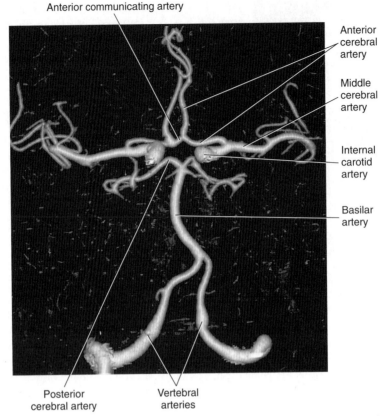

FIG. 4.19 Volume-rendered three-dimensional reformation of the circle of Willis (COW). This anterior perspective is produced from a CT angiographic acquisition through the brain. *(From Fig. 3.98 in Kelley L, Peterson C: Sectional Anatomy for Image Professionals, 3rd ed. St Louis, 2013, Mosby.)*

distance traveled between arterial inflow and venous outflow for a particular area.

5. The *central volume principle* illustrates the relationship between these factors as follows:

$$CBF = \frac{CBV}{MTT}$$

6. The primary indication for CTP is for the evaluation of acute stroke.
7. The primary goal of CTP is to identify and differentiate the infarct core and the penumbra.
8. Brain tissue within the infarct core is beyond repair by thrombolytic therapy.
9. The penumbra is the ischemic yet still viable tissue immediately surrounding the infarct core.
10. Ischemic tissue demonstrates a greater than 34% decrease in blood flow in comparison with normal brain tissue.
11. The penumbra can be described as the region of ischemic brain parenchyma where CBV is still greater than 2.5 mL/100 g.
12. Brain parenchyma with a CBV less than 2.5 mL/100 g is identified as the infarct core.
13. CTP imaging of the brain generates quantitative maps of CBF, CBV, and MTT. These maps can help distinguish regions of ischemic penumbra from an infarct core.

14. The technical procedure for CTP brain acquisition and quantitative display includes:
    a. Bolus administration of 50 mL of a contrast agent at a rate of 4 to 7 mL/sec.
    b. Cine acquisition of at least 2 cm of applicable brain region over a period of 45 to 60 seconds to allow for complete tracking of the first pass of the contrast agent through the intracranial vasculature. Careful attention must be paid to ensure that patient dose is kept to a minimum during the extended cine acquisition required for a perfusion-CT examination.
    c. The acquisition may be broken down into multiple slabs for greater coverage. Each slab must contain a major intracranial artery for accurate CTP map reconstruction.
    d. The slice thickness and subsequent coverage area depend on the detector configuration and technical capabilities of the individual CT system.
    e. Region of interest (ROI) measurements are placed over a well-opacified artery and an area of venous outflow, for example, the anterior cerebral artery and superior sagittal sinus, respectively.
    f. Computer software utilizes the ROI information to generate color-coded CBF, CBV, and MTT maps.
    g. The mathematical technique utilized for generation of perfusion maps is referred to as *deconvolution*.

15. Xenon CT perfusion (Xe-CT) is performed with the inhalation administration of a nonradioactive isotope of xenon (Xe) gas. The xenon enters the bloodstream and can be used to calculate a brain perfusion map on the basis of CBF.

NECK

Technical Considerations

A. Soft Tissue of the Neck

1. Helical axial plane images of the soft tissue of the neck are acquired from the superior orbital rim inferiorly through the lung apex (Figs. 4.20 to 4.22).
2. The gantry should be angled to avoid streak artifact from dental hardware, as follows:
   a. From the superior orbital rim to the hard palate, the gantry may be angled superiorly, parallel to the hard palate.
   b. The remainder of the acquisition is acquired with the gantry angled parallel to the mandibular body.
   c. The two scan groups should overlap slightly to ensure complete coverage of the posterior skull base and neck.
3. The patient is supine with the arms relaxed caudally to reduce artifact from the thicker area of the shoulders.
4. ATCM will increase the mAs through the lower neck and thoracic inlet as the patient dimension increases towards the shoulders. In the absence of ATCM, mAs should be manually adjusted accordingly.

5. Slice thickness of 3 to 5 mm is adequate for most CT studies of the neck soft tissue. Thinner sections (0.5 to 2 mm) may be employed for detailed examinations of the larynx or CT angiographic studies of the neck vasculature.
6. A medium-to-large scan field of view (SFOV) is required to accommodate the variation in part size as the scan progresses from the skull base through the thoracic inlet.
7. The DFOV typically ranges between 18 and 25 cm and should be tailored to the individual patient size.
8. Sample WL and WW settings for optimal image display are:
   a. Soft tissue: WL 50, WW 400.
   b. Bone: WL 300, WW 2000.
9. Image quality degradation resulting from motion is a primary concern during CT examinations of the soft tissue of the neck.
10. The patient should be instructed to breathe quietly and to suspend swallowing during data acquisition.
11. Clinical indications for CT examination of the soft tissues of the neck include:
    a. Inflammation or swollen glands.
    b. Infection or abscess.
    c. Malignant neoplasms, such as carcinoma, sarcoma, and parotid gland tumor.
    d. Benign masses such as cysts and lipomas.
    e. Lymphadenopathy.
    f. Trauma.
    g. Endocrine pathology involving the thyroid and parathyroid glands.

B. Larynx

1. The patient is positioned supine with the head extended to place the long axis of the larynx perpendicular to the CT images acquired in the axial plane. In this position, the gantry angle is adjusted so that the axial

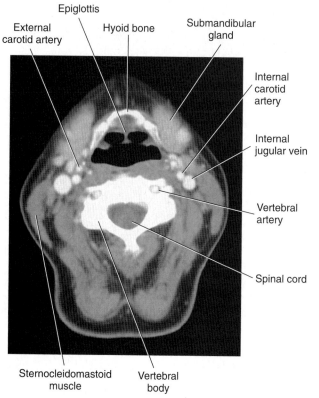

FIG. 4.20 Neck—axial image.

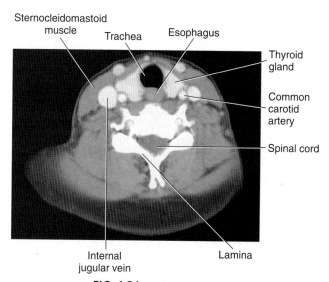

FIG. 4.21 Neck—axial image.

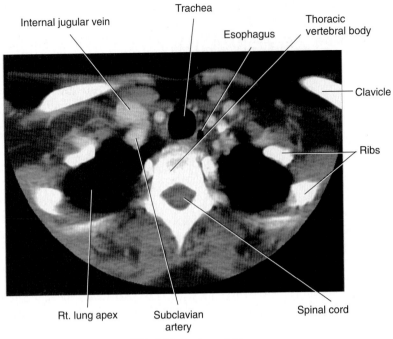

FIG. 4.22 Neck—axial image.

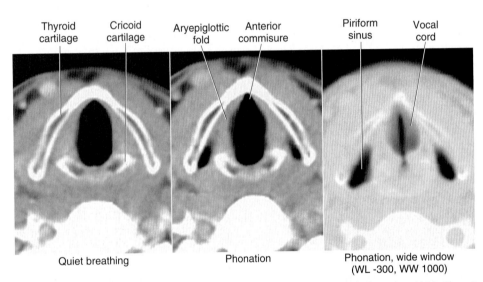

FIG. 4.23 Thin-section CT image of the larynx during quiet breathing and phonation. Wide "lung" windows may be used to demonstrate the vocal cords.

images are acquired parallel to the plane of the true vocal cords.

2. Thin-section (0.5 to 2.0 mm) helical acquisition extends from just above the hyoid bone inferiorly through the cricoid cartilage (Fig. 4.23).

3. Detailed examinations of the larynx may be obtained during suspended respiration (breath-hold) in an effort to improve visualization of the true vocal cords.

4. Phonation may be used to demonstrate abnormal mobility of the vocal cord(s).

5. After an initial acquisition through the larynx during quiet respiration, an additional sequence is obtained during which the patient is instructed to phonate a low, steady "EEE" sound during the entire scan length.

6. A wide window setting (WL −300, WW 1000) may be used to visually separate the small soft tissue vocal structures from the surrounding air-filled endolarynx.

7. MPR images in the coronal and sagittal planes may also be employed during MDCT examinations of the larynx, or any other applicable area of the neck.

8. Virtual endoscopic CT examinations of the nasopharynx and larynx may also be performed for evaluation of inflammatory processes, vocal cord lesions, and so on.

Contrast Media

1. Precontrast imaging of the soft tissues of the neck may be indicated to evaluate the enhancement pattern

of a suspicious mass or to identify salivary gland calculi.

2. CM should be employed for most other CT examinations of the soft tissues of the neck unless contraindicated. Contrast enhancement vastly improves differentiation of soft tissue structures such as lymph nodes, tumors, and vasculature.

3. Total volume of CM depends on clinical indication, CT system capabilities, and patient physiologic factors. It ranges from 50 to 150 mL.

4. Automated injection of a contrast agent is performed at 1 to 3 mL/sec with appropriate scan delays of 30 to 60 seconds.

5. Scan delay should be sufficient to prevent data acquisition through the thoracic inlet during active bolus administration. This delay avoids image degradation from dense contrast agent in the subclavian vein.

6. The bolus may be divided to accommodate any change in gantry angle necessary to reduce metal artifact.

7. The thyroid gland is hyperdense on CT because of its inherent iodine content. This density increases further with administration of iodinated contrast media.

Special Procedures

A. Carotid CT Angiography

1. Similar to the CTA of the brain, CT angiographic examinations of the neck involve imaging of the major neck vasculature, which has been opacified by IV administration of an iodinated contrast agent.

2. CTA of the neck is used primarily to evaluate the carotid arteries.

3. Indications for CTA of the carotids include:
   a. Stenosis.
   b. Occlusion.
   c. Aneurysm.
   d. Trauma.

4. Thin-section (0.5 to 1.5 mm) helical acquisition is performed in the caudocranial direction.

5. The MDCT carotid angiogram typically includes from the aortic arch to the skull base. If the intracranial vessels (circle of Willis) are to be evaluated, the acquisition proceeds to at least 1 cm above the dorsum sella. The scan extent may be limited as required by the clinical indication and the CT system capabilities.

6. The mA value is system dependent but should be kept at the minimal allowed to reduce patient radiation dose. The typical range is 300 to 400 mA for sub-second scan rotation.

7. Utilizing a reduced kVp setting of 80 to 100 can improve the visualization of vessel opacification by an IV contrast agent.

8. When possible, the gantry should be angled to avoid artifact from dental hardware.

9. The CTA spiral acquisition occurs during a rapid bolus infusion of iodinated contrast agent at a rate of 3 to 4 mL/sec.

10. When possible, rapid infusion of iodinated contrast should be performed in the patient's right arm to avoid perivenous streak artifact from dense contrast in the left vasculature.

11. Proper timing of the acquisition with regard to the contrast agent bolus is critical and may be accomplished by:
    a. Use of an empiric delay of 15 to 18 seconds.
    b. Performing a bolus-timing sequence, whereby multiple scans through a level of the carotid arteries are acquired during a test bolus. The proper delay can be determined by visually identifying the time at which peak vessel enhancement occurs.
    c. Use of automated triggering or bolus-tracking software that monitors vessel opacification during contrast agent administration. The scan automatically begins once a predetermined HU value of attenuation within the target vessel(s) is reached.

12. Thin sections are reconstructed with a minimum 50% overlap to maximize the quality of MPR and 3-D images.

13. The axial "source" images are reformatted into various coronal, sagittal, and oblique planes.

14. MIP, surface-rendered, and volume-rendered 3-D techniques are employed (Fig. 4.24).

15. Protocols for CTA of the neck depend on the technical capabilities of the CT system employed. Example technical parameters for a CTA of the neck (carotid arteries) using a 64-slice system are:
    a. Noncontrast helical axial neck images may first be acquired.
    b. Administration of 50 to 75 mL of a nonionic contrast agent at 4 mL/sec (12- to 15-second scan delay).
    c. Helical CTA acquisition with 0.625-mm collimation.
    d. 80 to 120 kVp/350 mA/0.8 sec.
    e. 0.75 mm × 0.5 mm (overlapping) source images are reformatted into coronal and sagittal MPR, MIP, and volume-rendered 3-D images.

CHEST

Technical Considerations

1. MDCT of the chest encompasses a variety of clinical areas, including:
   a. Interstitial lung disease.
   b. Evaluation of the mediastinum.
   c. Detection and differentiation of pulmonary nodules/masses.
   d. Oncologic staging
   e. CT angiography of the major vessels.
   f. Cardiac CT.
   g. Assessment of the airways.

2. Speed is one of the key attributes of helical MDCT. The acquisition of volumetric data for the entire lungs within a single breath-hold is now routine.

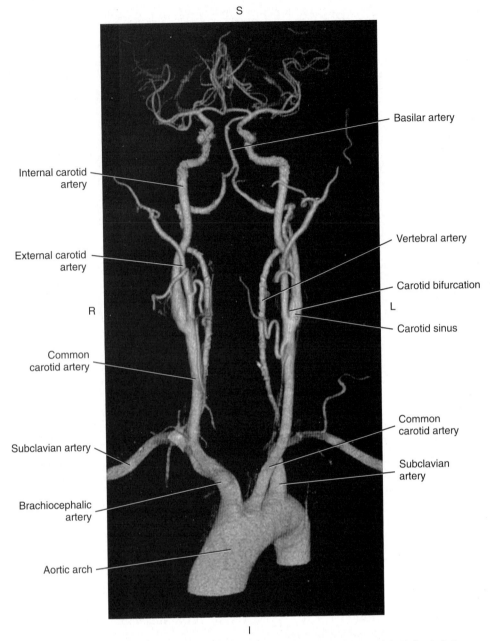

FIG. 4.24 CT angiogram of intracranial and extracranial arteries. *(From Fig. 5.85 in Kelley L, Peterson C: Sectional Anatomy for Image Professionals, 3rd ed St Louis, 2013, Mosby.)*

3. Some MDCT systems possess sufficient scanning speeds to allow for motion-free image acquisition without the need for suspended respiration by the patient.

4. Reduction of respiratory motion has all but eliminated the misregistration artifacts historically encountered during single-slice CT (SSCT) of the chest. This development has dramatically improved the quality of CT chest imaging.

5. The ability to retrospectively reconstruct thin-section images is another distinct advantage of MDCT. Better visualization and differentiation of small pulmonary nodules, high-quality MPR and 3-D techniques, and simultaneous high-resolution CT (HRCT) imaging are just a few of the technical improvements made possible by MDCT.

A. Lungs and Mediastinum

1. The patient is positioned supine with the arms brought above the head to reduce artifact from the shoulder area.

2. Axial plane helical images are acquired from above the lung apices through at least the costophrenic angles.

3. Oncologic CT surveys of the chest to evaluate for disease progression should extend through the adrenal glands, which are a common site for metastatic deposit.

4. Data acquisition is typically performed at the end of a patient's full inspiration.

5. Scanners with detector configurations of 64 rows or more typically acquire CT data through the chest with very narrow detector width, on the order of 0.5 to 2 mm. These data are then reconstructed into thicker sections (3 to 5 mm) for easy review, with the potential for thin sections to be used in MPR or 3-D applications.

6. Settings are 80 to 120 kVp with automatically modulated exposure in the range of 40 to 300 mA at rotational scan times of 0.33 to 1.0 seconds.

7. Low-dose CT of the chest should be considered for all patients when clinically possible, particularly in the pediatric or potentially pregnant patient. Reduced kVp settings and very low mA (down to one-quarter of the routine setting) may still produce images of sufficient quality for interpretation.

8. Pitch varies greatly according to the configuration of the SSCT or MDCT helical system. Overall pitch selection should strike a balance between the requirement for high-quality images and the lowest patient radiation dose possible. Pitch must also be set in accordance with the patient's ability to hold the breath for the length of the scan.

9. A standard reconstruction algorithm (kernel) is used for evaluation of the mediastinum and soft tissues (Figs. 4.25 to 4.29). A given CT system may also have specific algorithms available for review of the lung parenchyma.

10. Additional retrospective reconstructions utilizing a high spatial frequency algorithm (bone, edge) may be used for indications such as small airways disease, bone metastases, and fractures of the thorax.

11. High spatial frequency algorithms should not be utilized for the evaluation of small pulmonary nodules because of the risk of a false-positive demonstration of nodule calcification.

12. The chest consists of a wide range of anatomic structures and, subsequently, of CT densities: lung, mediastinum, bone, and so on. Images must be viewed in multiple window settings for proper evaluation.

13. Sample WL and WW settings for optimal display are:
    a. Lung parenchyma: WL −450, WW 1400.
    b. Mediastinum: WL 40, WW 350.
    c. Bone: WL 300, WW 2000.

14. MPR and 3-D techniques are often valuable tools for diagnosis during CT imaging of the thorax. For example, pulmonary vessels displayed in cross-section can be mistaken for pulmonary nodules. MIP reconstructions assist in differentiating surrounding pulmonary vasculature from true nodules.

15. Thin sections are reconstructed with a minimum 50% overlap to maximize the quality of MPR and 3-D images.

Contrast Media

1. Because of the inherently high contrast of the anatomic structures of the thorax, use of IV iodinated CM is often not necessary.

2. However, there are several indications for contrast agent administration, including:
   a. Evaluation of the mediastinum and/or major vessels.
   b. Hilar or pleural abnormalities.
   c. Assessment of lymphadenopathy (Fig. 4.30).
   d. CTA of the chest.

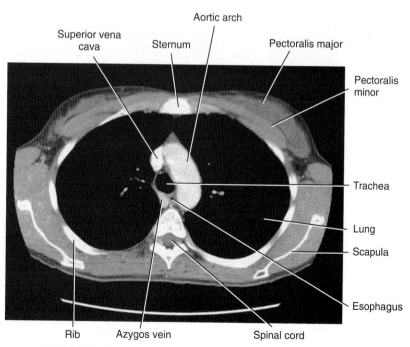

FIG. 4.25 Chest—axial image displayed with a soft tissue window.

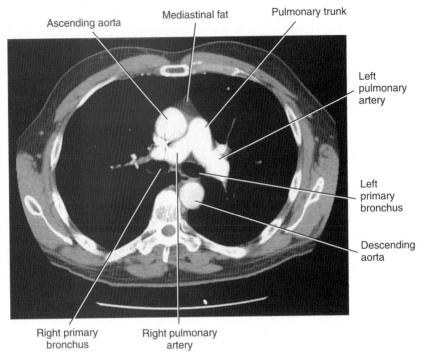

Ascending aorta

Mediastinal fat

Pulmonary trunk

Left pulmonary artery

Left primary bronchus

Descending aorta

Right primary bronchus

Right pulmonary artery

FIG. 4.26 Chest—axial image displayed with a soft tissue window.

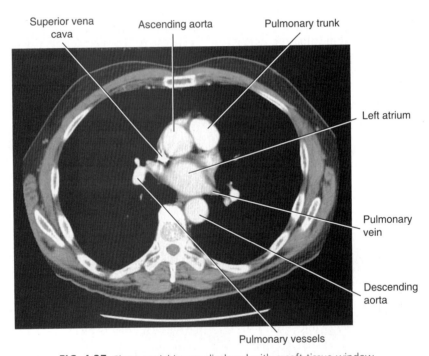

Superior vena cava

Ascending aorta

Pulmonary trunk

Left atrium

Pulmonary vein

Descending aorta

Pulmonary vessels

FIG. 4.27 Chest—axial image displayed with a soft tissue window.

3. Contrast enhancement of a lung mass or nodule can indicate tumor vascularity and malignancy (Fig. 4.31).

4. Sufficient opacification of vascular structures can be typically obtained with injection rates of 2.5 to 4.0 mL/sec.

5. The delay utilized before scanning is specific to the vessel(s) of interest and must be coordinated with the injection rate.

6. Contrast agent dose ranges from approximately 50 to 150 mL. The total dose depends on the patient's condition and the clinical indication for the study. The rapid acquisition of MDCT makes it possible to greatly reduce CM volume during CT of the chest.

7. There is often significant artifact within the mediastinum from high concentrations of iodine in the superior vena cava. It may be alleviated by administering a

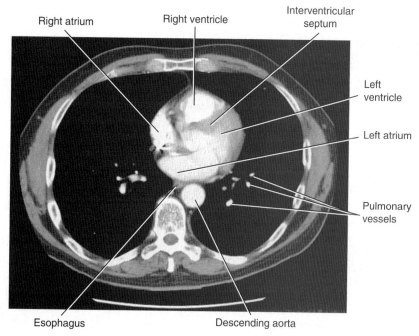

FIG. 4.28 Chest—axial image displayed with a soft tissue window.

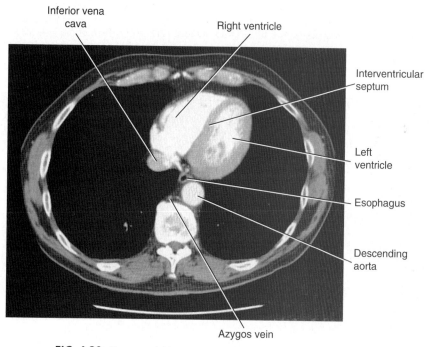

FIG. 4.29 Chest—axial image displayed with a soft tissue window.

bolus of contrast agent with reduced iodine concentration, which is achieved by diluting the full-strength contrast agent with saline. Another option is to scan in the inferior-to-superior direction so that acquisition of the superior mediastinum occurs after the period of peak contrast density within the superior vena cava.

8. An oral contrast agent such as barium sulfate paste may be administered to improve visualization of the esophagus when necessary.

A. High-Resolution CT of the Lungs

1. HRCT is used in the chest to demonstrate diffuse lung disease (Figs. 4.32 to 4.34).
2. Indications for HRCT of the lungs include:
   a. Emphysema.
   b. Bronchiectasis.
   c. Sarcoidosis.
   d. Cystic fibrosis.
   e. Chronic obstructive pulmonary disease (COPD).

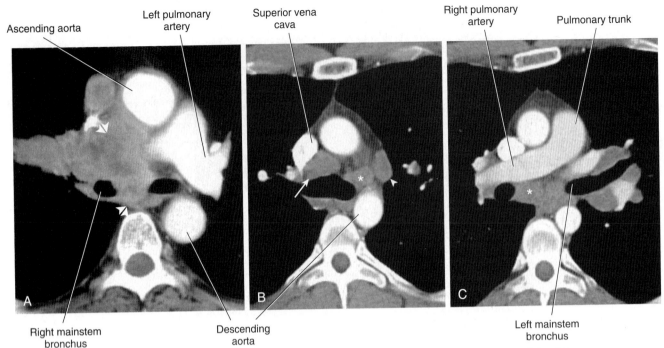

Ascending aorta   Left pulmonary artery   Superior vena cava   Right pulmonary artery   Pulmonary trunk

Right mainstem bronchus   Descending aorta   Left mainstem bronchus

FIG. 4.30 Chest—axial IV contrast enhanced image with mediastinal lymphadenopathy. (A) Axial enhanced chest CT at the level of the carina shows confluent soft tissue with areas of low attenuation (*double arrowheads*) occupying the right paratracheal and subcarinal spaces, extending toward the right peribronchial region. (B and C) Axial enhanced chest CT shows discretely enlarged lymph nodes in the right paratracheal space (*arrow,* B), left tracheobronchial angle (*, B), aortopulmonary window region (*arrowhead,* B), and subcarinal space (*, C). (*Adapted from* Murray and Nadel's Textbook of Respiratory Medicine, *2015, eFigure 53.20.*)

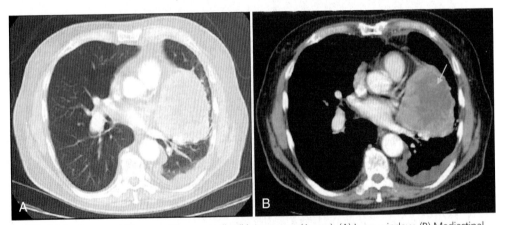

FIG. 4.31 Chest—axial image with non-small cell lung cancer (Arrow). (A) Lung window. (B) Mediastinal window. (*Adapted from Fig. 72-10 in Abeloff's Clinical Oncology, 2014*)

  f. Asbestosis.
  g. Asthma.
 3. HRCT of the lung incorporates the following technical parameters to maximize resolution:
  a. Axially acquired thin slices (0.6 to 2 mm).
  b. Reconstruction with a high spatial frequency algorithm.
  c. Reduced (targeted) DFOV to include only the lung parenchyma.
 4. Although the slices acquired are narrow to improve resolution, image spacing can be considerably wider (10 to 15 mm), accounting for the diffuse nature of interstitial disease.
 5. HRCT imaging of the lung is a sampling technique that is often performed as an adjunct to a general helical CT examination of the lungs.
 6. The patient is typically scanned in the supine position. Data acquisition occurs with suspension of respiration at full inspiration.
 7. HRCT images with the patient in the prone position can be acquired to differentiate the dependent edematous changes often seen in the lung bases.

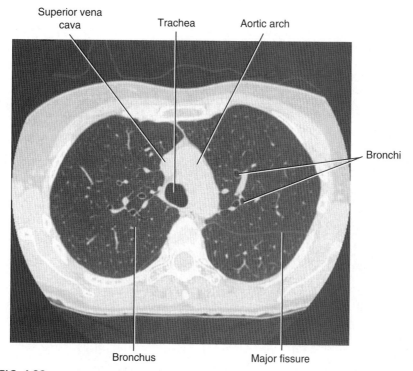

FIG. 4.32 High-resolution CT of the chest—axial image displayed with a lung window.

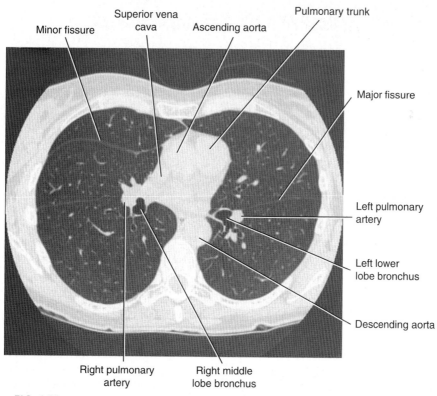

FIG. 4.33 High-resolution CT of the chest—axial image displayed with a lung window.

8. Suspension of breathing at the end of forced expiration (static expiratory HRCT) may be utilized to demonstrate air trapping in patients with suspected small airways disease.

9. MDCT scanners allow for retrospective reconstruction of helically acquired data utilizing high-resolution parameters. Additional images with a targeted DFOV or zoom factor, a high-resolution algorithm or kernel, and a width down to 0.6 mm can be reconstructed. This may be an alternative to direct HRCT imaging in some applications, thus eliminating the need for additional scanning.

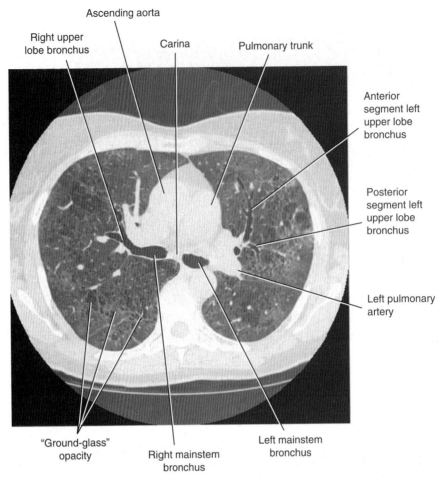

FIG. 4.34 High-resolution CT of the chest—axial image displayed with a lung window.

10. MDCT volumetric HRCT of the lungs also offers the added benefit of high-quality MPR and 3-D techniques using the acquired isotropic data.

11. In the minimum intensity projection (min-IP) technique, displayed pixels represent the minimum attenuation value encountered along each sampled ray. This type of multiplanar volume reconstruction (MPVR) can be applied to a volume of the thorax to demonstrate air trapping within the trachea and bronchial tree.

Special Procedures

A. CT Pulmonary Angiography

1. A pulmonary embolism occurs when a thrombus (blood clot) breaks free from elsewhere in the venous system (usually the lower extremities) and migrates into a pulmonary artery. The pulmonary artery becomes blocked, causing reduced blood flow to the lung tissue (Fig. 4.35).

2. A saddle pulmonary embolus refers to a large clot that straddles the main trunk of the pulmonary artery as it bifurcates into the left and right pulmonary arteries (Fig. 4.36).

3. The main tenets of chest CTA for evaluation of the pulmonary arteries (CTPA) are:

a. Helical scan through the thorax with thin-slice reconstruction ranging from 0.5 to 1.25 mm.

b. Short scan acquisition time performed during patient's shallow breathing to avoid the Valsalva effect and to improve pulmonary opacification.

c. Acquisition during the period of peak contrast enhancement of the pulmonary arteries.

4. The scan progresses from the diaphragm superiorly to the lung apex.

5. Scanning is best performed in the caudocephalad direction, for two reasons:

a. If the patient is unable to hold the breath for the entire scan, motion artifacts are reduced higher in the chest.

b. There is less streaking artifact from dense contrast agent in the superior vena cava as the scan progresses.

6. Iodinated contrast agent is administered as a bolus injection at a rate of 4 to 5 mL/sec through an 18- or 20-gauge catheter.

7. Low-osmolarity or iso-osmolar nonionic contrast agents are preferred to increase patient comfort and cooperation.

8. Contrast agent volume ranges from 80 to 150 mL, on the basis of patient physiologic factors and CT system capabilities.

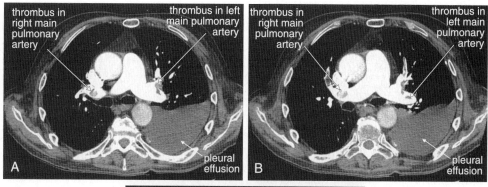

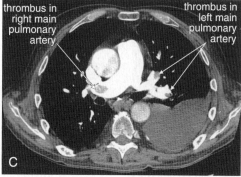

FIG. 4.35 (A) CT pulmonary angiography. (B) Pulmonary emboli *(From Broder, J: Imaging of pulmonary embolism and nontraumatic aortic pathology: diagnostic imaging for the emergency physician, pp 373–443, 2011.)*

9. Care must be taken to ensure that scan acquisition occurs during peak contrast enhancement of the pulmonary arteries. The previously mentioned test bolus and automated bolus-tracking methods are available for study optimization.

10. An injection of saline immediately after administration of the contrast agent bolus can increase enhancement within the pulmonary vessels. The saline flush makes use of any contrast agent remaining in the injector tubing and peripheral veins. This maneuver improves contrast agent utilization efficiency and may allow for an overall reduction in contrast agent dose for the patient.

11. The use of a saline flush also reduces artifact from dense contrast agent in the superior vena cava. It may also work to decrease the incidence of nephrotoxicity from administration of contrast media.

12. Protocols for CTPA strictly depend on the technical capabilities of the CT system employed. Example technical parameters for CTPA with a 64-slice MDCT system are:
    a. 100 mL of nonionic contrast agent at 4 mL/sec (20- to 25-second empiric scan delay or use of automated bolus tracking).
    b. Helical CTA acquisition with 0.625-mm detector collimation.
    c. 80 to 120 kVp/400 mA/0.8 sec.
    d. Overlapping 0.6-mm source images are reformatted into coronal and sagittal MPR, MIP, and volume-rendered 3-D images (Fig. 4.37).

13. MPR and MIP images in the coronal, sagittal, and para-axial planes may aid in the identification of pulmonary embolism or other pathology.

14. Electrocardiogram (ECG) gating can be utilized to eliminate pulsation artifacts caused by cardiac motion during the study.

15. *Prospective gating* or *triggering* is the synchronization of the data acquisition process with the cardiac cycle. Data are acquired only during the periods when the heart is at rest (diastole).

16. *Retrospective gating* involves scanning throughout the entire cardiac cycle. Only data from specific user-determined portions of the ECG waveform are reconstructed into images.

17. During a CTPA study, CTV of the lower extremities for the identification of deep vein thrombosis may also be performed.

18. After the CTPA acquisition, a delay of 2 to 3 minutes is employed. An additional acquisition is made from the iliac crest to the ankles using a 5.0- to 7.5-mm slice thickness.

B. Cardiac CT

1. *Cardiac CT* is a general term that covers several clinical applications:
   a. Coronary artery calcium (CAC) quantitation.
   b. Coronary CTA (CCTA).
   c. Noncoronary cardiac imaging.
2. The primary clinical indication for MDCT CAC quantitation is the assessment of atherosclerotic disease.

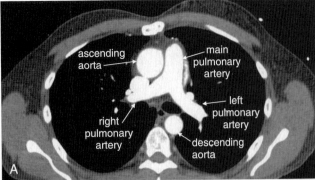

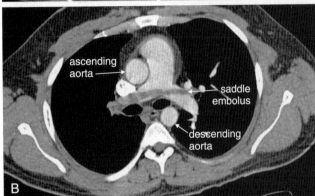

FIG. 4.36 Computed tomography (CT) pulmonary angiography: Axial images. (A) A normal pulmonary artery fills completely with contrast. There are no filling defects to suggest pulmonary embolus. (B) The stream of contrast is interrupted by a filling defect. This fully obstructs the right pulmonary artery and crosses through the left pulmonary artery—a "saddle" pulmonary embolus. An unenhanced CT cannot be used to identify pulmonary emboli, as the densities of thrombus and liquid blood are nearly identical without the use of injected contrast. *(Adapted from Broder J: Imaging of pulmonary embolism and nontraumatic aortic pathology. diagnostic imaging for the emergency physician. pp 373–443, 2011.)*

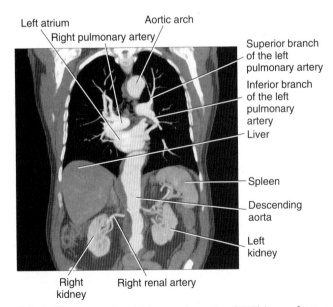

FIG. 4.37 A coronal multiplanar reformation (MPR) image from a CT angiographic acquisition through the chest and abdomen.

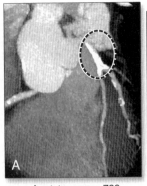
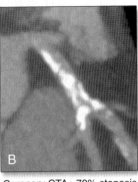

Agatston score 739   Coronary CTA >70% stenosis

FIG. 4.38 (A) Coronary CTA shows severe calcification of the left anterior descending artery (LAD) with a total Agatston score (AS) of 739. (B) Magnified view of coronary CTA showing 70% to 90% stenosis of the LAD and borderline stenosis of the first diagonal branch. *(Adapted from Nørgaard BL, Gaur S, Leipsic J et.al: Influence of coronary calcification on the diagnostic performance of CT angiography derived FFR in coronary artery disease. JACC 8[9];2015.)*

3. The presence of CAC is a specific indicator of atherosclerotic disease.
4. CAC quantitation by MDCT provides a measurement of calcified atherosclerotic plaque burden, a possible predictor of future cardiovascular events.
5. A limitation of this evaluation is the inability to measure and characterize noncalcified atherosclerotic plaque.
6. CAC quantification is often employed as the precontrast component of a more comprehensive cardiac CTA procedure.
7. MDCT for CAC quantitation typically employs a prospective gating approach for data acquisition:
   a. With simultaneous ECG monitoring, scanning occurs only during diastole, when the heart demonstrates the least motion.
   b. A user-defined percentage of the R-R interval is set as the trigger for data acquisition to occur during the T wave of the ECG.
8. Prospective gating reduces patient radiation dose and scan variability.
9. The Agatston scoring system quantifies the volume and density of calcium within the coronary arteries (Fig. 4.38).
10. Areas of calcium are identified as those greater than 1 mm² in area with HU values above 130.
11. The scores are characterized and compared on the basis of the patient's age and sex.
12. CAC scores can be graded as follows:
    a. 1 to 10: minimal.
    b. 11 to 100: mild.
    c. 101 to 400: moderate.
    d. >400: extensive.
13. MDCT for CAC quantitation is performed as a low-dose (80 to 120 kVp, <200 effective mAs) cine-axial examination.

14. Contiguous 2.5- to 3.0-mm axial sections are sequentially acquired from the aortic arch through the cardiac base.

15. The prospectively gated scans are obtained in a cine mode during diastole with fast gantry revolution times (0.35 second) to maintain excellent temporal resolution and provide motion-free images (Fig. 4.39).

16. CAC studies of patients with elevated heart rates are subject to motion artifact because such patients are typically imaged without the administration of β-blockers for heart rate control.

17. In an effort to reduce motion, some CT systems may have the ability to obtain multiple images at each axial location at set time intervals. For example, three images are obtained at each axial position, separated by 50-msec intervals. The user then chooses the image with the least motion artifact.

18. System software yields measurements of calcium volume, mass, and Agatston score.

19. Dual-energy MDCT technology allows voltage switching within the same scan from 80 kVp to 140 kVp. The system is then able to differentiate calcified plaque from iodinated contrast agent during CTA of the coronary arteries. This capability may eliminate the need for a separate CAC quantitation scan, thereby saving time and patient radiation dose.

20. Dual-energy scanning is also available on dual-source MDCT systems, which consist of two separate x-ray tubes and detector arrays mounted 90 degrees from each other on the rotating gantry.

21. The development of MDCT, particularly 64-slice and beyond, has enabled CT to assume a primary role in the noninvasive evaluation of the arterial blood supply to the heart known as *coronary CTA (CCTA)*.

22. The coronary arteries consist of a right coronary artery (RCA) and a left coronary artery (LCA), both arising from the aorta (Fig. 4.40).

23. The main branches of the RCA, in proximal to distal order, are:
    a. Conus artery.
    b. Sinus node artery.
    c. Right atrial branches.
    d. Right ventricular branches.
    e. Posterior descending artery (PDA); may also be referred to as the *posterior interventricular artery (PIV)*.
    f. Posterior left ventricular branches (PLBs).

24. The LCA typically has two main branches:
    a. Left anterior descending (LAD) artery.
    b. Left circumflex artery (LCX).

25. A normal variant may produce a third LCA branch, or trifurcation, known as the *ramus intermedius*. Such a variant is commonly called a *diagonal branch*.

26. The LAD divides further into left ventricular, right ventricular, and interventricular diagonal branches.

27. The LCX divides into obtuse marginal arteries to the left ventricle and left posterolateral branches (in codominant or left-dominant patients).

28. *Dominance* refers to the source of the PDA in a particular patient. It is an important consideration in the evaluation of the coronary artery anatomy during CCTA.

29. 85% of the population is said to be right dominant—the PDA branches from the RCA.

30. 8% is said to be left dominant—the PDA branches from the LCX.

31. In patients who have *codominant anatomy* (7%), the PDA is supplied by the RCA, and the left posterior ventricular branches arise from the LCX.

32. Indications for CCTA include:
    a. Coronary artery stenosis.
    b. Evaluation of coronary stents and bypass grafts.
    c. Coronary anatomic anomalies.

33. Contraindication to use of iodinated contrast agents is the only absolute contraindication to coronary CT.

34. Other relative contraindications are:
    a. Severe arrhythmia.
    b. Very densely calcified coronary artery plaque.
    c. Severe tachycardia that is not pharmaceutically controllable.
    d. Contraindication to β-blockers.

35. The major controlling factor of CCTA is the patient's heart rate. Stable, steady heart rates below 65 to 70 beats per minute (bpm) yield the best results.

36. Heart rate may be controlled pharmaceutically with the administration of oral or IV β-blockers before the study.

37. As MDCT technology improves (i.e., allows faster scanning), the need for low heart rates and pharmaceutical intervention is reduced.

38. The following technical attributes of MDCT allow for coronary artery CTA:
    a. High temporal resolution.
    b. High spatial resolution.
    c. ECG waveform synchronization.

39. The ability of an MDCT system to scan the heart quickly relies on its gantry revolution speed. Current CT systems have shorter gantry rotation times, as low as 0.25 sec (250 msec).

40. The *temporal resolution* of an MDCT system describes its ability to freeze the motion of the heart as well as the arterial motion velocity within the coronary vasculature.

41. The *gantry rotation time* is the technical parameter controlling a CT system's temporal resolution. For example, a gantry of rotation time of 400 msec results in a temporal resolution of 400 msec.

42. With gantry revolution times below 0.5 second, current state-of-the art MDCT systems employ additional modifications to achieve temporal resolution below 100 msec, as follows:

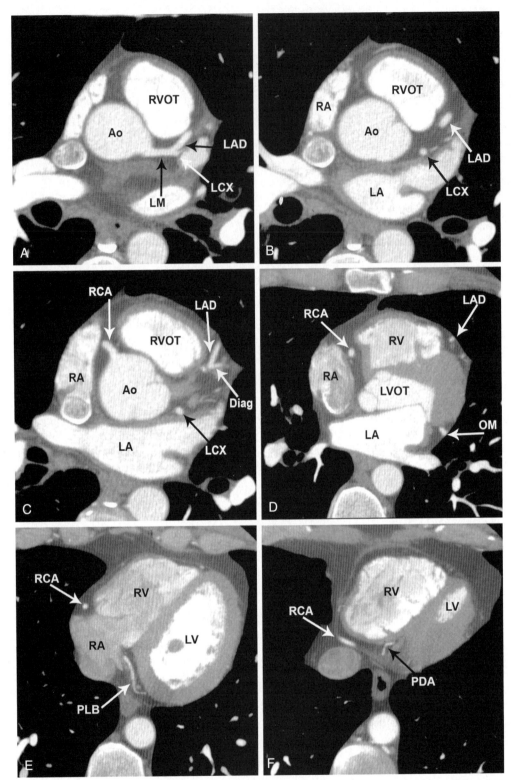

FIG. 4.39 Fig. 1 Normal axial anatomy on 64-slice CT coronary angiography at 0.625-mm collimation. AIVS – anterior interventricular septum; Ao – aortic root; AV – atrioventricular; Diag – diagonal; LA – left ventricle; LV – left ventricle; LAD – left anterior descending; LM – left main; LCX – left circumflex; OM – obtuse marginal; PDA – posterior descending coronary artery; PLB – posterolateral branch; RA – right atrium; RV – right ventricle; RCA – right coronary artery. (A) LM arising from the left sinus of Valsalva and giving rise to the LAD and LCX. (B) LAD and LCX, a couple of centimeters from the bifurcation of the LM. The LAD runs in the AIVS alongside the anterior interventricular vein. (C) RCA arising a little caudally from the anterior right sinus of Valsalva. Note the LAD giving rise to the diagonal. The LCX is just about to enter the posterior atrioventricular groove. (D) RCA in the anterior AV groove, the OM along the lateral margin of the heart, and the distal LAD in the AIVS. (E) The mid-RCA at the acute margin of the heart The PLB, a branch of the distal RCA, crosses the crux of the heart and runs in the left posterior AV groove. (F) The horizontal portion of the distal RCA is seen in the posterior right AV groove. The PDA came off the RCA and is running in the posterior interventricular septum alongside the middle cardiac vein. *(From Patel S: Normal and anomalous anatomy of the coronary arteries. Semin Roentgenol 2008;43[2]:100–112.)*

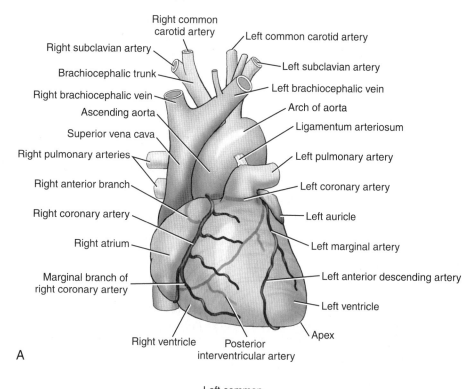

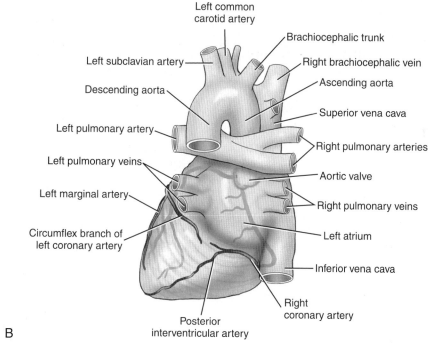

FIG. 4.40 Heart with coronary vessels. (A) Anterior view; (B) posterior view. *(From Fig. 6.103 in Kelley L, Peterson C: Sectional Anatomy for Image Professionals, 3rd ed. St Louis, 2013, Mosby.)*

a. *Half-scan reconstruction*: Single-segment reconstruction in which data from only half a gantry rotation are used, thereby halving the scan time. As a result, the temporal resolution equals one-half the gantry rotation time. Image reconstruction can be further reduced into two-segment and four-segment techniques for improved temporal resolution. For example, a CT system's minimum gantry rotation time is 400 msec. Single-segment reconstruction results in 200-msec temporal resolution (half-scan). Two-segment and four-segment reconstruction may also be available, providing temporal resolution of 100 msec and 50 msec, respectively.

b. The *multisegment reconstruction* method combines data from multiple heartbeats to form an image equaling 180 degrees of acquisition. The number of segments, and therefore the number of successive heartbeats scanned, is set by the user and determined by the patient's heart rate.

   c. For a *two-segment reconstruction*, two heartbeats are used for a single axial image. With this method, temporal resolution is reduced by one-half, allowing for a freezing of the heart motion even with heart rates up to 100 bpm.

   d. In *four-segment reconstruction*, data from four heartbeats is used (45 degrees of data per cycle), reducing the temporal resolution by a factor of 4. Four-segment reconstruction yields high-quality, motion-free CCTA images in patients with heart rates exceeding 100 bpm.

   e. Multisegment reconstruction requires a stable cardiac cycle, with the heart maintaining an equal size and shape during successive beats. Severe arrhythmia, premature contractions, and so on may be contraindications to CCTA.

   f. Dual-source CT systems utilize two separate sources of x-ray and two detector arrays. With each half-rotation of the system, temporal resolution may be reduced up to one-quarter.

43. The spatial resolution of a CT system describes its ability to image small objects. During CTA of the coronary arteries, the MDCT system must be capable of adequately demonstrating very small blood vessels with diameters averaging 2 to 5 mm in size.

44. Spatial resolution has two main components:

   a. *In-plane resolution*, which is controlled by factors related to the x- and y-axes of the CT image. A large (512×512) image matrix, small DFOV (18 to 22 cm), and smooth reconstruction algorithm (kernel) are preferred.

   b. *Z-axis resolution* is controlled by the minimum detector width. 64-slice MDCT systems utilize detectors between 0.5 and 0.625 mm wide.

45. If not contraindicated, administration of sublingual nitroglycerine immediately before the CTA procedure can improve spatial resolution by dilating the coronary vessels. Please consult the referring physician and/or department protocol for guidelines regarding medication administration.

46. Ventricular diastole is the portion of the cardiac cycle in which coronary artery motion velocity is slowest and cardiac motion is at its lowest.

47. Data used for reconstruction of CCTA images are synchronized with the ventricular diastolic portion of the cardiac cycle to eliminate motion artifact.

48. The R-R interval on ECG waveform corresponds to the entire cardiac cycle.

49. Diastole is the portion of the R-R interval (cardiac cycle) when the heart is at rest. During systole, the heart is in motion.

50. During retrospective ECG-gated MDCT, data acquisition and simultaneous ECG monitoring occur throughout the entire cardiac cycle for a predetermined number of heartbeats.

51. For evaluation of the coronary arteries, the MDCT system then includes only the portion of the acquisition attained during diastole in the reconstruction process.

52. The user selects the phase percentage of the R-R interval to reduce motion artifact and optimize image quality on a case-by-case basis as it relates to the patient's heart rate.

53. The least heart motion occurs from approximately 55% to 75% of the R-R interval, typically corresponding to the point of mid-diastole.

54. CTA acquisition is performed during suspension of respiration to reduce image degradation caused by breathing.

55. During prospective ECG-gated cardiac CTA, data are acquired in an axial step-and-shoot mode. The x-ray and data acquisition systems are activated only during the diastolic portion of the R-R interval.

56. Prospective ECG gating requires a steady heartbeat to limit motion artifact.

57. Evaluation of cardiac function is not possible because data are acquired only during diastole.

58. The main benefit of prospective ECG gating is the potential for up to a 70% reduction in patient radiation dose.

59. Administration of an iodinated contrast agent is a necessary component of CCTA. Proper timing of the contrast agent bolus is crucial to maximizing coronary artery opacification.

60. A test bolus technique can be used to determine timing delay, but the preferred method is to utilize system bolus tracking with the trigger ROI set in the ascending aorta.

61. 100 mL of a nonionic or iso-osmolar contrast agent is injected into an antecubital vein at a rate of 4 to 6 mL/sec.

62. Additional saline flush may also be employed to improve the efficiency of contrast agent utilization.

63. Protocols for CCTA depend strictly on the technical capabilities of the CT system employed. Example technical parameters for a CCTA using a 64-slice system are:

   a. Initial noncontrast CAC scoring scan or low-dose chest CT.

   b. Administration of 75 to 100 mL nonionic contrast agent at 4 to 6 mL/sec (automated bolus tracking).

   c. Helical CTA acquisition with 0.625-mm detector width.

   d. Scan extending from the carina through the base of the heart.

   e. 80 to 120 kVp/700 to 900 effective mAs (automatic mA modulation techniques may be employed).

   f. Pitch at 0.2 or less.

   g. Table feed/rotation of 3.8 mm.

   h. Reconstructed slice thickness of 0.75 mm; spacing at 0.5 mm.

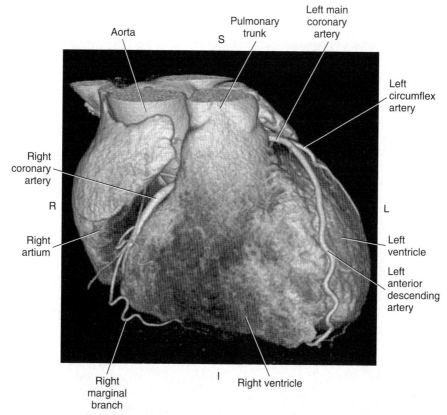

FIG. 4.41 3-D CTA of right coronary artery. *(From Fig. 6.108 in Kelley L, Peterson C: Sectional Anatomy for Image Professionals, 3rd ed. St Louis, 2013, Mosby.)*

i. Small DFOV or zoom factor (18 to 22 cm).

j. Sequences reconstructed at 10% intervals of R-R interval from 0 to 90%.

64. MPR, curved reformatted, and MIP images are used to evaluate the coronary arteries for stenoses. Volume-rendered and shaded-surface displays may also be of diagnostic value (Fig. 4.41 and Fig. 4.42).

65. Acquisition data from multiple phases may be demonstrated in a cine loop for four-dimensional (4D) evaluation (x-, y-, and z-axes + time = 4D).

66. In addition to the evaluation of the coronary arteries, retrospectively gated cardiac CT can be used to assess:

a. Morphology of the heart chambers and valves.

b. Myocardial perfusion.

c. Ventricular volume and ejection fraction.

d. Wall thickness and motion abnormalities.

67. Noncoronary cardiac imaging can also be performed for the identification and evaluation of pericardial disease and differentiation of cardiac masses.

68. Cardiac function can be assessed by collecting CT data throughout the entire cardiac cycle in what is termed a *multiphase data set*. A cine loop is then used to view the heart in motion from systole to diastole.

69. MPR images along the heart's long and short axes are also used to evaluate cardiac function, morphology, and pathology.

C. CT Angiography of the Aorta

1. MDCT angiography is a primary diagnostic tool in the evaluation of aortic aneurysm.

2. Aortic dissection occurs when an inner layer of the aorta tears and a false lumen is created. These lesions may be classified as follows:

a. Stanford type A, involving the ascending aorta.

b. Stanford type B, involving the descending aorta.

3. CTA acquisition should extend from the base of the neck inferiorly to include the celiac trunk.

4. When indicated, scan coverage may extend superiorly to include the carotid arteries or inferiorly through the bifurcation and iliac arteries.

5. Protocols are system specific, with detector collimation, gantry rotation time, and pitch adjusted to ensure that the entire acquisition is attained within a single breath-hold.

6. The guiding principle of contrast agent administration is that the bolus should last throughout the entire scan but not beyond it.

7. Total volumes of contrast agent range from 75 to 125 mL, determined by the flow rate and the scan duration.

8. Good venous access is required because flow rates in the range of 4 to 5 mL/sec are recommended.

9. An antecubital IV catheter should be placed in the right arm whenever possible. This practice helps avoid the streaking artifact that may obscure the main

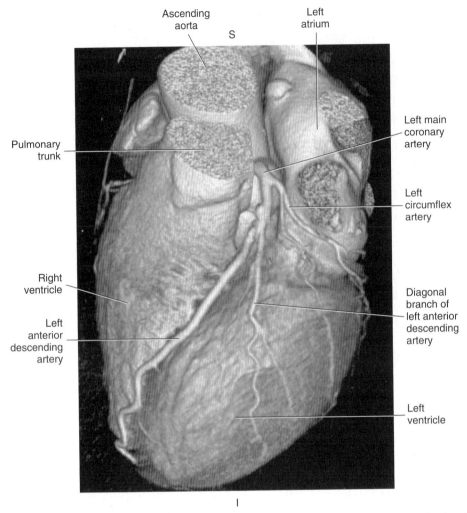

FIG. 4.42 3-D CTA of left coronary artery. *(From Fig. 6.111 in Kelley L, Peterson C: Sectional Anatomy for Image Professionals, 3rd ed. St Louis, 2013, Mosby.)*

branches off the aortic arch when contrast agent is administered in the arm and enters through the left brachiocephalic vein.

10. Scan delay is determined by test bolus or automated bolus tracking.

11. Thin-section images (0.5 to 1.5 mm) as well as thicker images (3 to 5 mm) may be reconstructed for MPR applications and general chest evaluation, respectively.

12. Pulsation artifacts, particularly in the ascending aorta, can be avoided with the use of retrospective ECG gating.

13. Protocols for CTA of the aorta depend strictly on the technical capabilities of the CT system employed. Example technical parameters using a 64-slice system are:

a. Initial noncontrast, low-dose, thick-slice (3 to 5 mm) acquisition through the chest to evaluate for calcium, intramural hematoma (IMH), and so on.

b. Administration of 75 to 125 mL of a nonionic contrast agent at 4 mL/sec (automated bolus tracking).

c. Helical CTA acquisition with 0.625-mm detector width.

d. Scan extending from the base of the neck through the celiac trunk.

e. 80 to 120 kVp/automatic mA modulation.

f. 0.33 to 0.35 second gantry rotation time.

g. Pitch <1.

h. Reconstructed slice thickness of 0.75 mm; spacing at 0.5 mm.

i. Small DFOV or zoom factor (18 to 22 cm).

j. Additional reconstruction at 5 × 5 mm with sufficient DFOV to evaluate entire thorax field.

k. MPR, MIP, and volume-rendering imaging techniques.

14. The "triple rule-out" MDCT procedure consists of a comprehensive evaluation of the chest for cardiac and noncardiac pain. Multiple clinical considerations are possible with a single MDCT procedure:

a. CCTA for coronary artery disease.

b. CTA of the aorta for aneurysm.

c. CTA of the pulmonary arteries for embolism.

15. To assess the thorax in its entirety, a full field of view is utilized to identify additional sources of chest pain, such as focal masses, pleural abnormalities, and pulmonary infiltrate.

D. CT Bronchography

1. *CT bronchography* is 3-D CT visualization of the tracheobronchial tree.
2. It consists of MPR and volume-rendered 3-D images reconstructed from thin, overlapping MDCT axial images acquired through the airways.
3. CT bronchography may also include "fly-through" endobrachial views, commonly known as *virtual bronchoscopy.*
4. Indications for CT bronchography and virtual bronchoscopy include:
   a. Airway stenosis.
   b. Foreign body aspiration.
   c. Trauma.
   d. Anatomic variants.
   e. Stent planning and evaluation.
   f. Bronchogenic carcinoma.
   g. Interventional guidance.

ABDOMEN AND PELVIS

1. The ability of MDCT to rapidly acquire large volumes (greater anatomic coverage) of extremely thin (isotropic) images has revolutionized the CT evaluation of the abdomen and pelvis.
2. Protocol selection and adaptation for MDCT of the abdomen and/or pelvis are vital to ensure that the scan produced meets the needs of the patient, referring physician, and radiologist.
3. Proper MDCT evaluation of the abdomen and pelvis is highly individualized. Great attention must be paid to the patient's history and the clinical indication.
4. Many vital considerations need to be tailored to any given examination, including:
   a. Extent of the area to be scanned.
   b. Necessity of IV and/or oral CM and the administration details.
   c. Phases of contrast enhancement required.
   d. Technical parameters, such as slice thickness, imaging planes, and 3-D applications.
5. The CT examination of the abdomen begins just above the diaphragm and extends through the aortic bifurcation at the general area of the iliac crest. An examination that includes the pelvis extends through at least the pubic symphysis.
6. The anatomic area scanned is based on the physician order and clinical concern—abdomen only; abdomen and pelvis; chest, abdomen, and pelvis; and so on.
7. The contents of the abdominal-pelvic cavity may be further divided as follows:
   a. The peritoneum forms a membranous sac called the *peritoneal cavity* that contains the following organs:

- Stomach.
- Small bowel, a small portion of the duodenum, and all of the jejunum and ileum.
- Transverse colon.
- Liver and gallbladder.
- Spleen.
- Ovaries.

   b. The peritoneal cavity is a closed sac in males but opens to the exterior in females through the fallopian tubes, uterus, and vagina.
   c. The peritoneum contains double layers and folds that surround and support the abdominal organs:
   - *Mesentery*: A thickened portion of the peritoneum that attaches portions of the intestines to the abdominal wall.
   - *Omentum*: A mesentery that is divided into lesser and greater components, each responsible for attaching portions of the stomach and intestines.
   d. *Retroperitoneum*: The space located between the peritoneum and the posterior abdominal wall. It includes the following organs and structures:
   - Duodenum.
   - Pancreas.
   - Adrenal glands.
   - Kidneys, ureters, and bladder.
   - Aorta and inferior vena cava.
   - Prostate.
   - Uterus.

Technical Considerations

General guidelines regarding the technical parameters for MDCT examinations of the abdomen and/or pelvis are outlined here. This section is followed by more specific technical details for the major organ systems of the abdomen and pelvis.

A. Examination Preparation

1. When possible, patients fast for 2 to 6 hours before the examination. Fasting results in an empty proximal GI tract, facilitating its evaluation and also limiting the potential hazard of aspiration of stomach contents in the event of GI upset because of IV administration of a contrast agent.
2. In most cases, an oral contrast agent is administered to distend the GI tract and clearly demonstrate the intestinal lumen. The agent used may be a dilute solution of an iodinated contrast medium, barium sulfate, or water. For general studies of the abdomen and pelvis, 750 to 1500 mL of oral contrast agent is administered 30 to 120 minutes before the examination.
3. Example protocol for oral contrast agent administration is:
   a. 450 mL given 90 to 120 minutes before the examination for opacification of the distal intestines.
   b. 300 to 450 mL given 30 minutes before the examination for opacification of the proximal intestines.

c. An additional volume of 150 to 250 mL given just before scanning for opacification of the stomach and duodenum.

B. Patient Position and Instructions

1. The patient is positioned supine with the arms placed overhead to eliminate scatter artifact.
2. Additional positions (prone, decubitus) may be employed to improve the demonstration of normal anatomy and the differentiation of pathologic processes.
3. Whenever possible, the patient is instructed to suspend respiration (hold the breath) during scan acquisition.

C. Scan Parameters

1. Detector configuration and section width: 64-detector row (or larger) MDCT systems allow for detector collimation as thin as 0.5 to 0.625 mm, with images reconstructed at widths based on the anatomy or pathology in question. For general survey studies, section widths of 3 to 5 mm are sufficient. Section widths of 1 to 2 mm or less may be preferable during multiphasic studies and in anticipation of 3-D and multiplanar reconstructions.
2. Table travel speed and pitch: The relationship among detector collimation, table travel speed, and pitch is important in determining the amount of data acquired per gantry rotation and the overall scan time. A state-of-the-art MDCT system is capable of long z-axis acquisitions in a short time, often within a single, comfortable breath-hold.
3. The detector configuration, table speed, and pitch should be optimized according to the clinical indications of the examination while keeping scan time and patient radiation dose to a minimum.
4. The mA and kVp settings should be based on patient size, yielding to the noise requirements of the particular examination.
5. Patient radiation dose may also be reduced with the utilization of automatic tube current modulation (ATCM) techniques, which are available on most CT systems.
6. DFOV is patient specific, being set as small as possible while still including the abdomen and pelvis in their entirety.
7. A standard soft tissue algorithm is used for reconstruction. When indicated, additional reconstruction with a high-resolution algorithm may be used to demonstrate bony detail.
8. Sample WL and WW settings for optimal display are:
   a. Soft tissue of the abdomen: WL 40, WW 350.
   b. Lung bases: WL –450, WW 1400.
   c. Bone: WL 300, WW 2000.

D. Administration of Intravenous Contrast Agents

1. When not contraindicated, the administration of an iodinated IV contrast agent improves the quality of abdominal and pelvic CT imaging by:
   a. Enhancing, or increasing the CT density of, abdominal organ parenchyma.
   b. Increasing the detectability of lesions from normal structures.
   c. Opacifying vascular structures.
   d. Providing assessment of organ perfusion and function.
2. There are also clinical indications for noncontrast or precontrast and postcontrast imaging, including:
   a. Characterizing the enhancement pattern of a lesion.
   b. Evaluation of calcifications within organ parenchyma.
   c. Assessment of unenhanced parenchymal attenuation values.
   d. Identification of calculi within the bile ducts, gallbladder, urinary tract, and appendix.
3. Contrast agent dose ranges from approximately 50 to 150 mL. The total dose depends on the patient's condition and the clinical indication for the study.
4. Injection rates vary between 2.0 and 5.0 mL/sec. The rate selected depends on the enhancement phase(s) to be acquired and the capacity of the venous access.
5. The delay between the initiation of contrast agent administration and scanning is tailored to the required phase of enhancement and coordinated with the injection rate.
6. Specific contrast agent injection rates, acquisition delays, and a description of the pertinent phases of contrast agent enhancement are described here for each anatomic region.

HEPATOBILIARY SYSTEM

1. The primary role of MDCT in evaluation of the liver is the identification and characterization of hepatic lesions.
2. When not contraindicated, most CT examinations of the liver involve the IV administration of an iodinated contrast agent to improve the differentiation between lesions and normal hepatic parenchyma.
3. However, noncontrast imaging may be indicated in cases of suspected hepatic calcifications, fatty infiltration, and visualization of hemorrhage or to characterize the enhancement pattern of hepatic lesions.
4. Normal unenhanced hepatic parenchyma is homogeneous in appearance, with CT densities in the range of 45 to 65 HU. The CT density of the unenhanced liver is normally slightly greater than densities of blood vessels and the splenic parenchyma.
5. Soft tissue masses may appear less dense (*hypodense*) or more dense (*hyperdense*) than the structures that surround them.
6. Upon enhancement with an IV contrast agent, a tumor may be described as *hypovascular* if it is lower in density than the surrounding organ parenchyma or *hypervascular* if it is higher in density.
7. The most common malignant hepatic neoplasms are metastases, which usually appear as hypodense.

8. Examples of hypervascular tumors are hemangiomas, hepatocellular carcinomas (HCCs), focal nodular hyperplasia (FNH), and hypervascular metastases.

9. Tumors with densities equal to those of surrounding tissue or structures are said to be *isodense*. These structures may not be well defined on the CT image. HCC is an example of a neoplasm that may appear isodense on routine contrast-enhanced CT. Scanning during multiple phases of contrast enhancement may improve the visualization of HCC and other tumors like it.

10. Benign neoplasms of the liver include:

   a. *Hemangioma:* Often an incidental finding, this commonly occurring vascular lesion is characterized by peripheral globular enhancement during initial postcontrast imaging. Progressive fill-in of enhancement occurs over time, until the mass becomes isodense with surrounding hepatic parenchyma (Fig. 4.43).

   b. *Focal nodular hyperplasia:* Another common vascular lesion often identified along the surface of the liver, FNH is characterized by intense homogeneous enhancement with contrast agent administration. There is usually a central scar that remains hypodense until delayed imaging, during which it may also enhance.

   c. *Hepatic cysts:* They appear as well-defined, thin-walled, round, or oval masses, with attenuation close or equal to that of water (0 to 20 HU). The hallmark feature is lack of enhancement with IV contrast agent administration.

11. Malignant neoplasms of the liver include:

   a. *Hepatocellular carcinoma:* The most common primary malignant neoplasm of the liver. HCC typically appears hypodense on noncontrast scans and hyperdense or hypervascular on arterial phase imaging (Fig. 4.44).

   b. *Metastases:* The liver is a common site for the metastatic spread of cancer. Primary neoplasms that commonly metastasize to the liver include those of the colon, lung, breast, pancreas, and stomach. The CT appearance of hepatic metastases

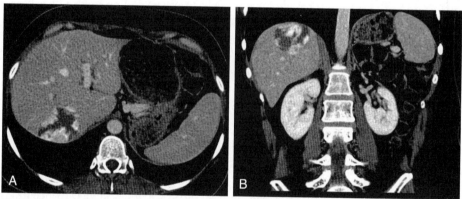

FIG. 4.43 Abdomen—axial and coronal MRP images demonstrating hepatic hemangioma with peripheral globular enhancement. *(From Shaked O, Siegelman E, Olthoff K, Reddy K, Rjander: Biologic and clinical features of benign solid and cystic lesions of the liver.* Clin Gastroenterol Hepatol *2011;9[7]:.)*

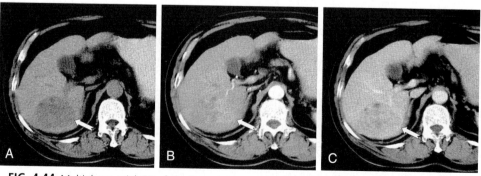

FIG. 4.44 Multiphase axial CT of the liver demonstrating hepatocellular carcinoma (HCC) tumor. (A) Noncontrast hypodense appearance; (B) hyperdense appearance during arterial phase; (C) portal venous phase. *(From Gao S-Y et al: Tumor angiogenesis-related parameters in multi-phase enhanced CT correlated with outcomes of hepatocellular carcinoma patients after radical hepatectomy. Eur J Surg Oncol 42[4]:538–544.)*

varies greatly and is nonspecific. They may appear as solitary or multiple, hypodense or hyperdense, necrotic or calcified, and so on.

12. Additional indications for MDCT of the liver include:
    a. Diffuse liver disease:
       - *Fatty liver (steatosis):* Normal liver parenchyma exhibits a CT density approximately 10 HU greater than that of the spleen. A liver with fatty infiltration demonstrates an overall density that is at least 10 HU less than that of the spleen. Areas of focal sparing of fatty infiltration appear hyperdense to surrounding tissue and may mimic hepatic neoplasm.
       - *Cirrhosis:* Chronic destructive disease characterized by a variety of features, including hepatomegaly, fatty infiltration, irregular nodular contour, enlargement of the left and caudate lobes of the liver, and portal hypertension. Common causes of cirrhosis are hepatitis and chronic alcoholism.
    b. Trauma: The liver is the second most commonly injured abdominal organ (after the spleen). Hematoma, hemorrhage, and laceration are typical signs of traumatic liver injury.
    c. Infection or abscess.
    d. Preoperative and postoperative assessments of the patient who may undergo hepatic transplantation.

13. The liver has a dual blood supply, receiving 75% of its supply from the portal vein and the remaining 25% via the hepatic artery. The dual nature of this blood supply has important ramifications with regard to IV contrast agent administration and scan timing.

14. There are three distinct phases of hepatic contrast enhancement:
    a. *Arterial phase:* The period of peak arterial enhancement typically occurs at 25 to 35 seconds after the initiation of contrast agent administration. During this phase, hypervascular tumors, or tumors supplied by the hepatic artery, undergo maximal enhancement. The lesions are made conspicuous by the relatively unenhanced hepatic parenchyma surrounding them.
    b. *Portal (or hepatic) venous phase:* The period of peak hepatic parenchymal enhancement during which contrast material redistributes from the blood into the extravascular spaces. Typically occurring at 60 to 70 seconds after the initiation of contrast agent administration, this is the phase during which hypovascular lesions are most conspicuous because of their density difference from the enhancing hepatic parenchyma.
    c. *Equilibrium phase:* Usually occurs at 2 to 3 minutes after the initiation of contrast agent administration. During this phase, hepatic parenchymal enhancement dissipates, and there is minimal difference in contrast enhancement between the intravascular

and extravascular spaces. Many hepatic lesions become indistinguishable from their surroundings. The rapid acquisition made possible by MDCT helps avoid scanning during this phase.

15. An *early arterial phase*, occurring at 15 to 20 seconds after the initiation of contrast agent administration, has also been identified. During this phase the hepatic arterial supply is well opacified with little or no parenchymal enhancement. This is the optimal phase for angiographic applications of liver CT.

16. The *delayed phase* of hepatic data acquisition occurs approximately 5 to 20 minutes after contrast agent administration. This phase is used primarily to demonstrate the complete "fill-in" of a hemangioma as it becomes isodense with surrounding parenchyma.

17. The timing of each of these phases depends on a number of factors:
    a. Cardiac output: As it is reduced, peak arterial and parenchymal enhancement is delayed.
    b. Injection duration: A function of the total contrast agent volume and the injection rate. A short duration, via smaller volume, faster injection rate, or a combination thereof, results in a faster delivery of the iodine load and earlier peak arterial and parenchymal enhancement. Rapid injection rates also provide a greater temporal separation between the arterial and venous enhancement phases.
    c. Iodine concentration of contrast agent: The use of media with higher iodine concentrations (at or above 350 mgI/mL) results in a higher administered iodine load, which helps widen the window of peak arterial and parenchymal enhancement.

18. The degree of hepatic parenchymal enhancement depends on the overall dose of iodine delivered. Iodine dose may be increased directly, with the use of contrast agents with a higher concentration, or indirectly, through using a higher injection rate.

19. Lesion detectability improves as parenchymal enhancement improves. Care must be taken to ensure that CT scanning of the liver is performed during the highest level of enhancement possible.

20. Automated bolus-tracking software can be utilized to improve the timing accuracy of multiphasic acquisitions of the liver.

21. Current MDCT technology allows for scanning of the liver during multiple phases of contrast enhancement. This improves characterization of both hypovascular and hypervascular lesions.

22. Protocol considerations for a multiphasic MDCT scan of the liver are department specific but may include any or all of the following:
    a. Noncontrast survey of the liver to evaluate baseline lesion density, fatty infiltration, calcifications, and so on.
    b. Early arterial phase (15 to 20 seconds) for assessment of the hepatic arterial supply. Important in cases of preoperative planning for resection,

transplantation, or placement of a chemotherapy infusion pump.

c. Arterial phase (25 to 35 seconds) for optimal visualization of hypervascular hepatic lesions such as hemangioma and HCC.

d. Portal venous phase (60 to 70 seconds) for evaluation of the maximally enhanced hepatic parenchyma and demonstration of hypovascular lesions such as hepatic metastases.

e. Delayed phase (5 to 20 minutes) for demonstration of hemangioma fill-in, FNH central scar, and so on.

f. Reconstructed images 3 to 5 mm thick from data obtained with detector collimation as low as possible. Section width may range from 2.5 mm in a 4-slice MDCT system to 0.6 mm in a 64-slice system.

g. Thinner (0.5 to 2.5 mm), overlapping reconstructions may be used for angiographic, MPR, and 3-D applications.

23. In an effort to keep patient dose to a minimum, the number of contrast enhancement phase acquisitions should be limited to only those that are vital to the diagnostic process, as indicated by the clinical history and the suspected pathology.

24. The gallbladder is demonstrated as a bile-filled (near water density) oval sac positioned within a fossa along the inferior surface of the liver.

25. CT is not usually the modality of choice for evaluation of the gallbladder. However, MDCT is capable of adequately demonstrating many pathologic etiologies of gallbladder symptoms in the patient who is undergoing CT evaluation of the abdomen and pelvis:

a. *Cholelithiasis* (gallstones): The ability of CT to demonstrate gallstones depends primarily on the stone composition. Cholesterol stones may exhibit

a CT density less than that of the surrounding bile. Calcified gallstones are easier to identify. Mixed-composition stones may be obscured on CT (Fig. 4.45).

b. *Cholecystitis:* Inflammation of the gallbladder is nonspecific but may be characterized on CT by a thickened and contrast-enhancing wall, distention, gallstones, and/or pericholecystic fluid.

c. Neoplasms of the gallbladder such as benign adenoma and malignant carcinoma.

26. Components of the biliary tract commonly demonstrated on CT examination include:

a. Common hepatic duct (CHD).

b. Common bile duct (CBD).

c. Intrahepatic bile ducts (IHBDs).

27. Common clinical indications for CT examination of the biliary tree include:

a. Biliary dilatation or obstruction.

b. *Choledocholithiasis* (bile duct stones).

c. *Cholangitis* (inflammation of the bile ducts).

d. Biliary duct neoplasms.

28. Optimal CT demonstration of the gallbladder and biliary tree requires thin-section (0.5 to 2.0 mm), dual-phase (arterial and portal venous) acquisition.

29. Water is used as an oral contrast material to eliminate the streak artifact that may occur from the positive contrast agent within the duodenum.

30. Precontrast imaging may be performed initially to look for stones.

SPLEEN

1. The spleen is evaluated concurrently with the remaining organs and structures of the abdomen on CT examination (Fig. 4.46).

2. The CT density of the unenhanced spleen is between +40 and +60 HU, which is approximately 10 HU less than that of the unenhanced liver.

3. The spleen is optimally imaged after administration of a contrast agent.

4. On arterial phase imaging, the spleen demonstrates a heterogeneous enhancement pattern. The preferred timing for CT acquisition of the spleen is the portal venous phase (60 to 70 seconds), when a more homogeneous pattern of enhancement is demonstrated.

5. Common indications for CT evaluation of the spleen include:

a. Trauma: The spleen is the most common site of organ injury resulting from blunt abdominal trauma. Hematoma, hemorrhage, and laceration are typical signs of traumatic splenic injury.

b. Focal lesions: Benign masses such as cysts and hemangiomas and malignant lesions, including those from lymphoma and metastatic disease.

c. Splenomegaly: An enlargement of the spleen with numerous etiologies, including lymphoma, cirrhotic portal hypertension, and infection.

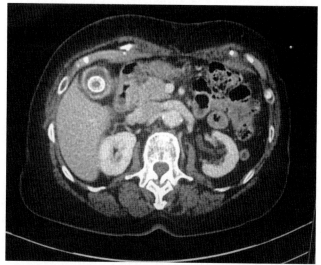

FIG. 4.45 Postcontrast axial CT of the abdomen demonstrating cholelithiasis. Note abnormal thickening of the enhanced gallbladder wall, indicting cholecystitis. *(Image courtesy of Steven Ahrenstein, BS, RT[R][CT].)*

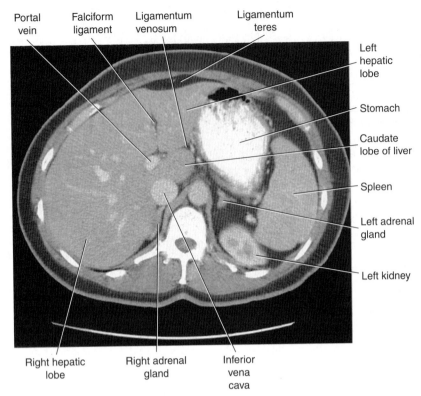

FIG. 4.46 Abdomen—axial image.

6. Accessory spleens (splenules) are common incidental findings on CT examinations of the abdomen. They appear as small nodules of splenic tissue just adjacent to the main spleen. They usually have little clinical significance but may be mistaken for other types of abdominal masses.

PANCREAS

1. MDCT is capable of thin-section acquisition through the entire pancreas, in a single breath-hold, during multiple phases of contrast enhancement (Fig. 4.47).
2. The isotropic nature of current MDCT acquisition also allows for high-quality reformation of the pancreas in multiple planes and volume-rendered techniques, further improving its diagnostic capabilities.
3. Indications for CT of the pancreas include:
   a. Evaluation of pancreatitis: The role of CT is to assess pancreatic and peripancreatic inflammatory changes and to identify the presence of pancreatic necrosis.
   b. Identification of pancreatic neoplasms, including:
      • Adenocarcinoma, the most common pancreatic neoplasm.
      • Cysts or pseudocysts.
      • Endocrine masses, such as islet cell tumors.
   c. Trauma.
   d. Complications of cystic fibrosis.
4. Most pancreatic tumors appear hypodense in comparison with surrounding contrast-enhanced pancreatic parenchyma.

5. Imaging the pancreas during the phase of peak parenchymal enhancement vastly increases the conspicuity of most pancreatic neoplasms.
6. The pancreatic phase of contrast enhancement is a delayed arterial phase occurring approximately 35 to 45 seconds after the start of contrast agent administration, assuming that an adequate volume is injected at a rate of 3 mL/sec or higher.
7. Protocol considerations for a multiphasic MDCT scan of the pancreas are department specific but may include any or all of the following:
   a. Water as an oral contrast agent to distend the proximal GI tract without the streaking artifact possible when positive CM are used.
   b. Injection of 100 to 150 mL of iodinated contrast agent at 3 to 5 mL/sec.
   c. Precontrast imaging for localization of the pancreas and identification of calcifications.
   d. Arterial phase acquisition through the pancreas after a 20- to 25-second delay from the start of the injection. During this period there is maximum opacification of the surrounding vasculature, including the aorta and superior mesenteric artery. An important goal of pancreatic CT is to evaluate the involvement of surrounding vessels by pancreatic neoplasm.
   e. Pancreatic (delayed arterial) phase acquisition after a 35- to 45-second delay from the start of injection. This is the phase of optimal pancreatic parenchymal enhancement.
   f. Venous phase acquisition through the entire abdomen after a 60- to 70-second delay from the start of

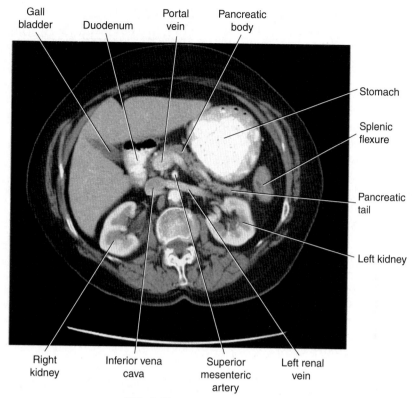

Gall bladder · Duodenum · Portal vein · Pancreatic body · Stomach · Splenic flexure · Pancreatic tail · Left kidney · Right kidney · Inferior vena cava · Superior mesenteric artery · Left renal vein

FIG. 4.47 Abdomen—axial image.

injection. This phase provides imaging during portal opacification and optimal hepatic enhancement.

  g. Images 1 to 3 mm thick are reconstructed from data obtained with detector collimation as low as possible. The detector collimation may range from 1.25 mm in a 4-slice MDCT system to 0.5 mm in a 64-slice system, or higher.

  h. Thinner (0.5 to 1.25 mm) overlapping reconstructions may be used for angiographic, MPR, and 3-D applications.

8. The primary goal of multiphasic CT evaluation of a pancreatic mass is the determination of tumor resectability. Several factors determine the potential for surgical removal of a pancreatic tumor, including:

  a. Vascular involvement of the mass.

  b. Local tumor spread.

  c. Metastases.

9. Patients who have been determined to be candidates for surgical intervention typically undergo a resection of the pancreas and duodenum known as a *Whipple procedure.*

ADRENAL GLANDS

1. CT is the primary imaging modality for the evaluation of the adrenal glands.

2. The *adrenal glands* are small, soft tissue structures with a CT density similar to that of muscle (25 to 40 HU).

3. They lie in the space just superior to each kidney and are surrounded by fat, a feature that improves

their inherent contrast and subsequent visualization by CT.

4. During routine abdominal CT imaging, the adrenal glands are usually adequately imaged with slice thicknesses in the 3- to 5-mm range.

5. Specific CT assessment of the adrenal glands benefits from thinner slice widths, in the range of 0.5 to 2.0 mm, depending on the CT system's capabilities.

6. When not contraindicated, both precontrast and postcontrast imaging are usually necessary to fully characterize adrenal pathology.

7. Acquisition is made routinely during the portal venous phase of contrast enhancement. Delayed imaging (10 to 15 minutes) may also be employed for tumor characterization.

8. Beyond assessment during routine scanning of the abdomen, there are several indications for specific CT evaluation of the adrenal glands, including:

  a. Endocrine abnormality, to rule out an adrenal mass.

  b. Oncologic staging; the adrenal gland is a common location for metastatic disease from lung carcinoma.

  c. Characterization of an adrenal lesion identified on another study/modality (adrenal "incidentaloma").

9. Adrenal hyperplasia is an enlargement of the adrenal gland(s), usually associated with a disorder of endocrine function.

10. The majority of focal adrenal masses are benign adenomas.

11. Differentiation between a metastatic lesion and a benign adenoma is an important goal of the CT evaluation of an adrenal mass:

a. On precontrast imaging, ROI measurements of a mass that are less than 10 HU indicate a benign process.

b. On delayed postcontrast imaging, metastatic lesions of the adrenal gland remain enhanced longer than adrenal adenomas.

c. The extent of the dissipation of enhancement, or "washout," can be calculated during delayed (10 to 15 minutes) imaging of the adrenal glands.

12. The pancreatic tail, tortuous vasculature, splenules, bowel loops, and so on may appear as pseudotumors on axial CT images. The utilization of MPR (coronal, sagittal) images improves differentiation of pseudo-tumors from true adrenal masses.

GENITOURINARY SYSTEM

1. CT is the primary imaging modality for the evaluation of the *urinary tract*, which consists of the kidneys, ureters, and bladder.

2. The kidneys are enveloped and supported by a sheath of connective tissue called *Gerota's fascia*.

3. The renal parenchyma consists of the internal medulla surrounded by the renal cortex.

4. The renal pelvis contains the minor and major calyces, which lead inferiorly into the ureters.

5. The epithelial lining of the urinary tract is called the *urothelium*.

6. General indications for CT assessment of the urinary tract include:
   a. Identification of urinary calculi.
   b. Evaluation of the kidney, ureters, and/or bladder for tumor, infection (pyelonephritis), and trauma.
   c. Assessment of renal vasculature.

7. Unenhanced helical CT of the urinary tract has become the standard for the investigation of urinary tract lithiasis (stones).

8. Thin-section (3 to 5 mm) acquisition is made from above the kidneys through the base of the bladder.

9. Per specific department protocol, the scan may begin above the diaphragm to include the entire abdomen. CT holds a distinct advantage over other imaging modalities in its ability to identify nongeni-tourinary pathology—pancreatitis, cholelithiasis, appendicitis, diverticulitis—in patients with abdominal pain.

10. No patient preparation is typically required because this is a noncontrast study. However, better patient hydration through the ingestion of water before the study can help eliminate small hyperdensities of the renal pyramids that can mimic stones.

11. When there is a question of stones within the bladder or at the uterovesical junction (UVJ), additional imaging with the patient in the prone position may be used to improve differentiation between UVJ stones and calcifications (phleboliths) within the pelvic veins (Fig. 4.48).

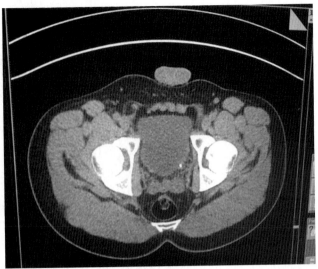

FIG. 4.48 Axial pelvis with patient in the prone position. Note the calcification at the left uretovesical junction (UVJ) that does not change position in the prone patient, indicating that this stone is not in the bladder. *(Image courtesy of Steven Ahrenstein, BS, RT[R] [CT].)*

12. Patient radiation dose should be kept at a minimum through either weight-based manual or automated modulation techniques.

13. In a further effort to reduce overall patient radiation dose, all noncontrast renal stone survey studies may be performed in the prone position. This alternative may help reduce the need for additional sequences by initially differentiating UVJ stones and pelvic *phleboliths* (calcifications within pelvic veins).

14. The diagnosis of distal ureteral stones may be complicated by the presence of phleboliths, regardless of patient position. An IV contrast agent may be administered to better distinguish the ureter from adjacent phleboliths.

15. Administration of an iodinated contrast agent also aids in demonstrating the inflammation of the renal fascia and obstruction of the collecting system that are often associated with urinary lithiasis.

16. The characterization of most renal masses also requires the IV administration of an iodinated contrast agent.

17. Cystic renal masses are common, are usually benign, and may be identified before the administration of contrast agent, as follows:
   a. *Simple cysts:* Smooth, round, thin-walled masses with homogeneous near-water CT density (<20 HU).
   b. *Hyperdense cysts:* Complicated cystic masses with CT densities in the range of 25 to 90 HU on unenhanced scans. Because of infection or hemor-rhage, these masses have CT densities greater than the density of surrounding normal renal parenchyma and therefore appear "hyperdense."
   c. *Polycystic kidney disease (PKD):* A genetic disorder characterized by the formation of numerous renal cysts.

d. *Parapelvic cysts:* Instead of arising from the renal cortex as most simple cysts do, parapelvic cysts occur within the renal pelvis. They can sometimes appear as hydronephrosis, or distention of the pelvis and calyces, which would be secondary to renal obstruction. Delayed imaging after IV administration of a contrast agent opacifies the renal pelvis, clearly differentiating hydronephrosis from parapelvic cysts.

18. After administration of a contrast agent, a renal cyst should not "enhance," or exhibit a significant increase in CT density.

19. *Pseudoenhancement* describes the minimal "enhancement" of a renal cyst after contrast agent administration. This apparent increase in attenuation, of 15 to 20 HU, likely results from volume averaging primarily caused by dense cortical enhancement of the kidneys. The occurrence of pseudoenhancement has increased with the advent of MDCT.

20. An *angiomyolipoma* of the kidney is a benign mass of blood vessels (angio-), muscle tissue (myo-), and fat (lipoma). An ROI measurement of less than −10 HU characterizes a renal mass as an angiomyolipoma.

21. Malignant masses of the kidney include:
    a. Renal cell carcinoma (RCC): The most common primary renal malignancy. RCC is typically characterized by marked contrast enhancement (>20 to 25 HU).
    b. *Transitional cell carcinoma* (TCC): A tumor originating in the urothelium. Most TCCs arise in the bladder, with the possibility of additional masses in the ureters, renal pelvis, or both. On precontrast imaging, TCC usually appears as a hypodense lesion within the renal collecting system that has a CT density greater than that of urine but less than that of renal parenchyma (<40 HU). TCC significantly enhances after administration of a contrast agent.
    c. Metastases: Lung, colon, and breast cancers are primary malignancies that commonly result in renal metastases.

22. Like other abdominal organs, the kidneys undergo distinct phases of contrast enhancement. The described phases are transient in nature, and their reported times assume a contrast agent bolus of adequate volume administered at a rate of 2 mL/sec or higher:
    a. *Corticomedullary phase:* A late arterial phase beginning 30 to 40 seconds after the initiation of contrast agent administration. Optimal enhancement of the renal cortex and renal veins occurs during this period. The renal medulla is minimally enhanced, allowing for its maximum differentiation from the renal cortex.
    b. *Nephrographic phase:* Time between 70 and 90 seconds after the start of injection. Enhancement differences between renal cortex and medulla reach equilibrium, providing optimal sensitivity for parenchymal lesions. Imaging during the nephrographic phase also allows for portal opacification and optimal hepatic enhancement, which are important for the assessment of disease spread (Fig. 4.49).
    c. *Excretory phase:* A delayed imaging phase that begins approximately 3 minutes after the initiation of contrast agent administration. During this phase, the contrast agent has been excreted into the renal

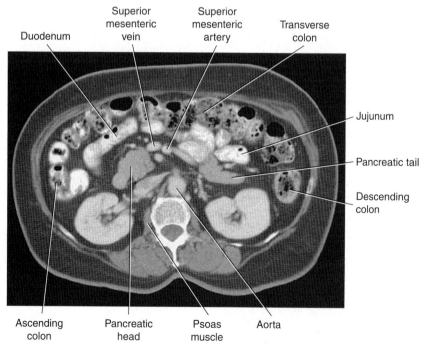

FIG. 4.49 Abdomen—axial image.

calyces, opacifying the renal pelvis and the remainder of the urinary collecting system (ureters, bladder). The excretory phase best demonstrates the filling defects and the potential lesions involving the urothelium.

23. A *CT urogram* (CT intravenous pyelogram [IVP]) is a comprehensive, multiphasic evaluation of the urinary tract. Although variation in specific protocols exists, the key components to a CT urogram are:
    a. Noncontrast image acquisition of the urinary tract.
    b. Postcontrast image acquisition of the abdomen and pelvis.
    c. Thin-section delayed (excretory phase) imaging of the urinary tract.
    d. Coronal MIP and volume-rendered images for CT urographic display.

24. Opacification of the urinary tract may be improved by the IV drip administration of approximately 250 mL of normal (0.9%) saline during the delay before the excretory acquisition.

25. Another approach combines axial CT with 2-D excretory urography. Postcontrast CT sequences are followed by an appropriate delay (5 to 15 minutes). Conventional radiographs are then obtained with or without compression to form a combination CT-radiography urogram.

26. Protocol considerations for a multiphasic MDCT scan of the kidneys and urinary tract are department specific but may include any or all of the following:
    a. Use of water as oral contrast agent to distend the proximal GI tract while avoiding interference from positive CM during MPR and 3-D techniques. A positive oral contrast agent (iodine or barium) may be utilized to simultaneously evaluate the GI tract for alternative etiologies, assess lymphadenopathy, and so on.
    b. Precontrast imaging through the kidneys, ureters, and bladder for identification of calculi.
    c. Injection of 100 to 150 mL of iodinated contrast agent at 3 to 5 mL/sec.
    d. Arterial phase image acquisition through the kidneys and renal vasculature after a 20- to 25-second delay after the start of injection. During this period there is maximum opacification of the aorta and renal arteries.
    e. Corticomedullary (late arterial) phase acquisition through the kidneys after a 30- to 40-second delay after the start of injection. This phase best demonstrates the interface between renal cortex and medulla as well as the potential vascular involvement of a renal mass.
    f. Nephrographic (parenchymal) phase acquisition through the entire abdomen after a 70- to 90-second delay after the start of injection. The nephrographic phase best demonstrates parenchymal renal masses.
    g. Excretory (delayed) acquisition through the kidneys, ureters, and bladder after a 3- to 15-minute (or longer) delay. This phase allows for optimal opacification of the renal collecting system. The excretory acquisition is utilized in MPR, volumetric rendering (VR), and MIP techniques for the production of a CT urogram. This is also the phase that best demonstrates TCC of the urothelium.
    h. Images 1 to 3 mm thick reconstructed from data obtained with detector collimation as low as possible. Detector collimation may range from 1.25 mm in a 4-slice MDCT system to 0.6 mm in a 64-slice system.
    i. Thinner (0.5 to 1.25 mm) overlapping reconstructions may be used for angiographic, MPR, and 3-D applications (Figs. 4.50 and 4.51).
    j. Selection of acquired phases of enhancement should balance the clinical needs of the examination while reducing patient radiation dose to a minimum.

27. The most common abnormality of the ureters is a dual collecting system, or ureteral duplication. This condition is often an incidental finding characterized by the appearance of a second ureter descending from an individual kidney.

28. Ureteral duplication is more symptomatic in the pediatric patient and may present as urine reflux or obstruction.

29. TCC and obstruction from stones are two additional pathologic conditions of the ureters demonstrated on CT examination.

30. The bladder varies in size and appearance according to the amount of urine held. The unenhanced CT density of urine is similar to that of water.

31. Nephrographic (70 to 90 seconds) imaging provides an enhanced bladder wall used to evaluate the extent of tumor infiltration.

32. The additional delayed phase (>5 minutes) imaging of CT urography can be helpful in displaying the filling defects associated with bladder cancer.

33. Additional sequences with the patient in a prone and/or decubitus position may improve visualization of bladder wall tumors.

GASTROINTESTINAL SYSTEM

1. The *gastrointestinal tract* consists of the esophagus, stomach, small intestine, and large intestine.
2. Anatomic structures of the GI system are evaluated on all CT studies of the abdomen and/or pelvis (Figs. 4.52 and 4.53).
3. Although its findings are often nonspecific, CT plays an important role in the identification of disease within the GI tract.
4. General indications for CT evaluation of the GI system include:
    a. Inflammatory disease.
    b. Identification, evaluation, and staging of GI neoplasm.

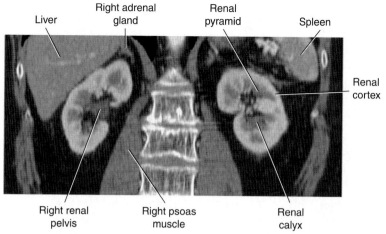

FIG. 4.50 Abdomen—coronal multiplanar reformation (MPR) image.

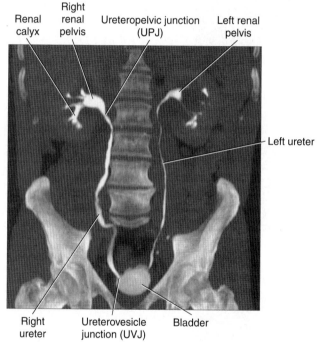

FIG. 4.51 Coronal maximum intensity projection (MIP) image of the abdomen and pelvis. This image was produced from a delayed (excretory) phase acquisition during a CT urogram.

c. Trauma.

d. Vascular disease.

5. CT imaging is also extremely valuable in the evaluation of various complications of GI disease processes, such as:

a. *Perforation:* Puncture in the wall of the GI tract. Contents within the stomach or intestine may then spill into the abdominal cavity, with the potential to cause infection known as *peritonitis.*

b. *Fistula:* An abnormal connection between the intestine and an adjacent structure. Fistulas are commonly associated with inflammatory bowel disease (IBD).

c. *Abscess:* A collection of pus caused by an infectious or inflammatory process within the GI tract.

6. The most important identifying sign of GI pathology on CT examination is wall thickening. The ability to evaluate the gastric and bowel walls is a crucial component of successful CT evaluation of the GI system.

7. Historically, CT evaluation of the bowel wall has been hampered by the muscular digestive motion of peristalsis. The acquisition speed of MDCT effectively eliminates peristaltic motion artifact and greatly improves the CT evaluation of intestinal wall pathology.

8. Distention and opacification with oral media, coupled with contrast enhancement through IV administration, offer the best level of GI wall demonstration.

9. The factors governing optimal bowel opacification and distention from oral contrast agents are:

a. Contrast agent type: Dilute barium and water-soluble iodine oral CM are available as positive contrast agents. Water may serve as a negative oral contrast agent, providing bowel distention without the artifact possible with denser material. Air and gas are negative contrast agents used for stomach or bowel distention.

b. Contrast agent volume: 750 to 1500 mL of oral contrast agent is typical for general studies of the abdomen and pelvis.

c. Timing: Delay of scanning after the administration of oral contrast agent is based on the area of clinical concern. Opacification of the stomach and proximal small bowel may take only 30 minutes, whereas proper evaluation of the large intestine requires a delay of at least 90 minutes. Delays of up to 24 hours are not uncommon for complete opacification of the distal large intestine. Transit time varies with the patient's physiologic condition.

d. Route of administration: Direct and immediate opacification of the distal large colon is possible

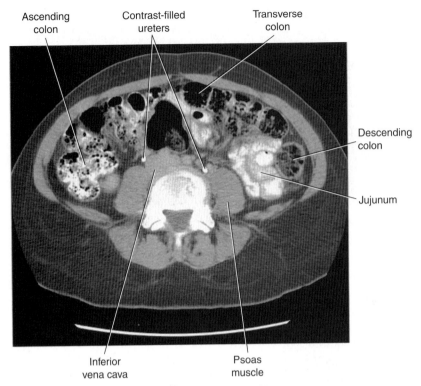

FIG. 4.52 Abdomen—axial image.

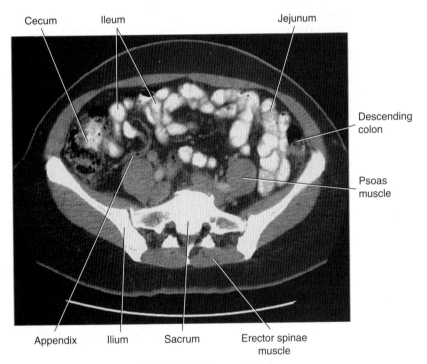

FIG. 4.53 Pelvis—axial image.

with an enema of 150 to 250 mL of a positive contrast agent.

e. Patient position: CT of the abdomen and/or pelvis is performed predominantly with the patient in the supine position. Additional positions may be used to improve opacification and distention of a particular portion of the GI tract.

10. Bowel wall enhances with the IV administration of an iodinated contrast agent. Enhancement improves demonstration of bowel wall thickening, mass lesions, inflammatory processes, and vascular perfusion abnormalities such as bowel ischemia.

11. Injection techniques for studies of the GI system are similar to those for general abdominal indications.

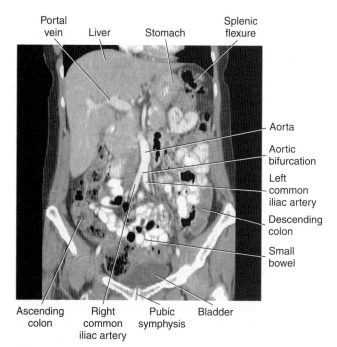

Portal vein   Liver   Stomach   Splenic flexure

Aorta

Aortic bifurcation

Left common iliac artery

Descending colon

Small bowel

Ascending colon   Right common iliac artery   Pubic symphysis   Bladder

FIG. 4.54 Coronal multiplanar reformation (MPR) image of the abdomen and pelvis.

100 to 150 mL of nonionic contrast agent administered at a rate of 2 to 4 mL/sec provides adequate wall enhancement.

12. Acquisition is typically obtained during the portal venous phase for optimal gastric and intestinal wall enhancement.

13. Contiguous 3- to 5-mm sections through the abdomen and pelvis, from above the diaphragm to the pubic symphysis, are acquired for complete evaluation of the GI system.

14. MDCT systems may utilize a narrow detector collimation (0.5 to 1.25 mm) for optimal MPR quality when clinically indicated (Fig. 4.54).

15. For evaluation of potential esophageal pathology, the acquisition may begin more superiorly as dictated by the area(s) of clinical concern.

16. The esophagus appears as an air- or contrast-filled cylindrical structure on axial CT imaging.

17. In addition to oral and IV contrast agents, a thick barium paste may be given immediately before scanning to further outline the esophagus.

18. CT of the esophagus is performed predominantly for evaluation of a neoplasm and staging of esophageal malignancy.

19. Inflammation of the esophagus, or *esophagitis*, is characterized on CT by uniform cylindrical thickening of the esophageal wall. Esophagitis is often secondary to gastroesophageal reflux disease (GERD).

20. Other abnormalities demonstrated during CT of the esophagus include:
    a. Foreign bodies.
    b. *Esophageal varices*, which are dilated veins of the esophagus that result from portal hypertension.

They are often seen in patients with cirrhosis of the liver.
    c. *Hiatal hernia*, defined as a protrusion of the gastroesophageal junction through the diaphragm into the thorax.

21. The stomach must be distended with a positive or negative oral contrast agent, or both, for CT evaluation.

22. 150 to 250 mL of dilute barium or iodine contrast agent is administered immediately before scanning. Alternatively, use of water as an oral contrast agent improves visualization of the enhancing gastric mucosa when an IV contrast agent is administered.

23. The stomach may be further distended with the administration of effervescent granules.

24. Placing the patient in the prone or decubitus position may also improve the demonstration of gastric pathology. A positive oral contrast agent distends the dependent portion of the stomach, whereas gasforming crystals provide distention of the side facing upward.

25. Patients should have fasted for 4 to 6 hours before the study to ensure that the stomach is empty of food, which otherwise may mimic abnormality.

26. Common indications for specific CT evaluation of the stomach include benign and malignant gastric neoplasms, lymphoma, hiatal hernia, and assessment of complications resulting from bariatric (weight loss) surgery.

27. The *small intestine* is divided proximally to distally as the duodenum, jejunum, and ileum.

28. The duodenal bulb connects to the stomach's pyloric sphincter. The ileum leads to the large intestine at the ileocecal valve.

29. The duodenum is suspended from the diaphragm by the ligament of Treitz.

30. Opacification with an oral contrast agent is typically necessary for CT evaluation of the small intestine.

31. An oral contrast agent should be administered in sufficient volume (>750 mL) and at least 30 minutes before scanning for the duodenum and jejunum. Opacification of the ileum and proximal large intestine may take an hour or more, depending on the individual patient.

32. Water as an oral contrast agent improves visualization of the enhancing enteral wall when an IV contrast agent is administered.

33. MPR and 3-D techniques may aid in visualization of the small bowel in its entirety.

34. External hernia of the small intestine is a common occurrence. There are many types of external hernias, including:
    a. *Inguinal:* Lower anterior abdominal wall in the region of the groin.
    b. *Umbilical:* Near the umbilicus; umbilical hernia is most common in pregnant women and obese patients.
    c. *Incisional:* A complication of surgery.

35. *Small bowel obstruction* (SBO) is a serious and potentially fatal pathologic condition amenable to CT assessment.

36. SBO is typically characterized by loops of dilated proximal small bowel terminating abruptly at an area of collapsed bowel. Oral contrast agent does not pass beyond the obstruction.

37. Causes of SBO include adhesions, hernia, and tumor.

38. *Intussusception* describes the condition whereby a portion of the small intestine collapses or telescopes into itself. It is a rare occurrence that may result in obstruction.

39. *Ileus* is an area of intestine that has lost normal contractile motion, resulting in obstruction.

40. *Crohn's disease* is an inflammatory condition that often affects the small intestine. It is usually characterized on CT by wall thickening, edema, and haziness of the fat surrounding the affected bowel. Also referred to as *stranding,* this increase in density of fat usually indicates inflammation. Crohn's disease may also affect the large colon and the remainder of the GI tract.

41. Other conditions of the small intestine that are evaluated by CT are benign and malignant neoplasm, lymphoma, edema, and trauma.

42. The *large intestine* begins with the cecum at the ileocecal valve and progresses to the ascending, transverse, and descending portions; the sigmoid colon; and rectum.

43. The appendix appears in most patients as a tubular structure extending from the cecum, near the ileocecal valve.

44. Anatomic location, haustral markings, and the presence of fecal matter help identify the large intestine on CT cross-section.

45. Opacification with an oral contrast agent is typically a necessity for CT evaluation of the large intestine.

46. Oral contrast agents should be administered in sufficient volume (>750 mL) and at least 90 minutes before scanning. Opacification of the distal large intestine may take as much as 24 hours, depending on the individual patient.

47. Direct and immediate opacification of the distal large intestine is possible with an enema of 150 to 250 mL of a positive contrast agent.

48. Insufflation with air or gas distends the rectum and distal colon, allowing for improved visualization of wall pathology.

49. Clinical indications for CT evaluation of the large intestine include:
    a. Neoplasm: Polyps (adenoma): precancerous growths of the colon.
       • Colorectal carcinoma: CT is used primarily for staging of the disease and assessment for reoccurrence.
    b. Inflammation:
       • *Diverticulitis* refers to the inflammation of *diverticula,* which are pouches that develop outward from the colon wall. It is most common in the sigmoid and is characterized on CT by wall thickening and stranding of the surrounding fat (Fig. 4.55).
       • *Inflammatory bowel disease* (IBD) is a general term used to describe conditions of inflammation of the colon, or colitis:
       • *Crohn's colitis* is similar to Crohn's disease, which affects the small intestine.
       • *Ulcerative colitis* (UC) is characterized on CT by wall thickening and narrowing of the intestinal lumen.
       • Appendicitis, inflammation of the appendix, is characterized on CT by distention, a thickened contrast-enhancing wall, and periappendiceal fat stranding. CT examinations to diagnose appendicitis should be optimized with thin-section (<5 mm) imaging through the entire abdomen and pelvis to identify potential causes of abdominal pain that are unrelated to the appendix. IV administration of a contrast agent may improve visualization of the appendix in the patient with limited intra-abdominal fat. Oral or rectal administration of a contrast agent can also improve identification of the appendicitis and its associated inflammatory changes (Fig. 4.56).

50. Focused CT for appendicitis reduces patient radiation dose by limiting the acquisition to the area of the cecum and appendix only. Although the radiation dose is significantly reduced with this technique, the chances of detection of alternative diagnoses are also lower. Focused CT for appendicitis is usually employed in pediatric patients.

51. An *appendicolith,* a calcification within the appendix, is often associated with appendicitis.

52. An *enterovesical fistula* is an abnormal communication between the bowel and the bladder. It typically results from inflammatory processes of the colon such as diverticulitis. The role of CT in suspected fistula is to identify the entry of oral or rectal contrast agent into the bladder through the fistula. It is important that the bladder not be opacified. Therefore acquisition of sections before the administration of an IV contrast agent is crucial.

PELVIS AND REPRODUCTIVE SYSTEM

1. Clinical indications for CT evaluation of the pelvis include:
   a. Identification of primary pelvic cancers, including those of the colon, bladder, and reproductive organs.
   b. Oncologic staging, which includes evaluation of pelvic adenopathy for metastatic spread of primary cancer to the pelvic lymph nodes and assessment of local tumor recurrence.
   c. Assessment of soft tissue and bony trauma.

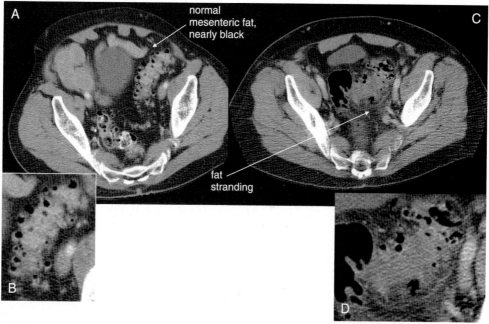

FIG. 4.55 Diverticulosis compared with diverticulitis, CT. Compare the axial image in (A) showing uninflamed sigmoid diverticuli, with that in (C) showing sigmoid diverticulitis. The normal fat surrounding the sigmoid colon appears nearly black with a soft-tissue window in A, whereas the inflamed fat in C shows stranding, giving it a gray or smoky appearance. Whereas the borders of the uninflamed sigmoid colon are quite distinct in A, the margins of the sigmoid are blurred in C, reflecting inflammation of the bowel wall and surrounding fat. (B and D) Close-ups from A and C, respectively. *(Adapted from Broder J:* Imaging of nontraumatic abdominal conditions in diagnostic imaging for the emergency physician, *2011, pp. 445–577.)*

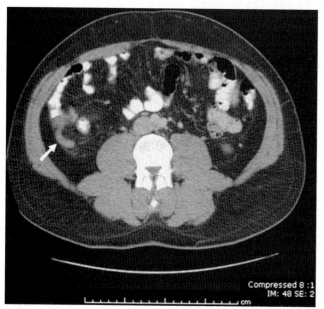

FIG. 4.56 Axial CT of the lower abdomen showing an enlarged appendix with a diameter greater than 1 cm (arrow), consistent with acute, uncomplicated appendicitis. *(Adapted from Horn A, Ufberg J: Appendicitis, diverticulitis, and colitis.* Emerg Med Clin North Am *2011; 29[2]:347–368.)*

2. The male reproductive organs are not commonly imaged by CT. However, the internal location of the prostate gland and seminal vesicles allows for their visualization during a routine examination of the male pelvis (Fig. 4.57).

3. The external penis and testicles are not routinely evaluated by CT but may be included on scans that proceed inferiorly beyond the pelvic floor.

4. Ectopic or undescended testes appear internally within the pelvis. They are usually atrophic in appearance and have a greater propensity for malignancy.

5. A *hydrocele* of the testes is an abnormal accumulation of fluid around a testicle.

6. On axial CT, the prostate gland is positioned between the pubic symphysis anteriorly and the rectum posteriorly. It lies just inferior to the base of the bladder.

7. *Benign prostate hyperplasia (BPH)* is an increase in prostate volume, which can result in constriction of the urethra and interference with urination. It typically occurs in middle-aged to elderly men and is similar in CT appearance to prostate carcinoma.

8. CT findings in prostate carcinoma include prostatic enlargement and pelvic adenopathy. The primary role of CT in the diagnosis and treatment of prostate cancer is one of staging.

9. The pair of seminal vesicles forms a "bow-tie" shape between the prostate and the base of the bladder.

10. The *female reproductive organs* are routinely demonstrated on CT because of their internal location. They are the uterus, cervix, ovaries, and fallopian tubes (Figs. 4.58 and 4.59).

11. The uterus is typically demonstrated as an oval, homogeneous, soft tissue mass positioned between the bladder and rectum.

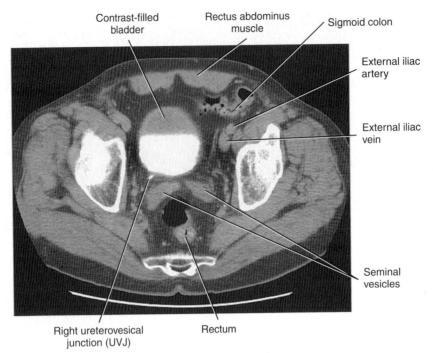

Contrast-filled bladder — Rectus abdominus muscle — Sigmoid colon — External iliac artery — External iliac vein — Seminal vesicles — Right ureterovesical junction (UVJ) — Rectum

FIG. 4.57 Male pelvis—axial image.

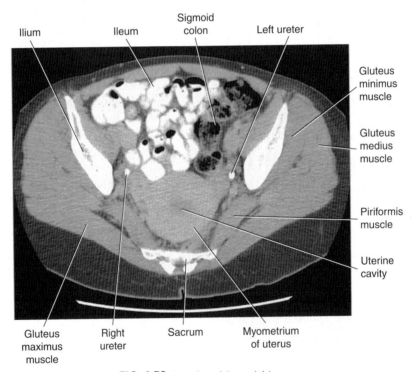

Ilium — Ileum — Sigmoid colon — Left ureter — Gluteus minimus muscle — Gluteus medius muscle — Piriformis muscle — Uterine cavity — Gluteus maximus muscle — Right ureter — Sacrum — Myometrium of uterus

FIG. 4.58 Female pelvis—axial image.

12. The uterine wall is divided as follows:
    a. *Perimetrium:* Outer layer.
    b. *Myometrium:* Middle layer.
    c. *Endometrium:* Inner layer.
13. The myometrium enhances brightly after IV administration of a contrast agent, because of its highly vascular composition.

14. The cervix extends inferiorly from the uterus and may also enhance after IV administration of a contrast agent.
15. *Adnexa* is used to describe an appendage of an organ; the ovaries and fallopian tubes constitute the uterine adnexa.
16. The ovaries may demonstrate a soft tissue or cystic CT density and are located in close proximity to the

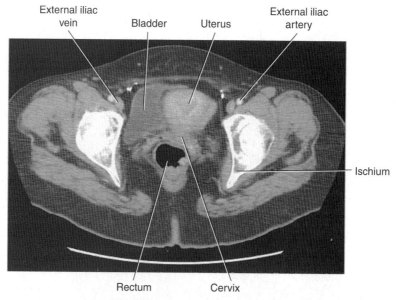

External iliac vein   Bladder   Uterus   External iliac artery

Ischium

Rectum   Cervix

FIG. 4.59 Female pelvis—axial image.

uterus. The ovaries are often not visualized in post-menopausal women.

17. The primary clinical indications for CT of the female pelvis and reproductive organs are the evaluation of pelvic pain and the identification or staging of gynecologic masses.

18. Benign masses of the uterus and adnexa include:
   a. *Leiomyoma,* or fibroid uterus.
   b. Ovarian cysts.
   c. *Cystic teratoma,* a dermoid mass consisting of various CT densities, including those of soft tissue, fat, teeth, and bone.

19. Malignant masses of the uterus and adnexa include:
   a. Cervical cancer.
   b. Uterine cancer; endometrial carcinoma is the most prevalent gynecologic malignancy.
   c. Ovarian cancer, the CT appearance of which may be uniformly solid or cystic, or a combination of the two.

20. For the evaluation of a gynecologic mass, the insertion of a tampon assists in identifying the vaginal canal.

Special Procedures

A. Body CT Angiography

1. MDCT systems with detector configurations of 16-slice and above are readily capable of scanning the entire abdomen with submillimeter collimation in less than 20 seconds. With careful bolus timing, the abdominal vasculature may be imaged during a single breath-hold and at peak arterial enhancement.

2. Isotropic data acquisition allows for high-quality vascular imaging in any plane, including volumetric 3-D display.

3. Body CTA includes the CT angiographic evaluation of the following structures:

   a. Aorta.
   b. Renal arteries.
   c. Mesenteric arteries.
   d. Hepatic arteries.

4. The technical considerations for body CTA are similar to those outlined in previous sections on CT angiography. Additional information specific to each anatomic area is summarized in this section.

5. Protocols are CT system specific, being adjusted according to the clinical area of concern. Detector collimation, gantry rotation time, and pitch are adjusted to ensure that the entire acquisition is attained during a single breath-hold.

6. The guiding principle of contrast agent administration for CTA is that the bolus should last throughout the entire scan, but not beyond it.

7. Total volumes of contrast agents used range from 75 to 125 mL, being determined by the flow rate and the scan duration.

8. Good venous access is required because flow rates in the range of 4 to 5 mL/sec are recommended.

9. Scan delay is determined by a test bolus or automated bolus tracking.

10. Arterial phase imaging is performed for arterial vascular mapping, and portal venous phase imaging for venous vascular mapping.

11. A positive oral contrast agent is not given because of its interference with MPR and 3-D imaging techniques.

12. The primary indications for CTA of the aorta are aneurysm and dissection.

13. MDCT technology allows for scanning of the entire aorta in a single breath-hold from above the arch through the common iliac arteries. The extent of acquisition is determined by the clinical indication (Fig. 4.60).

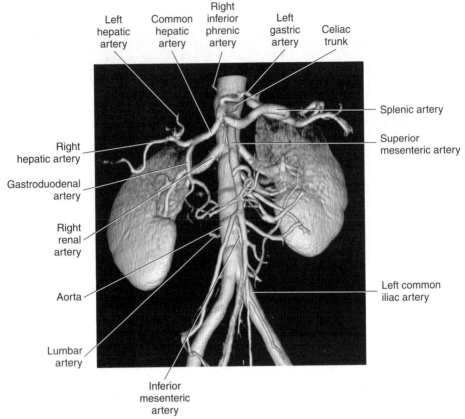

Left hepatic artery · Common hepatic artery · Right inferior phrenic artery · Left gastric artery · Celiac trunk

Splenic artery

Superior mesenteric artery

Right hepatic artery

Gastroduodenal artery

Right renal artery

Aorta

Left common iliac artery

Lumbar artery

Inferior mesenteric artery

FIG. 4.60 CT angiogram of the abdominal aorta. *(From Kelley L, Peterson C: Sectional anatomy for image professionals, 3rd ed. St Louis, 2013, Mosby. Fig. 7.141.)*

14. The abdominal aorta divides into the right and left common iliac arteries at approximately the level of L4.
15. Additional technical considerations for CTA of the aorta may be found earlier, in the section on chest CTA.
16. The primary indications for CTA of the renal arteries are stenosis, aneurysm, and renal transplant evaluation.
17. The renal arteries, which are small structures, are optimally visualized with MDCT section widths of 1.25 mm or less.
18. The general rule for CTA in all body areas is that the section width should be no wider than the diameter of the smallest vessel to be evaluated.
19. CTA evaluation of the mesenteric vasculature includes the superior mesenteric artery (SMA), inferior mesenteric artery (IMA), superior mesenteric vein (SMV), and inferior mesenteric vein (IMV).
20. Also evaluated are the branches of the celiac axis:
    a. Left gastric artery.
    b. Common hepatic artery.
    c. Splenic artery.
21. Dual-phase imaging, which consists of the arterial (20 to 30 seconds) and portal venous (60 to 70 seconds) phases, is typically performed for complete evaluation of the mesenteric vasculature.

22. Indications for CTA evaluation of the mesenteric vasculature include:
    a. Assessment of neoplastic invasion (primarily from pancreatic cancer).
    b. Bowel ischemia; occlusion or thrombosis of the mesenteric vessels can result in decreased blood supply to bowel.
    c. Unexplained GI bleed.
23. CTA of the hepatic arteries is performed primarily for assessment of the hepatic transplant patient. Additional indications are aneurysm and pretherapy planning for hepatic carcinoma.
24. Protocols for body CTA depend strictly on the area(s) of clinical concern and the technical capabilities of the CT system employed. Example technical parameters using a 64-slice system are:
    a. Water as an oral contrast agent to distend the proximal GI tract.
    b. Initial noncontrast, low-dose acquisition through the area(s) of interest to localize vasculature, evaluate for calcium, intramural hematoma (IMH), or other pathology.
    c. Injection of 75 to 125 mL of a nonionic contrast agent at 4 mL/sec.
    d. Administration of a saline flush to improve contrast agent dose efficiency.

e. Test bolus or automated bolus tracking measured at the celiac artery.

f. Helical CTA acquisition with 0.625 mm detector width.

g. Scan extent is determined by the area(s) of clinical concern.

h. 80 to 120 kVp, auto mA modulation.

i. 0.5- to 0.8-second gantry rotation time.

j. Reconstructed slice thickness of 0.6 to 0.75 mm with 50% overlap.

k. Use of MPR, MIP, and VR imaging techniques.

B. CT Enteroclysis

1. *CT enteroclysis* is a specialized evaluation of the small bowel whereby a nasogastric catheter is placed into the duodenum under fluoroscopic guidance. 1.5 to 2.0 L of enteral contrast agent is administered directly into the small intestine for maximal opacification.

2. Non-IV contrast, thin-section (0.6 to 1.25 mm) CT images are acquired through the abdomen and pelvis.

3. Coronal and sagittal MPR images are used to visualize the small intestine in its entirety.

4. Alternatively, CT enteroclysis can be performed with a neutral enteral contrast agent such as water or 0.1% barium sulfate (VoLumen) infused through a nasogastric tube. 125 to 150 mL of an iodinated IV contrast agent is administered at a rate of 3 to 5 mL/sec. CT acquisition occurs at a delay of 45 to 50 seconds, corresponding to the early portal venous phase of optimal intestinal wall enhancement.

5. Clinical indications for CT enteroclysis include Crohn's disease, obstruction, and neoplasms of the small intestine.

C. CT Enterography

1. *CT enterography* is an MDCT scan specifically of the small intestine that is less invasive than CT enteroclysis.

2. Opacification of the small intestine is achieved by the oral administration of a large volume (1.5 to 2.0 L) of low-density (0.1%) barium sulfate solution (VoLumen).

3. Example protocol for oral contrast agent administration is:

a. 500 mL 60 minutes before scan.

b. 500 mL 40 minutes before scan.

c. 250 mL 20 minutes before scan.

d. 250 mL 10 minutes before scan.

4. An iodinated IV contrast agent is administered at a rate of 3 to 5 mL/sec to a total volume of 125 to 150 mL. CT acquisition occurs at a delay of 45 to 50 seconds, corresponding to the early portal venous phase of optimal intestinal wall enhancement.

5. Thin-section (0.6 to 1.25 mm) acquisition is made through the abdomen and pelvis.

6. Coronal and sagittal MPR images are used to visualize the small intestine in its entirety.

7. CT enterography avoids the necessity of a nasogastric catheter. However, it may not consistently achieve the level of small bowel distention and opacification possible with CT enteroclysis.

D. CT Colonography

1. *CT colonography* (CTC) is a primarily screening MDCT examination of the large intestine with the main goal to identify adenomatous polyps.

2. Beyond routine screening for polyps or malignancy, additional indications for CTC include:

a. Failed conventional colonoscopy.

b. Patient contraindication to conventional colonoscopy.

3. The properly prepared bowel is distended and scanned utilizing MDCT technology. Dedicated CTC software displays the acquired slice data as a 2-D or 3-D model with an endoscopic perspective. The viewer has the ability to "fly through" the colon to identify polyps.

4. Proper bowel preparation is crucial to the success of a CTC examination. The components of bowel preparation may be itemized as:

a. Diet: The patient is restricted to low-residue diet for 2 to 3 days before the examination. On the day before the examination, only clear liquids may be ingested.

b. Catharsis: Bowel cleansing agents include the standard colonoscopy preparations of polyethylene glycol and magnesium citrate. Please consult your department protocol for details regarding bowel cleansing agents and procedures.

c. Tagging: A dual-agent method consisting of the oral administration of both barium and a water-soluble iodine contrast agent. The barium tags residual stool and coats the surface of polyps. The iodine contrast agent tags residual fluid. Tagged fluid and fecal matter exhibit high CT density and appear "white" on the CTC image. Tagging allows for differentiation of polyp from fecal matter and improves the visualization of polyps that may be surrounded by residual fluid.

5. Adequate distention of the colon is the second important component of a successful CTC examination.

6. Colon insufflation involves the introduction of room air or carbon dioxide (CO_2) into the colon for the purpose of bowel wall distention.

7. Insufflation occurs after a small catheter has been inserted into the rectum with the patient in the left lateral decubitus position.

8. In the manual technique of colon insufflation, room air is manually introduced into the large intestine via rectal catheter.

9. Automated CO_2 delivery also accomplishes insufflation with the use of a mechanical pump that dispenses CO_2 into the colon.

10. The advantages of automatic CO_2 insufflation include better overall distention and lower risk of perforation. Also, because of the faster absorption rate of CO_2, there is less postprocedural discomfort for the patient.

11. Once insufflation is complete, the patient is placed in the supine position, and a scout (topogram) image is obtained. Additional air or CO_2 is administered until the desired level of distention is reached.

12. Thin-section (1.0 to 1.25 mm) acquisition of the colon is obtained with the patient supine. Detector collimation ranges between 0.6 mm and 2.5 mm, depending on the capabilities of each particular MDCT system.

13. The patient is then turned prone, and the scan is repeated.

14. If the patient is unable to tolerate the prone position, a decubitus or oblique position may be substituted.

15. Two positions are necessary to ensure maximal distention of the various segments of the colon and to differentiate between fixed polyps and mobile feces and fluid.

16. Dedicated CTC software reformats the acquired data into 2-D and 3-D endoluminal displays of the interior walls of the colon.

17. Electronic stool extraction software may be employed to remove retained fecal matter from the display and reduce false-positive interpretations.

18. Images are best displayed in a "lung-type" window setting, for example, WL –400, WW 1600.

19. Screening CTC is typically performed without the use of an iodinated IV contrast agent.

20. Dose reduction is vital for the screening CTC examination. Because of the high-contrast nature of soft tissue polyps surrounded by air, very low mA settings are possible with minimal image quality loss caused by noise. Effective mAs can be manually set at 50 or lower. Automated tube current modulation techniques may also be used to limit patient radiation dose during CTC.

E. CT Cystography

1. *CT cystography* is a specialized CT examination of the bladder in which an iodinated contrast agent is directly administered under gravity into the bladder via Foley catheter.

2. Indications include:
   a. Trauma.
   b. Fistula formation between the bladder and adjacent organs.
   c. Postoperative leakage.
   d. Neoplasms.

3. Technical considerations for CT cystography include:
   a. An iodinated contrast agent, mixed with normal saline, is introduced to fully distend the bladder. Total volume of fluid ranges between 250 and 300 mL.
   b. Thin-section (<1 mm) acquisition is performed through the bladder.
   c. Multiple acquisitions—contrast administration, postcontrast administration, and postdrainage—may be obtained.
   d. Sagittal or coronal MPR and 3-D volume-rendered reconstructions are performed.

MUSCULOSKELETAL SYSTEM

1. Despite the superiority of MRI in most clinical applications, CT of the musculoskeletal system remains a valuable modality option.

2. Mainly because of its superior speed, CT remains the primary imaging choice for evaluation of the patient with trauma. CT has become the first choice for assessment of spinal injury in the emergency setting. Fractures and dislocations of the complex components of the spine, joints, and so on, are imaged superbly with MDCT. The cortex of bony structures is particularly well demonstrated on CT.

3. Also, patients with orthopedic hardware, incompatible implanted devices, or other contraindications to MRI may benefit from CT evaluation of the musculoskeletal system.

4. Each CT examination of the musculoskeletal system must be individualized to meet the clinical needs of the patient. Many vital considerations need to be tailored to any given examination, including:
   a. Optimal patient position.
   b. Extent of the area to be scanned.
   c. Necessity of IV contrast agent and the administration details.
   d. Technical parameters such as slice thickness, imaging planes, and 3-D applications.

Technical Considerations

A. Spine

1. The articulation between successive vertebrae consists of the intervertebral disc and two posterior facet (zygapophyseal) joints.

2. An intervertebral disc separates each two vertebrae, beginning at the C2 to C3 space. There is no disc space between C1 and C2.

3. Each disc consists of a soft center called the *nucleus pulposus*, which is surrounded by the firmer, outer *anulus fibrosus*. The disc is connected to the superior and inferior surfaces of the respective vertebral bodies at the end plate.

4. The *spinal cord* extends inferiorly from the brain's medulla and terminates at approximately the level of T12 to L1. At its distal end, the spinal cord tapers into the *conus medullaris*. The *cauda equina* is the nerve bundle extending inferiorly from the spinal cord.

5. The intervertebral discs are homogeneous in appearance with attenuation values ranging between 50 and 100 HU.

6. Clinical indications for CT evaluation of the spine include:
   a. Trauma: CT of the spine has become routine and has replaced radiographic evaluation in many trauma centers. The lower cervical spine (C6 to C7) and the thoracolumbar junction (T12 to L2) are the most common sites of spine fracture.

b. Degenerative disease, including the evaluation of neck or back pain and the associated neurologic symptoms of degenerative disc disease. Degenerative processes include:

- *Herniated disc*: Disc herniation may appear as a slight bulge, a moderate protrusion, or a more severe disc extrusion, whereby the nucleus pulposus tears through the anulus fibrosus. A *sequestered disc* or *free fragment* occurs when a portion of the disc's nucleus completely breaks free and migrates from its normal position.
- *Facet joint disease*: The *facet (zygapophyseal) joints* are formed by the articulation between the inferior articular processes of one vertebra and the superior articular processes of the next. Degenerative changes caused by arthritis or abnormal facet growth (hypertrophy) are common.
- *Spondylosis*: A condition of hypertrophy (overgrowth) of the facets that can lead to spinal stenosis.
- *Spinal stenosis*: Consists of narrowing of the bony canals that contain the spinal cord, nerve roots, or both. Compression of the spinal cord or nerve roots may result in the referred limb pain commonly referred to as *sciatica*. Additional causes are disc herniation, tumor, and the formation of osteophytes (abnormal bone growths).
- *Spondylolysis*: A defect in the pars interarticularis commonly caused by osteophyte formation. The *pars interarticularis* is the area of a vertebra between in the inferior and superior articular processes (the neck of the "scotty dog").
- *Spondylolisthesis*: Forward "slipping" of an upper vertebral body over the lower caused by degenerative changes of the facet joints. This disorder is best demonstrated on sagittal MPR images of the spine.

c. Neoplasm: Although primary tumors readily occur, the majority of neoplasms involving the spine are metastatic in origin. Metastatic spinal lesions from breast, lung, or prostate cancer are the most prevalent.

d. Infectious processes such as osteomyelitis and abscess.

e. Inflammatory disorders, including rheumatoid arthritis and ankylosing spondylitis.

f. Postoperative assessment: In general, CT undergoes less image degradation from metallic hardware compared with MRI.

7. The patient is positioned supine and head-first for CT examinations of the cervical, thoracic, or complete spine. During CT evaluation of the lumbar spine only, positioning the patient supine and feet-first may improve comfort by limiting how much of the patient's body enters the gantry.

8. For the nontraumatic CT examination of the cervical spine, the patient should be instructed to relax the shoulders downward to reduce streak artifact from the broad upper trunk. The patient's hands may be positioned underneath the body or stabilized with appropriate, comfortable immobilization straps.

9. For nontraumatic examinations of the thoracolumbar spine, the legs should be slightly elevated and flexed at the knees and supported on pillows or an appropriate positioning cushion to alleviate pressure on the lower back.

10. The trauma patient undergoing CT evaluation of the musculoskeletal system must be positioned with minimal manipulation.

11. Acquisition with 16-detector row (or higher) MDCT systems typically utilize detector collimation within the range of 0.625 to 1.25 mm, with images reconstructed at widths based on the anatomy or pathology in question.

12. For general studies of the thoracic and lumbar spines, slice reconstruction at widths of 3 to 5 mm are sufficient. Section widths of 1 to 2 mm or less are preferable for imaging the cervical spine. For trauma situations and in anticipation of 3-D and multiplanar reconstructions, the thinnest possible detector collimation should be utilized, with overlapping slices at thicknesses ranging from 0.75 to 1.25 mm.

13. Cervical spine acquisition usually includes at least C3 through T1 for general indications; the cervical spine in its entirety (C1 to C7) should be included for trauma (Figs. 4.61 and 4.62).

14. For CT evaluation of the thoracic spine, the specific area of clinical concern is acquired, including at least one vertebral level both above and below. The entire thoracic spine may be covered, offering the availability of comprehensive sagittal and coronal reformation for evaluation of vertebral alignment, degenerative disease, and so on.

15. Most degenerative disease processes affect the lumbar spine beginning at the level of L3 to L4. Scanning from L2 to S1 is typically sufficient, with expansion of coverage for trauma situations (Figs. 4.63 to 4.65).

16. All CT examinations of the spine should consist of a contiguous, volumetric acquisition. Individually angled scans through each disc space are unnecessary because of the isotropic nature of MDCT.

17. ATCM techniques should be utilized to minimize patient radiation dose.

18. Acquisition is performed with a large SFOV (48 to 50 cm). Targeted reconstructions are made using a DFOV between 10 and 15 cm. Larger DFOV reconstructions may be used to retrospectively display a greater anatomic area as the clinical indication dictates.

19. Separate data reconstructions using soft tissue and bone algorithms (kernels) may be required to display pathology optimally.

20. Dual window settings are used for bone and soft tissue evaluation. Sample WL and WW settings for optimal image display are:

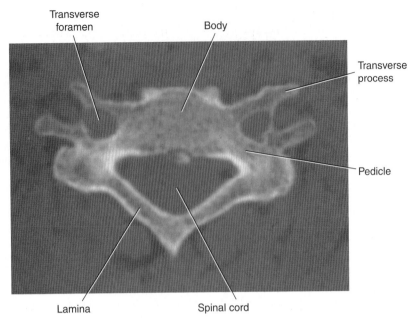

FIG. 4.61 Cervical spine—axial image.

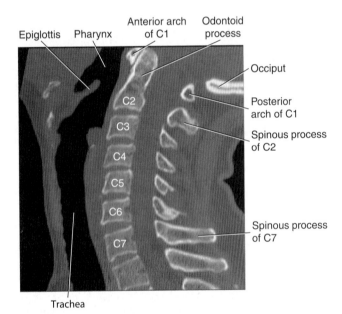

FIG. 4.62 Cervical spine—sagittal multiplanar reformation (MPR) image.

    a. Soft tissue: WL 50, WW 400.
    b. Bone: WL 300, WW 2000.
21. IV administration of a contrast agent is typically not indicated for CT examination of the spine. Exceptions include assessment for metastatic disease, soft tissue mass, infection, or abscess. An IV contrast agent may also be indicated in the patient with a history of prior spine surgery in an effort to differentiate scar tissue from recurrent disc disease.
22. When indicated, 100 to 125 mL of a nonionic contrast agent may be administered at a rate of 2 to 3 mL/sec with scanning during the portal venous phase.

23. For trauma settings, injury to the vertebral arteries may be evaluated with administration of an IV contrast agent and the inclusion of a CT angiographic study of the affected spinal area. Higher injection rates (4 to 5 mL/sec) are used, and arterial phase or dual-phase imaging is performed.
24. MPR, MIP, and 3-D volume-rendered techniques are routinely used for CT spine evaluation.
25. Thin-section MDCT offers less streak artifact from metallic hardware than conventional single-detector CT, leading to better imaging of the postoperative spine.

B. Upper and Lower Extremities

1. Trauma is the primary indication for CT evaluation of the musculoskeletal system. CT provides demonstration of fractures and identification of bony fragments.
2. CT of the musculoskeletal system is used to identify and characterize bony neoplasms such as cysts, benign and malignant tumors, and metastatic deposits.
3. Benign tumors of the skeletal system include enchondroma, chondroblastoma, osteoid osteoma, and osteochondroma.
4. Malignant tumors of the skeletal system include osteosarcoma, chondrosarcoma, and multiple myeloma.
5. Multiple myeloma is the most common malignant primary tumor of the skeletal system. It is a systemic malignancy involving the plasma cells found within bone marrow.
6. The degenerative changes to bone resulting from arthritis are well demonstrated on CT.
7. Infection of a bone, or *osteomyelitis*, may be assessed with CT imaging.
8. Inflammatory and infectious processes involving the soft tissues of the extremities, such as cellulitis,

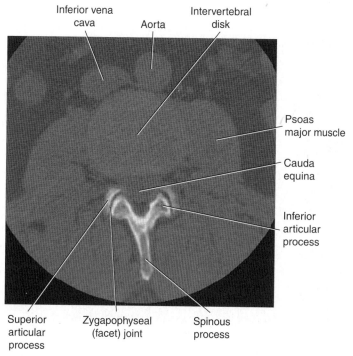

FIG. 4.63 Lumbar spine—axial image displayed using a bone window.

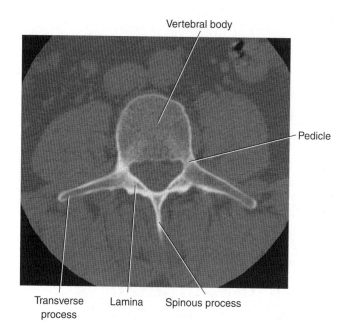

FIG. 4.64 Lumbar spine—axial image displayed using a bone window.

fasciitis, and abscess, may also be amenable to CT assessment.

9. Isotropic data acquisition allows for the production of high-quality MPR images. Isotropic multiplanar imaging is the hallmark of quality MDCT evaluation of the musculoskeletal system and is accomplished by applying two key concepts:

   a. Choose the thinnest detector collimation available to produce the thinnest slices available.

   b. Reconstruct the acquired data with the smallest DFOV possible for the part of interest.

10. Thin section acquisition and the use of reduced DFOV settings may result in an increase in patient radiation dose. In cooperation with the interpreting physician, the CT technologist must balance the image quality requirements of the study against the responsibility to reduce patient dose to a minimum.

11. Thin-section (<1.25 mm) volumetric acquisition is made in the axial plane. The scan is acquired perpendicular to the long axis of the part to maximize the number of slices obtained. The extent of the scan is determined by the clinical indication.

12. Images are reconstructed using at least a 50% overlap to improve the quality of 3-D and MPR images.

13. With isotropic data acquisition, resolution of the MPR images is equal to that of the axial scan. This capability eliminates the need for an additional scan in a second plane for most clinical situations.

14. A high spatial frequency algorithm (kernel) is used for image reconstruction to maximize bony detail. Additional reconstruction with a soft tissue algorithm can be utilized as clinically warranted.

15. Dual window settings are used for bone and soft tissue evaluation. Sample WL and WW settings for optimal image display are:

    a. Soft tissue: WL 50, WW 400.

    b. Bone: WL 300, WW 2000.

16. Scout (topogram) images should be acquired in both anteroposterior (AP) and lateral projections. Scout images are carefully evaluated to ensure proper patient position and minimize the scanning coverage.

17. Patient positioning during CT studies of the extremities varies with the part to be scanned and the clinical

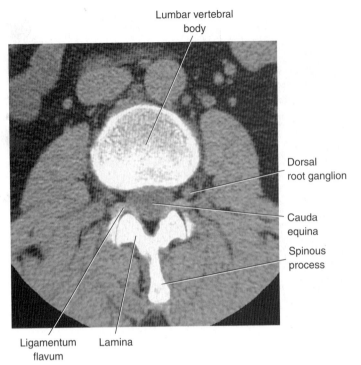

FIG. 4.65 Lumbar spine—axial image displayed using a soft tissue window.

indication. The challenge is to obtain the proper position while maintaining a sufficient level of comfort for the patient throughout the examination.

18. Ensuring patient comfort is vital because movement severely compromises scan quality.

19. The primary goal of patient positioning during scanning of the upper extremity is to comfortably place the part of interest free of superimposition with the rest of the body.

20. The "superman" position places the patient prone with the affected arm above the head. This position allows the hand, wrist, forearm, and elbow to be scanned without superimposition with the patient's head and trunk.

21. The patient's hand is usually pronated for studies of the hand, wrist, and forearm. When not contraindicated, the patient's hand is supinated for scans of the elbow, a position that places the humeral epicondyles parallel to the CT table.

22. When the "superman" position is unattainable, acquisition may be obtained with the patient supine and the affected arm at the side in a neutral position. This position results in unavoidable streaking artifact from the patient's body.

23. Assessments of fracture and dislocation are the primary indications for CT of the elbow, forearm, wrist, and hand.

24. The wrist's scaphoid bone is a common location for complex fracture. Axial CT imaging with coronal and sagittal MPR images of the scaphoid are extremely valuable in their ability to demonstrate small fractures

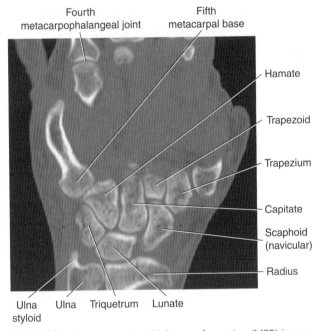

FIG. 4.66 Wrist—coronal multiplanar reformation (MPR) image.

and nonunion, which may not be easily identified on conventional radiographs (Fig. 4.66).

25. The foot may be clinically divided as:
    a. *Forefoot:* Metatarsals and phalanges.
    b. *Midfoot:* Navicular, cuboid, cuneiforms.
    c. *Hindfoot:* Talus and calcaneus.

26. Imaging planes for the foot and ankle for both direct acquisition and MPR reconstruction may be described as follows:

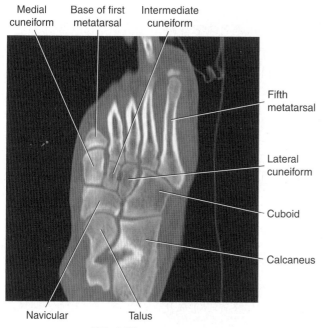

FIG. 4.67 Foot—axial image.

Medial cuneiform · Base of first metatarsal · Intermediate cuneiform · Fifth metatarsal · Lateral cuneiform · Cuboid · Calcaneus · Navicular · Talus

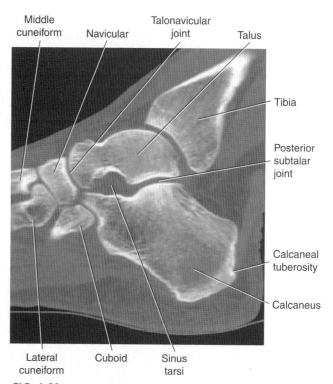

FIG. 4.68 Ankle—sagittal multiplanar reformation (MPR) image.

Middle cuneiform · Navicular · Talonavicular joint · Talus · Tibia · Posterior subtalar joint · Calcaneal tuberosity · Calcaneus · Lateral cuneiform · Cuboid · Sinus tarsi

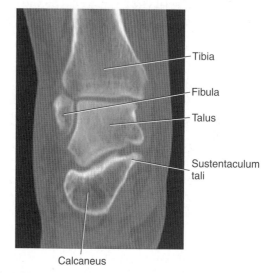

FIG. 4.69 Ankle—coronal multiplanar reformation (MPR) image.

Tibia · Fibula · Talus · Sustentaculum tali · Calcaneus

a. Direct axial: The plane parallel to the foot's plantar surface. Scanning in the direct axial plane is performed with the patient's foot flexed and the toes pointing straight up. Gantry angulation may be used to achieve correct scan plane when it is not otherwise possible (Fig. 4.67).

b. Oblique axial: Parallel to the metatarsals, approximately 20 to 30 degrees caudal from the direct axial plane. MPR images along this plane are used to assess the tarsal-metatarsal joint.

c. Sagittal: Divides the foot and ankle from medial to lateral. Sagittal MPR images provide detailed visualization of the tarsal and metatarsal bones and joints (Fig. 4.68).

d. Coronal: Divides the foot and ankle from posterior to anterior. Provides visualization of the ankle joint with an AP perspective (Fig. 4.69).

27. Examinations of the midfoot and forefoot are usually performed with the patient supine, knee slightly flexed, with the affected foot flat on the scan table. The unaffected foot should be removed from the scan plane through greater flexing of the unaffected leg. Removing the other extremity from the field allows for DFOV optimization and minimizes streak artifact.

28. Thin-section (<1.5 mm) volumetric acquisition is made in the oblique coronal plane. The scan plane is perpendicular to the long axis of the metatarsals to maximize the number of slices obtained. The gantry may be angled to achieve the proper scan acquisition plane. The extent of the scan is determined by the clinical indication.

29. The ankle and hindfoot are typically scanned with a thin-section (<1.5 mm) volumetric acquisition in the direct axial plane, perpendicular to the tibia. The

patient's feet are flexed 90 degrees (toes up) and supported on a box or cushion. The scan should begin above the syndesmosis—the articulation between the distal tibia and fibula—and should extend through the entire calcaneus.

30. *Tarsal coalition* refers to the abnormal union of adjacent bones of the ankle. It is most common at the talocalcaneal and calcaneonavicular joints.

31. The *Lisfranc joint* is the articulation between the tarsals and metatarsals. CT is used to evaluate fractures, subluxations, and dislocations of the Lisfranc joint.

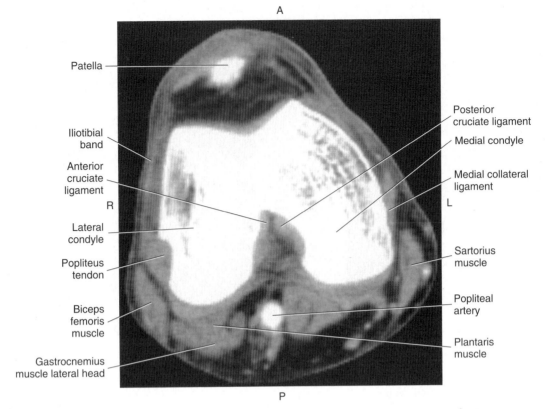

FIG. 4.70 Knee—axial with contrast. *(From Kelley L, Peterson C: Sectional Anatomy for Image Professionals, 3rd ed. St Louis, 2013, Mosby, Fig. 10.97.)*

32. Examinations of the distal femur, knee, and proximal tibia are performed with the patient in a relaxed, supine position. When possible, the other leg may be flexed at the knee and/or raised to bring it out from direct superimposition with the part of interest (Fig. 4.70 and 4.71).

33. CT examinations of the knee may also be performed at varying degrees of flexion (0, 30, 45, 60, and 90 degrees) to demonstrate patellar tracking abnormalities.

34. Tibial plateau fractures are particularly well suited to evaluation by CT.

35. The *bone length study* involves the use of the CT system to acquire digital scout radiographs of the lower extremities. Both AP and lateral scout views are obtained using a low-dose technique. Scout views include from above the hip joint through the ankle joint. Analytical system software is used to measure and compare the length of each extremity for size discrepancy.

36. Most CT studies of the musculoskeletal system do not require IV administration of a contrast agent.

37. The indications for the use of an IV contrast agent are:
    a. Identification of bony or soft tissue infection and abscess.
    b. Inflammatory processes involving muscle, which may be better demonstrated with a contrast agent

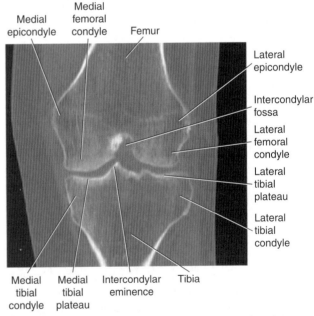

FIG. 4.71 Knee—coronal multiplanar reformation (MPR) image.

because of the tendency of infected muscle to enhance to a lesser degree than normal musculature.
    c. Assessing the vascularity of a musculoskeletal neoplasm.
    d. CTA evaluation in trauma situations.

C. Shoulder Girdle and Sternum

1. The *shoulder girdle* consists primarily of the glenohumeral, acromioclavicular, and sternoclavicular joints.
2. The clinical indications for and technical aspects of CT studies of the shoulder girdle are similar to those for studies of the distal extremities.
3. The patient is typically positioned supine with the arms down at the side.
4. Studies of patients with wide shoulders may suffer from *out-of-field artifacts,* in which the shoulders extend beyond the limits of the SFOV. This streaking artifact can be avoided by positioning the side of interest more toward the center of the gantry. The out-of-field artifact will still occur but will not appear in the small DFOV chosen to target the shoulder of interest.
5. When not contraindicated, the unaffected arm may be raised above the head to reduce streaking caused by the dense shoulder area.
6. The patient should be instructed to suspend respiration during CT acquisition through the sternum, sternoclavicular joints, or clavicle to avoid motion artifact.
7. For the shoulder, thin-section (<1.25 mm) axial scans are volumetrically acquired through the glenohumeral joint, extending from above the humeral head inferiorly through the proximal humerus (Fig. 4.72).
8. The isotropic data set may then be reformatted into coronal and sagittal images through the glenohumeral joint. Surface- and volume-rendered 3-D images may be reconstructed.
9. The scan prescription for studies of the clavicle, acromioclavicular joints, sternoclavicular joints, clavicle, sternum, scapula, and humerus is adjusted accordingly.

D. Pelvic Girdle

1. Bony structures of the *pelvic girdle* include the sacrum, coccyx, sacroiliac joints, and hips.
2. The clinical indications for and technical aspects of CT studies of the sacrum and coccyx are similar to those in the remainder of the spine.
3. Trauma is the chief clinical indication for CT evaluation of the articulation between the femoral head and acetabulum (hip joint). Dislocations and fractures of the hip joint are well demonstrated on CT.
4. The *acetabulum* comprises the ischium, the ilium, and the pubis.
5. MPR and 3-D reconstructions provide excellent views of the acetabulum and femoral head. CT is an important imaging tool for the diagnosis of fracture in these areas (Figs. 4.73 and 4.74).
6. Additional clinical indications for CT of the hips include:
   a. Postoperative evaluation of prosthesis for hip fracture.
   b. Developmental dysplasia of the hip.
7. The technical considerations for CT studies of the pelvic girdle are similar to those for studies of the distal extremities.
8. The patient is scanned in the supine position, feet-first in the gantry. The hands and arms are raised above the acquired field.
9. Contrast-enhanced MDCT acquisitions of the post-traumatic pelvis may include CTA evaluation for vascular injury as well as assessment of the bladder via CT cystography.

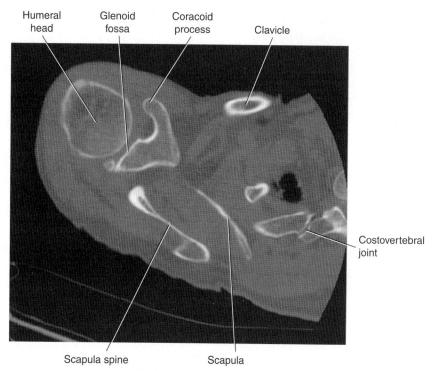

FIG. 4.72 Shoulder—axial image.

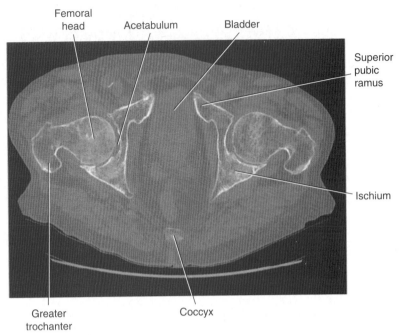

FIG. 4.73 Hips—axial image.

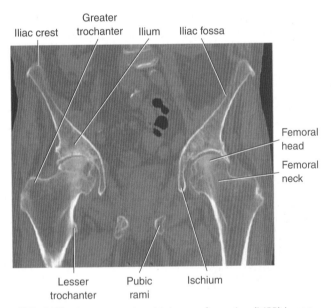

FIG. 4.74 Hips—coronal multiplanar reformation (MPR) image.

Special Procedures

A. CT Arthrography

1. *CT arthrography* is CT evaluation of a joint after the intra-articular injection of an iodinated contrast agent.
2. This evaluation offers additional detail of the soft tissue structures of the joints, including ligaments, tendons, cartilage, and menisci.
3. The single-contrast technique involves the direct administration into the joint space of a small amount (approximately 0.5 to 10.0 mL, depending on the joint) of a contrast agent diluted with saline before thin-section CT acquisition.

4. In the double-contrast technique, a small amount of room air is also introduced into the joint along with the contrast medium.

B. CT Myelography

1. The intrathecal administration of a contrast during a myelogram improves visualization of the spinal cord, nerve roots, and surrounding soft tissue structures. An iodinated contrast agent is administered directly into the subarachnoid space surrounding the spinal cord.
2. Postmyelography CT examinations of the spine are commonly performed to take advantage of the intrathecal contrast agent administration.

C. Peripheral CT Angiography

1. Peripheral CTA the angiographic assessment of the peripheral arterial tree from the renal arteries through the feet, is commonly referred to as a *CT runoff*.
2. The speed, greater volume coverage, and isotropic spatial resolution of MDCT make the acquisition of the entire peripheral arterial system of the lower extremities possible.
3. The abdominal aorta bifurcates into the left and right common iliac arteries at about the level of L4.
4. Each iliac artery further bifurcates at about the level of L5 to S1 into internal and external iliac arteries.
5. The internal iliac arteries are the major blood suppliers to the pelvis. The external iliac arteries supply blood to the lower limb as the femoral arteries (Fig. 4.75).
6. Appropriate IV contrast agent administration is the key to performing high-quality peripheral CTA examinations. Acquisition must occur during the period of peak opacification of the arterial tree:

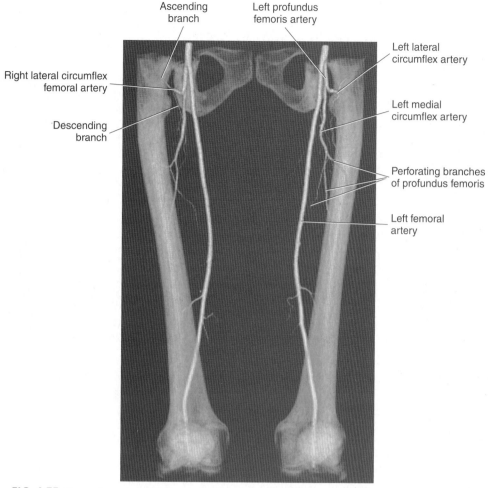

Ascending branch

Left profundus femoris artery

Right lateral circumflex femoral artery

Left lateral circumflex artery

Descending branch

Left medial circumflex artery

Perforating branches of profundus femoris

Left femoral artery

FIG. 4.75 Three-dimensional CT angiography of the femoral arteries. *(From Kelley L, Peterson C: Sectional Anatomy for Image Professionals, 3rd ed., St Louis, 2013, Mosby, Fig. 10.173.)*

a. The time it takes for contrast agent to reach the peripheral arteries from the injection site varies widely among patients. The CM transit time—the time needed for an IV contrast agent to reach the aorta—in patients with vascular disease ranges from 12 to 40 seconds. Accurate scan delay should be obtained by either a test bolus or automated bolus-tracking techniques.

b. Acquisition speeds range from 35 mm/sec in 4-slice MDCT systems to upwards of 92 mm/sec or greater with 64-slice systems and beyond. The scan delay chosen must coincide with the acquisition time to ensure that scanning occurs during the period of peak arterial opacification. Faster scanners run the risk of "outrunning" the bolus by completing the acquisition before the entire contrast agent volume has been administered. Faster scanners, therefore, require longer preparation delays.

c. The duration of scan acquisition is based on the anatomic length of the study and the capabilities of the particular CT system in use. The following formula may be used as a guide to determine injection rate and contrast agent volume specific to the required scan time:

$$\text{Bolus duration} = \text{Scan time} - 5 \text{ seconds}$$

d. The subtraction of 5 seconds allows the scanner to keep pace with the contrast agent as the latter moves down the aorta and results in the cessation of contrast agent administration just (5 seconds) before the end of data acquisition.

e. The calculated bolus duration is attained with injection rates between 3 and 5 mL/sec for total contrast agent volumes between 125 and 175 mL (2 mL/kg maximum).

f. A biphasic injection technique, in which a higher rate is followed by a lower rate, may be used to widen the period of optimum peripheral arterial enhancement.

g. The use of a saline flush may also assist in broadening the peak enhancement window and improving the efficiency of contrast agent utilization.

7. The technical parameters of peripheral CTA vary according to departmental protocol. A few generalizations can be outlined as follows:

a. The patient is positioned supine and feet-first into the gantry. The feet are immobilized with the legs carefully aligned in a neutral, comfortable position to limit motion.

b. The detector collimation and subsequent slice thickness values depend on scanner capability. For systems at 16 slices and above, 0.6 to 0.75 mm detector collimation with 0.75 to 1.0 mm reconstructions is used.

c. Overlapping reconstructions are used for high-quality volume-rendered 3-D and MIP images.

d. Acquisition is made from just below the diaphragm to below the ankles (approximately 1200 to 1400 mm of coverage) in a single scan.

e. Reduction of kVp to 100 and the utilization of the ATCM technique effectively manage patient radiation dose levels. Lowering the kVp setting from the standard 120 down to 100 also has the added benefit of increasing the image contrast provided by the iodine administration.

f. The minimum kVp setting should be determined after consideration of the patient size, tolerable image noise level, degree of pathologic conspicuity and preference of the interpreting independent licensed practitioner.

g. DFOV is kept as small as possible to improve resolution of the peripheral vasculature while including the wider-appearing abdominal vessels in the display.

h. Evaluation of peripheral artery disease is the primary indication for peripheral CTA.

i. *Claudication* refers to the condition of intermittent cramping pain in the legs caused by poor circulation. Arterial stenosis and occlusion are typically the causes of the vascular insufficiency.

j. Additional indications for peripheral CTA include:
   • Acute ischemia from thrombosis.
   • Vascular trauma.
   • Lower extremity aneurysm.
   • Postoperative evaluation of endovascular repair.

D. Interventional CT

1. CT provides precise localization for interventional procedures, such as percutaneous biopsy, abscess drainage, and radiofrequency ablation.

2. CT interventional guidance is used during procedures involving the lungs, mediastinum, adrenals, liver, pancreas, kidneys, retroperitoneum, and pelvis (Fig. 4.76).

3. The most common indication for CT-guided percutaneous biopsy is to confirm the malignancy of a mass.

4. Protocol and procedures for CT-guided biopsy are department specific. Details regarding the technical aspects of any given CT-guided biopsy vary greatly, depending upon the clinical indication, anatomic area of interest, and individual physician preferences.

5. Generalizations regarding the role of CT during percutaneous biopsy procedures are as follows:

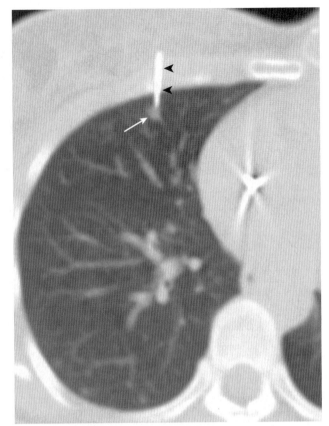

FIG. 4.76 Transthoracic percutaneous lung biopsy to diagnose pulmonary malignancy. The biopsy needle (arrowheads) has been advanced to biopsy a nodule (arrow). *(From Murray and Nadel's Textbook of Respiratory Medicine, 2015, eFigure 53.15.)*

a. Diagnostic CT examination of the area is performed and reviewed to determine the optimal patient position for the biopsy.

b. The patient is positioned (supine, prone, decubitus) according to plan, and the area of interest is scanned for relocalization of the mass.

c. The z-axis location for biopsy is determined and marked through use of the laser lighting system of the CT unit.

d. CT system software is used to measure the distance between the lesion and skin entrance point and determine the optimum angle for needle insertion.

e. Once the biopsy pass is made, additional scans are obtained to ensure proper location of the needle tip within the lesion. The needle tip is often readily identified as an area of black shadow artifact in the immediately adjacent soft tissue of the lesion.

f. Upon removal of the biopsy sample, additional CT acquisition is performed through the area to detect postprocedural complications such as pneumothorax and hemorrhage.

g. CT guidance for fluid aspiration and drainage is similar in concept to that for percutaneous needle biopsy.

h. Abscess drainage and cyst aspiration are the most common indications for CT imaging guidance.

i. Percutaneous abscess drainage often involves the placement of a catheter within the fluid collection for drainage.

j. Before catheter removal, a repeat CT scan is typically performed to confirm resolution of the fluid collection.

k. CT-guided radiofrequency ablation (RFA) involves the placement of a probe into a tumor under CT imaging guidance.

l. Once the probe is positioned precisely within a tumor, radiofrequency waves are passed through the probe to heat and destroy malignant tissue.

m. The most common indication for CT-guided RFA is treatment of a hepatic neoplasm.

E. CT Fluoroscopy

1. *CT fluoroscopy* is the use of real-time CT imaging for CT-guided interventional procedures.

2. It allows for continuous monitoring of needle insertion to ensure proper path, angle, and depth.

3. A disadvantage of CT fluoroscopy is the added radiation dose for both patient and staff.

4. The patient dose can be reduced by employing the lowest possible mA station and minimizing the fluoroscopic time of the procedure.

5. Techniques employed to reduce occupational exposure during CT fluoroscopy–guided interventional procedures include:

   a. Low mA and kVp, limited CT fluoroscopy time, and increased distance from source.

   b. Use of the "last-image hold" feature to reduce the need for continuous CT fluoroscopy.

   c. Use of appropriate lead shielding, including apron, thyroid shield, glove, and glasses.

   d. Draping of a lead shield over the patient area that is not involved in the interventional procedure, to reduce scatter radiation.

   e. Use of a needle holder to keep the operator's hands out of the CT fluoroscopy field.

F. CT and Positron Emission Tomography

1. *Positron emission tomography* (PET) is a functional nuclear medicine study utilizing fludeoxyglucose F 18 (FDG) as a radiopharmaceutical.

2. Malignant cells demonstrate an increase in metabolic activity and glucose utilization. Once administered, FDG mimics glucose and is taken up by normal and abnormal tissues. The amount of FDG uptake is directly proportional to an area's metabolic activity. Malignant cells take up a disproportionate amount of FDG in comparison with metabolically normal tissue.

3. Annihilation photons are emitted from the radionuclide FDG that has been taken up by the tumor cells. PET detectors absorb the emitted photons, measuring the activity of a given area of potential malignancy.

4. The emitted photons are attenuated as they travel along their path toward exit from the patient. Photons that travel longer distances undergo greater attenuation and a reduction in energy. The process of *attenuation correction* utilizes the transmission data acquired in the corresponding CT analysis to account for this change in energy.

5. PET provides a map of normal and abnormal tissue function. It offers excellent sensitivity for malignancy but suffers from an inability to accurately localize tumor activity. Fusion of PET with CT provides such precise anatomic localization.

6. The PET-CT scanner provides a single image data set, from the combined technologies. Hybrid PET-CT yields cross-sectional images displaying functional abnormalities and accurately registered to precise anatomic locations.

7. A combined PET-CT system contains separate CT and PET hardware within a single gantry.

8. Patients have usually fasted for 6 to 12 hours before a PET-CT examination to maximize FDG tumor uptake. Fasting is necessary to control the blood glucose level.

9. The patient's blood glucose level may be measured before the injection of FDG. It should be below 150 mg/dL to prevent inhibition of FDG uptake by glucose circulating in the bloodstream.

10. A typical dose is 10 to 15 millicuries (mCi) of FDG administered intravenously.

11. Strenuous physical activity can cause abnormal physiologic uptake of the FDG in muscle. Therefore the patient is instructed to avoid such activity before the injection and during the delay for imaging. In addition, all patient activity and speech are limited for up to 60 minutes after the injection of FDG.

12. After this 1-hour uptake period, the patient is positioned within the scanner.

13. Scout (topogram) images are obtained for the region(s) of clinical interest after the patient is given the appropriate instructions regarding limiting motion, breath-holds, and so on.

14. CT images are first acquired, both for anatomic localization of structures and to provide the attenuation correction information necessary for accurate PET data.

15. PET scan acquisition for the same area along the z-axis is then obtained after automatic translation of the patient table into the PET portion of the gantry apparatus.

16. Once the scans are completed, images are available for review either separately or fused together.

17. The major clinical applications for PET-CT are in oncology and neurology.

18. PET-CT now plays an important role in the diagnosis and management of cancers of the head, neck, lung, breast, and GI system. Patients with lymphoma and melanoma are also monitored with PET-CT.

19. The characterization of solitary pulmonary nodules is an additional important clinical application of PET-CT.
20. Neurologic disorders such as Alzheimer's disease, dementia, and epilepsy may be evaluated by PET-CT.

G. Radiation Therapy Planning

1. Advanced imaging may be used to provide volume and localization information for tumors to improve the accuracy of radiation delivery for therapy purposes.
2. 3-D tumor localization aids planning in shaping the dose to maximally irradiate the tumor volume while reducing the radiation dose to the surrounding normal tissue.
3. CT *simulation, or virtual simulation,* describes the process of obtaining anatomic information with CT imaging that is used to calculate the beam arrangement during radiotherapy.
4. The CT simulator consists of a standard CT system with the following additions and modifications:
   a. A flat tabletop, similar to that used during radiotherapy.
   b. Immobilization devices to position the patient in a fashion equal to the therapy procedure.
   c. A large-bore dimension to accommodate multiple patient positions and to ensure the inclusion of the entire patient anatomy utilizing a large SFOV.
   d. Virtual simulation software for treatment planning.

Review of Image Production in Computed Tomography

CHAPTER OUTLINE

CT SYSTEM PRINCIPLES, OPERATION, AND COMPONENTS

1. The fundamental principle of computed tomography (CT) may be summarized as follows: an image of an object may be reconstructed on the basis of the attenuation that occurs as x-radiation is transmitted through it.
2. The x-ray beam is rotated around the patient, exposing a given volume of tissue from all directions. Detectors measure the radiation that is transmitted through the patient. An image is reconstructed on the basis of the magnitude of x-ray attenuation that occurs at spatially distributed points within the patient.
3. The general process of CT imaging may be divided into several steps:
   a. *Data acquisition*—the measurement of the attenuation that occurs along each path through the patient from x-ray tube to detector.
   b. *Data reconstruction*—the computerized processing of the transmission measurements into the CT image.
   c. *Multidimensional image display*—display of the reconstructed grayscale image in two-dimensional (2-D) and/or three-dimensional (3-D) format; a representation of the attenuation that occurred across the scanned volume of tissue.
   d. *Image archival and communication*—display as well as storage, both short-term and long-term (archival), of images on computer workstations (Fig. 5.1).

A. Scan Modes

1. The most basic scan mode utilized by a CT system is scout image acquisition (Fig. 5.2). This survey scan is a digital radiograph obtained by keeping the x-ray

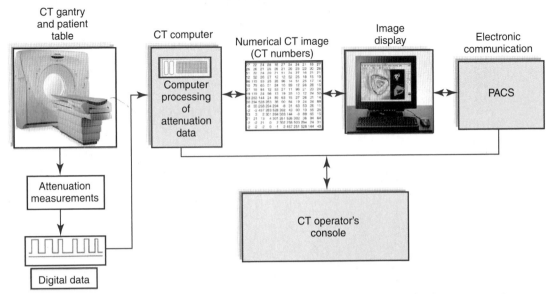

FIG. 5.1 The main components of CT image production, display, and archival. *(From Seeram E: Computed tomography: physical principles, clinical applications, and quality control, ed 4, St Louis, 2016, Saunders, Fig. 1.5.)*

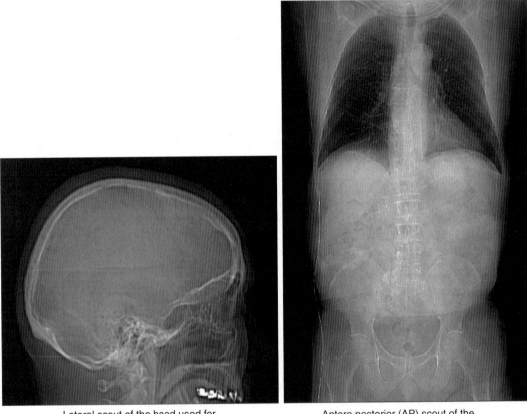

Lateral scout of the head used for CT examinations of the brain, sinuses, orbits, mastoids, and so on.

Antero posterior (AP) scout of the chest, abdomen, and pelvis used for various CT examinations of the trunk.

FIG. 5.2 The CT scout image or scanogram is typically the first image acquired during any CT examination.

tube and detector array in a fixed position while the patient bed is translated through the gantry.

2. Also referred to as a scanogram or localizer, a scout image may be produced in the anteroposterior, posteroanterior, lateral, or oblique projection through

adjustments in the positions of the x-ray tube and detectors.

3. The angle of the tube and detectors in relationship to the patient position during scout acquisition is referred to as the *azimuth*.

4. The scout image, the initial image acquired during a CT examination, is used as a localizer for the prescription of the subsequent cross-sectional CT acquisition(s).

5. Historically, conventional axial, or step-and-shoot, CT scanning consisted of the complete revolution of the x-ray tube around the patient, acquiring a single data set at a precise anatomic location. During the data acquisition process, the patient table would not move. The data would then be mathematically reconstructed into a single image. The thickness of the reconstructed image was controlled by the extent to which the beam was collimated. To acquire the next CT image, the table would translate (index) a predetermined amount to the next anatomic position, and the system would again rotate around the patient. This process would repeat until the area of clinical interest was completely evaluated.

6. The CT system itself is generally composed of a powerful computer and display system, a patient bed, and the gantry components (Fig. 5.3).

7. The CT gantry houses the majority of the mechanical components of CT system operation, including the generator, x-ray tube, assorted collimators, the data acquisition system (DAS), slip-rings, and the detectors.

8. The x-ray and detector components of a CT system were originally limited by hardwired cables, which prevented continuous rotation within the gantry. At the end of each rotation of the x-ray tube and/or detectors, the system would need to reverse course and travel in the opposite direction because the cables were of finite length.

9. *Slip-ring technology* eliminates the need for cables by utilizing a system of contact brushes that supply electricity to power the system and enable the passage of transmission data to the computer system.

10. The addition of slip-ring technology allows for the continuous helical acquisition that has become the standard in modern CT imaging.

11. The technical elements of helical CT acquisition include:
    a. Continuous rotation of the gantry components (slip-ring technology).
    b. A powerful x-ray tube capable of long exposure output.
    c. Continuous movement of the patient bed.
    d. Specialized mathematical reconstruction techniques.

12. Helical geometry allows for volumetric data acquisition. The reconstruction of CT sections at any point along the scanned volume is possible. The section width must be the same, however, and is controlled by the collimation (slice thickness) chosen before data acquisition.

13. The development of multidetector CT (MDCT) advanced the helical acquisition principle. Multidetector arrays enable CT sections of varying widths to be reconstructed at any point along the acquired volume.

B. X-Ray Tube

1. CT employs a metal-enclosed x-ray tube consisting of a cathode and a rotating anode disc.

2. Dual filaments allow for a choice of two focal spot sizes ranging from 0.5 to 1.2 mm in diameter. Depending on the vendor, the choice of foci may be controlled by the user through the selection of milliamperage (mA) setting, scan field of view (SFOV), and so on.

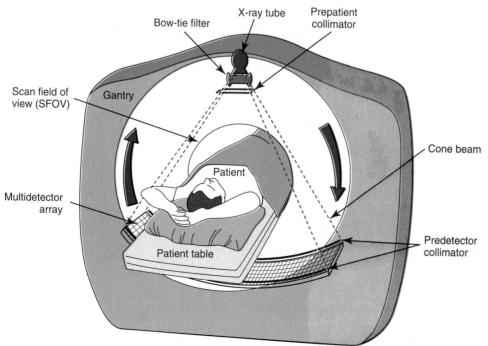

FIG. 5.3 General schematic diagram of a multidetector CT (MDCT) system.

3. Smaller focal spots improve the geometric efficiency of the x-ray beam, leading to greater spatial resolution.

4. *Flying focal spot technology* involves the electromagnetic steering of the electron beam emitted from the cathode. The beam of electrons is directed toward two separate locations on the rotating anode, resulting in two sources of x-radiation.

5. As the tube rotates around the patient, the number of data samples is essentially doubled because of the electronic switching between the two focal spots. This oversampling technology can be used to improve the system's temporal and spatial resolution.

6. The long acquisition times and relatively high exposure rates of helical single-slice CT (SSCT) and MDCT require an x-ray tube with very high heat storage capacity.

7. The x-ray tube must be very efficient at dissipating the tremendous heat generated during a CT examination. Several methods, including oil and air cooling, increased anode diameter, and conduction by tube rotation, have been utilized to improve heat capacity.

8. The modern CT x-ray tube has specific characteristics that enable it to achieve the performance demanded by state-of-the-art MDCT:
   a. High heat rating—must have the ability to absorb tremendous heat, while dissipating it quickly.
   b. Small size, lightweight—must be capable of rotating within the CT gantry at a high rate of speed.
   c. Stable and long lasting—must be capable of withstanding huge centrifugal forces with an extended useful life.

9. Milliampere (mA) setting can vary widely from 30 mA to upwards of 800 mA. Selection of mA setting depends on a number of factors, including the clinical indication for the CT study, patient size/density, and required signal-to-noise ratio (SNR) for adequate examination quality.

10. The mA setting for a given study may be manually selected on the basis of the aforementioned criteria. Automatic tube current modulation (ATCM) programs adjust the mA throughout an acquisition to reduce patient radiation dose to a minimum. ATCM automatically alters the applied mA according to a predetermined noise index that is acceptable for appropriate image quality.

11. Exposure time for a given CT acquisition varies and is determined by anatomic extent, detector configuration, table speed, and so on. Each acquisition may reach upwards of 30 to 60 seconds in length, with total scan times equal to the sum of all acquisitions occurring during the study.

12. The mA setting in coordination with the scan time (seconds) gives the constant milliampere-seconds (mAs) value for a CT acquisition. The mAs value directly controls the quantity of x-radiation, or *photon fluence*, directed toward the patient.

13. The rate at which the photon fluence passes through a unit area over unit time is termed the *photon flux*.

14. The mAs value for a given acquisition is directly proportional to patient radiation dose and inversely proportional to image noise.

15. *Effective mAs* describes the calculated mAs value per acquired slice. The main controlling factor of effective mAs is table speed. The pitch selected for a given acquisition determines the speed at which the patient translates through the gantry for each tube revolution, as shown by the following formula:

$$\text{effective mAs} = \frac{\text{mAs}}{\text{pitch}}$$

16. As illustrated by the formula, as pitch increases, the mAs applied to each acquired slice decreases.

17. *Peak kilovoltage* (kVp) controls the quality of the x-ray beam with regard to its overall penetrating capabilities. Higher kVp settings produce x-ray beams with greater penetrating power.

18. The use of lower kVp decreases the patient radiation dose and may improve contrast, particularly during CT angiography (CTA) procedures.

19. Higher kVp settings are utilized to decrease the streak artifact that may occur as the beam passes through very dense parts, such as those found in the posterior fossa during head imaging.

20. The CT x-ray tube is extremely efficient and capable of generating an x-ray beam using peak voltages typically within the range of 70 to 150 kVp.

21. Automated tube voltage selection (ATVS) is an advanced feature that may be available on some modern CT systems. Similar to ATCM, this software automatically modulates the tube potential based upon the changing patient attenuation along the scan acquisition range.

22. Dual-energy CT systems are capable of applying multiple x-ray energies during a single CT acquisition. Transmission data are acquired from tissue interaction with both high- and low-kVp radiation. Differentiation and characterization of tissue composition are made possible by the difference in attenuation between the two x-ray spectra.

23. Complex voltage-switching systems may be employed to achieve *dual-energy CT scanning*. As the single tube rotates around the patient, the applied peak kVp is switched at an extremely high rate for each successive projection.

24. Alternatively, *dual-source CT systems* utilize two completely separate x-ray tubes and detector arrays positioned 90 degrees from each other within the gantry. The two x-ray tubes acquire data simultaneously at different kVp values.

25. Dual-energy CT has expanded clinical opportunities, including:
   a. Improved resolution of soft tissue structures (ligaments, tendons) during musculoskeletal imaging.

b. The ability to visualize atherosclerotic plaque within contrast-enhanced vasculature during cardiac CT studies.

c. Contrast medium subtraction techniques for the demonstration of precontrast images from a single scan acquired after the IV administration of iodinated contrast media.

d. Characterization of the biochemical composition of urinary tract calculi.

26. The beam that emerges from the CT system x-ray tube consists of photons with varying energy.

27. The half-value layer (HVL) of the CT beam may be measured by a radiation physicist or other appropriate CT personnel. The HVL of an x-ray tube is defined as the thickness of material that is capable of reducing the intensity of the x-ray beam to one-half of its original value. HVL is used as a measure of the overall quality of the beam and is helpful in determining the amount of beam filtration necessary for a given CT system.

28. The polyenergetic (heterogeneous) x-ray beam undergoes filtration in an effort to remove low-energy x-ray photons. These are photons with insufficient energy to complete the path from source to patient to detector and would go unmeasured, adding solely to patient radiation dose.

29. Additionally, a filtered beam that is more homogeneous (monoenergetic) is less susceptible to artifacts from a process known as *beam hardening*. As the beam traverses the patient, low-energy photons are absorbed first, increasing the average intensity of the beam as it travels along its path. This change in the beam quality can have an artifactual result on the CT image.

30. The CT x-ray tube contains both inherent and added filtration in an effort to improve the energy quality of the x-ray beam.

31. The tube housing, cooling oil, and so on constitute the inherent filtration, which amounts to approximately to 3.0 mm of aluminum-equivalent filtration.

32. Minimal additional filtration in the form of thin (0.1 to 0.4 mm) copper sheets and bow-tie filters are also added to improve beam utilization efficiency.

33. *Bow-tie filters*, which are thicker at the ends than in the middle, help shape the beam to reduce patient radiation exposure. Because most body parts are circular or cylindrical, less radiation is necessary at the periphery than in the center. Bow-tie filters reduce beam intensity toward the outer margins, resulting in a lower patient radiation dose.

34. Each CT unit will have a proprietary standard procedure for proper tube warm-up before patient scanning. Tube warm-up prevents damage to the x-ray system and prolongs tube life.

35. This procedure will may also involve a series of calibration scans programmed to include a wide range of the many combinations of kVp, mA, and collimation settings available.

C. Generator and Transformers

1. Current CT scanners utilize high-frequency generators. These modern and efficient units are small enough to be housed within the CT gantry.

2. The CT generator includes a high-voltage transformer necessary to convert the low-frequency/low-voltage alternating current supplied to the unit into the high-frequency/high-voltage current required for efficient x-ray production.

3. Power output is vendor specific, within a typical range of 60 to 100 kilowatts (kW).

D. Collimation

1. Once straightforward, the concept of collimation has become more complex with the advent of MDCT.

2. CT collimation for MDCT can be divided into two distinct components:
   a. Beam collimation.
   b. Detector (section) collimation.

3. A review of detector collimation can be found later, in the section on detector configuration.

4. The general purpose of beam collimation in CT is to restrict the radiation exposure to the area of interest, reducing patient radiation dose and improving image quality.

5. SSCT incorporates a fan-shaped beam with a transverse (x-y) dimension corresponding to the size of the detector array and the maximum SFOV.

6. The length of detector coverage in the transverse dimension is determined by the fan angle of the emitted beam. A wider fan angle extends coverage of the detector array along the x- and y-axes.

7. Along the longitudinal, or z-axis, the beam is collimated to the anticipated slice thickness. Located just outside the tube housing, the mechanical aperture responsible for beam restriction is termed the *prepatient collimator*.

8. Prepatient beam collimation in SSCT directly controls the amount of tissue exposed to x-radiation as the tube rotates about the patient.

9. For example, acquisition of 5-mm slices during a SSCT examination is obtained with a beam collimation of 5 mm: the collimator aperture is mechanically set to an opening 5 mm wide along the z-axis. The width of tissue exposed at the center of beam rotation is 5 mm. Beam collimation of 5 mm results in the reconstruction of 2-D images that each represent 5 mm of tissue.

10. No further adjustments to slice thickness are possible after the slice data have been acquired (retrospectively) during SSCT.

11. SSCT beam collimation consists of:
    a. Prepatient collimation: A mechanical device controls the aperture dimension at the x-ray tube, directly limiting the beam to the desired section width.

b. Postpatient collimation: The radiation transmitted through the patient is controlled by predetector collimators. Postpatient (predetector) collimators are used to improve image quality by limiting scatter radiation before it reaches the detectors.

12. There are two components of prepatient collimation:
   a. The tube housing itself acts as an initial collimator. The tube aperture roughly shapes the primary beam into a fan or cone shape, for SSCT or MDCT, respectively. The beam emerges from the tube housing at a specific fan angle, corresponding to the in-plane length of the detector array.
   b. The primary prepatient collimator is positioned just beyond the tube housing. It restricts the beam along the z-axis, controlling slice thickness in the SSCT system.

13. MDCT systems also utilize prepatient and postpatient collimation for reasons similar to those described for SSCT.

14. During MDCT, the beam may be limited before reaching the patient, according to the desired section width and the number of detector rows to be utilized for image formation.

15. Postpatient collimation occurs through a high-resolution comb placed over the detector array. Functioning like a grid, this comb removes unwanted scatter radiation and off-axis photons that result from the more divergent nature of the MDCT beam.

16. MDCT utilizes a cone-shaped beam, which is incident upon an expanded array of detectors. The detector array consists of multiple rows of individual detector elements.

17. As the number of detector rows in an MDCT system increases, the divergence of the cone beam needed for coverage also increases.

18. The MDCT beam is collimated to the total width of the slices acquired with each gantry rotation.

19. At a maximum, the MDCT cone beam may be collimated to a dimension equal to the entire multirow detector array. For example, in a 64-slice system with 0.625-mm detectors, the cone beam is calculated as follows:

$$64 \times 0.625\,mm = 40\,mm$$

In this example, the primary beam is limited by prepatient collimators to a maximum dimension of 40 mm along the z-axis.

20. Beam collimation in the MDCT system may further restrict the field to expose a smaller portion of the detector array. However, this has only an indirect effect on section thickness, which is controlled primarily by detector configuration in the MDCT system.

21. The combination of user-defined beam width and detector configuration ultimately controls the number and thickness of the images acquired during an MDCT examination.

22. The relationship among beam collimation (width), detector size (collimation), and the number of detectors is described as follows:

$$d\,(mm) = \frac{D\,(mm)}{N}$$

where d is detector collimation, D is beam collimation (width), and N is number of detector rows. From the previous example, a 64-slice system with 0.625-mm detectors:

$$0.625 = \frac{40\,mm}{64}$$

23. Collimation of the beam in MDCT directly affects the volume of tissue measured for each rotation of the tube. Wider collimation results in greater anatomic coverage with each tube rotation. This allows for an increase in the overall acquisition volume over a given scan time.

24. Compared with SSCT, MDCT allows faster and more extensive coverage along the z-axis while also providing thinner section widths for each gantry rotation.

25. The *section width* (slice thickness) describes the amount of tissue in the longitudinal or z-axis that is represented by the 2-D CT image.

26. Section width is controlled directly by beam collimation during SSCT. During MDCT, section width is determined by a combination of beam collimation and detector collimation settings.

27. *Detector collimation* describes the process of determining section width in the MDCT system; it is covered further later, in the section on detector configuration.

28. *Section interval* describes the spacing between two adjacent CT images. It is measured as the distance between the center of one section and the center of the next adjacent section.

29. *Contiguous images* are those acquired with equal section thickness and interval. For example, 5-mm sections reconstructed every 5 mm will completely cover a given volume of tissue, with no unmeasured tissue.

30. *Noncontiguous images* are those acquired with an interval greater than the section width. For example, 1-mm sections reconstructed every 10 mm would not evaluate the intermittent 9 mm of tissue.

31. *Overlapping images* are reconstructed with a section interval that is less than the section width. A percentage value may be assigned to the extent of overlap. For example, 1.0-mm-thick images reconstructed every 0.5 mm are said to possess a 50% overlap.

32. Overlapping images are used predominantly to improve the quality of multiplanar reformation (MPR) and 3-D reconstructions.

33. Pitch is an important factor during helical SSCT and MDCT studies. *Pitch* describes the relationship between collimation and table movement during scanning (Fig. 5.4).

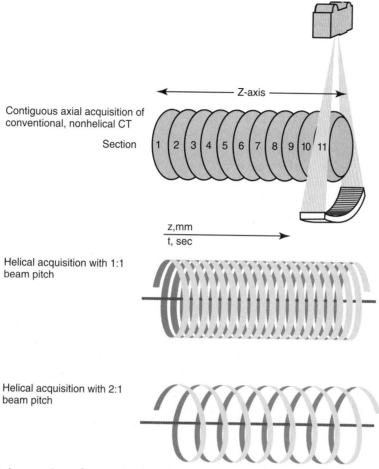

FIG. 5.4 A comparison of conventional axial CT acquisition and helical CT acquisition. The diagram also illustrates the geometric change in data acquisition as pitch increases during helical CT scanning.

34. The pitch of a helically acquired CT study characterizes the amount of longitudinal data acquired for every rotation of the gantry apparatus and the overall acquisition speed.

35. The original definition of pitch for single-slice helical CT (SSCT) was as follows:

$$\text{pitch} = \frac{\text{table feed per rotation}}{\text{section width}}$$

For example, with a section width of 5 mm and a user-defined pitch of 1.5, the table would move 7.5 mm for each gantry rotation.

$$1.5 = \frac{7.5\,\text{mm}}{5.0\,\text{mm}}$$

36. This original definition of pitch may now be referred to as *detector pitch*.

37. Increasing the detector pitch would result in greater table translation with each gantry revolution.

38. Higher detector pitch settings resulted in greater coverage along the z-axis with each revolution of the gantry, but at the cost of reduced image quality.

39. In the helical MDCT system, section width is no longer primarily controlled by beam collimation at the x-ray tube. Detector configuration plays a major role in the determination of reconstructed section width.

40. A new adaptation of the pitch principle, termed *beam pitch*, is required:

$$\text{beam pitch} = \frac{\text{table feed per rotation}}{\text{total collimation}}$$

41. Specific to MDCT, total collimation equals the combined thickness of all of the sections that are simultaneously acquired with each gantry rotation:

$$\text{total collimation} = \text{No. of sections} \times \text{section width}$$

42. For example, a given MDCT system has an array of 16 detectors, each 1.25 mm wide. The total length of the detector array (along the z-axis) equals 20 mm ($16 \times 1.25 = 20$). A beam pitch set at 1.75 will have the table move 35.00 mm for every gantry rotation:

$$\begin{aligned}
\text{beam pitch} &= \frac{\text{table feed per rotation}}{\text{total collimation}} \\
&= \frac{35.00\,\text{mm}}{(16 \times 1.25)} \\
&= \frac{35.00}{20} \\
&= 1.75
\end{aligned}$$

43. A pitch setting less than 1 reduces the table speed for each gantry revolution. This increases the acquired data and subsequently improves image quality.

44. However, lower pitch settings also result in higher patient radiation dose. Increasing pitch moves the patient through the gantry faster, exposing tissue to the beam for shorter periods and reducing dose.

45. Precise collimation of the MDCT x-ray beam along the z-axis also reduces added patient dose from *overbeaming,* as the cone beam extends beyond the range of the linear detector array. This unwanted extension of the cone-shaped beam may be referred to as *penumbra.* Complex beam-shaping collimation restricts radiation at the periphery of the beam, so that only the *umbra* (central) portion of the beam remains (Fig. 5.5).

46. The flying focal spot configuration of some CT systems may also be used to improve the accuracy of the cone beam, directing and restricting the radiation so that penumbra is minimized.

47. To acquire the data necessary for interpolation during helical image reconstruction, an additional half-rotation (180 degrees) of the gantry components may be necessary at the initial (prespiral) and final (post-spiral) portion of each acquisition. This may be referred to as *z-axis overscanning or overranging,* which results in unnecessary added radiation dose to the patient.

48. *Adaptive collimation* technology may also be employed in a modern CT system to reduce z-axis overscanning by blocking the portion of the beam that would potentially expose tissues outside of the desired acquisition volume.

E. Detectors: Design and Scan Geometry

1. The CT detector is responsible for measuring transmitted radiation and converting it into a proportionate electronic signal to be used for image reconstruction.

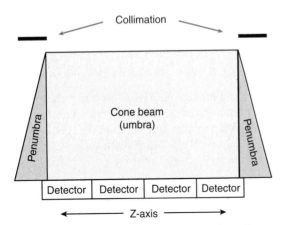

FIG. 5.5 Precise beam collimation reduces overbeaming so that only the center portion of the cone-shaped beam (umbra) remains. Restriction of the periphery (penumbra) of the beam, reduces unnecessary radiation exposure to the patient.

2. The signal emitted by a detector is proportionate to the intensity of the transmitted radiation incident upon and measured by the detector.

3. The desired qualities of a CT detector include:

    a. High efficiency: The CT detector material must be efficient at absorbing the transmitted x-ray photons and converting them into a proportionate signal. The detectors' absorption efficiency is controlled by factors such as the overall size of the detector and the density and atomic number of the material used. The geometric efficiency of a CT detector is primarily influenced by the amount of interspace material necessary between adjacent detectors. Although valuable in limiting interference (cross-talk) between adjacent detectors, the interspace material reduces geometric efficiency by absorbing transmitted x-ray energy. X-ray photons absorbed by interspace material do not add to the generated signal.

    b. Rapid signal decay: The detector must be capable of measuring transmitted x-ray photons with an excellent response time and limited afterglow. The *response time* of a detector is its ability to quickly measure x-rays and then recover before the next measurement. *Afterglow* refers primarily to the tendency of scintillation crystal detectors to continue to glow in response to x-rays once the exposure source has been terminated.

    c. High dynamic range: The CT detector must be sensitive enough to measure a broad range of x-ray transmission data and accurate enough to modulate signal in response to small changes in radiation transmission.

4. Historically, CT detectors were composed of either gas ionization chambers or scintillation crystals. Gas ionization detectors convert x-ray energy directly into an electrical signal. Solid-state scintillation crystal detectors convert x-ray energy first into light energy, which must then be converted into electrical signal.

5. Gas ionization detectors consist of small high-pressure chambers of xenon gas. Interaction with x-rays causes a proportional amount of ionization of the xenon gas, resulting in the discharge of a small electrical signal. An increase in absorbed x-ray energy would result in an increase in emitted signal.

6. Gas ionization detectors were used primarily for conventional third-generation CT systems, before the advent of helical technology.

7. All modern MDCT systems utilize solid-state detectors, consisting primarily of a scintillating crystal material.

8. The detector crystal emits a quantity of light energy proportional to the x-ray incident upon an individual detector (*scintillation*). The light is measured by a photodiode device and is converted to an electronic signal to be sent for processing by the CT computer system.

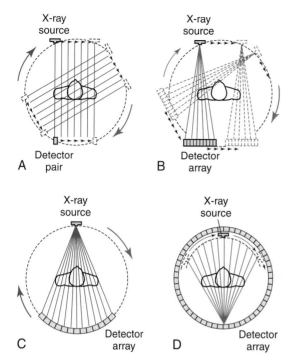

FIG. 5.6 The geometries of the first four generations of CT scanners. (A) First-generation scanners: pencil beam, translate and rotate. (B) Second-generation scanners: fan beam, translate and rotate. (C) Third-generation scanners: fan beam, rotate only. (D) Fourth-generation scanners: fan beam, stationary circular detector array. *(Modified from Seeram E:* Computed tomography: physical principles, clinical applications, and quality control, *ed 4, St Louis, 2016, Saunders.)*

9. Crystal materials employed as CT detectors include cesium iodide, cadmium tungstate, ceramic gadolinium oxysulfide, and scintillating gemstone (e.g., garnet) minerals.

10. Solid-state scintillation-type (nonxenon) detectors are preferred for MDCT because of their ability to accurately record incident x-ray energy from any angle. This flexibility is important because of the widened cone beam geometry inherent to MDCT systems.

11. The detector configuration or detector geometry is often used to delineate the major technologic advances in CT imaging. Each generation of CT system is identifiable by its detector geometry, as follows (Fig. 5.6):

    a. First generation: The prototypical, head-only CT system developed by Sir Godfrey Hounsfield who first put the technology to clinical use in 1972.

       • Consisted primarily of two detectors (paired adjacently along the z-axis) exposed to a tightly collimated pencil beam of x-rays.

       • The tube and detectors would translate across the patient's head, rotate by 1 degree, and then translate back in a method known as *rectilinear or translate–rotate scanning*.

    b. Second generation

       • Also utilizes a translate–rotate geometry, but with an increase in the number of detectors, allowing for greater increments of rotation between translations and a reduction in the overall scan time.

       • First use of fan beam to expose a wider detector array.

       • Expanded clinical capabilities beyond head imaging.

    c. Third generation

       • An expanded curvilinear array of detectors rotates with the x-ray tube around the patient.

       • Rotate–rotate geometry eliminates the need for translation.

       • Larger fan beam is used to expose the expanded detector array.

    d. Fourth generation

       • Co-evolved with third-generation systems and based upon a rotate–stationary geometry.

       • The gantry houses a stationary circular ring of detectors and the x-ray tube rotates around the patient.

12. Later developments in CT technology have not been consistently labeled as additional "generations." However, there have been substantial advances in detector configuration, which will be outlined next.

13. Electron beam CT (EBCT) utilizes a unique technical configuration devoid of moving parts (Fig. 5.7). As an adaptation of fourth-generation design, EBCT has a stationary–stationary geometry, with both the x-ray source and detectors fixed during scanning.

14. EBCT systems have no x-ray tube. A fan beam of x-radiation is produced by directing a beam of electrons toward stationary target rings of tungsten.

15. Each curved tungsten target emits radiation when bombarded by the electron beam, and x-rays are collimated toward the patient.

16. After passing through, and being attenuated by, the patient, the transmitted radiation is measured by a curvilinear array of stationary detectors, which lie opposite the target portion of each ring.

17. Without moving parts, an EBCT system is capable of extremely short exposure times, on the order of 50 msec or less.

18. Because of its high-speed capabilities, the primary application of EBCT is cardiac imaging.

19. As discussed earlier, helical or spiral CT scanners utilize slip-ring technology, which removes the necessity of cables to power the assembly and transmit data. With the resulting continuous rotation of the tube and/or detector array, a helix of data is obtained as the patient is transported through the gantry.

20. Helical SSCT systems may have third- or fourth-generation geometries. The helical acquisition is made possible by the addition of slip-ring technology, not by advancement in detector technology.

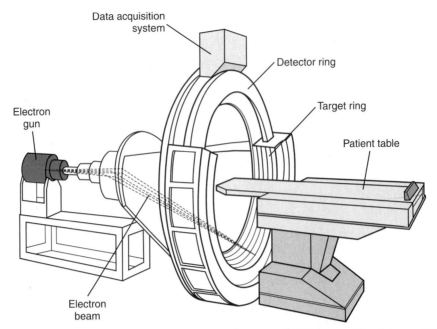

FIG. 5.7 The essential components of an electron beam CT (EBCT) system. The data acquisition geometry consists of a fan beam of x-rays produced by an electron beam that strikes a tungsten target ring. *(Modified from Seeram E:* Computed tomography: physical principles, clinical applications, and quality control *ed 4, St Louis, 2016, Saunders.)*

21. Most helical CT systems utilize solid-state detector arrays because of their improved efficiency and stability.

22. The introduction of MDCT was made possible through a complete redesign of the CT detector array. ·

23. All MDCT systems utilize third-generation geometry and solid-state scintillation detectors.

24. In contrast to the one-dimensional detector array of SSCT, the MDCT detector is said to be 2-D. An MDCT system utilizes a curvilinear detector array with multiple rows of individual detector elements segmented along the longitudinal axis, or z-axis.

25. Parallel rows of individual detectors allow for acquisition of multiple sections of scan data with each rotation of the x-ray tube around the patient. This results in a markedly larger coverage area over a given scan time.

26. Of equal importance is the ability of MDCT scanners to reconstruct images of varying thicknesses at any z-axis position within the volume of data acquisition.

27. From the same data set, both thin-section images for maximum resolution and thicker images for ease of display may be reconstructed without additional scanning.

28. In traditional SSCT, the section width was controlled by beam collimation. Prepatient collimators restricted the primary beam at the center of rotation equal to the desired section width.

29. With MDCT, detector collimation determines the width of the reconstructed section. By electronically adjusting the detector dimension, the operator can control the width of the x-ray beam contributing to a reconstructed section. Beam collimation no longer directly controls section width.

30. Beam collimation still has an important indirect effect on section width. The beam width must be wide enough to encompass the total thickness of the simultaneous sections to be acquired with each gantry revolution.

31. For example, as previously described in the section on collimation, a 64-channel MDCT system acquires 64 slices simultaneously, each 0.625 mm wide along the z-axis. The maximum coverage for each gantry revolution is 40 mm ($64 \times 0.625 = 40$). The beam width must therefore be collimated to 40 mm.

32. In summary, MDCT technology dictates that the width of a CT slice is no longer primarily controlled by prepatient collimation, but instead is controlled by electronic separation or combination of signals from the individual detector rows.

33. *Detector configuration* refers to the number, length, and organization of the individual detector elements in an MDCT system.

34. The three general formats of MDCT detector configuration are as follows (Fig. 5.8):

    a. Uniform matrix array: Utilizes multiple detectors in the longitudinal direction, each the same length. For example, a 4-slice MDCT system employs 16 detector elements, each 1.25 mm in length.

    b. Adaptive array: Detectors are configured with the thinnest widths at the center, surrounded by detectors of incrementally increasing widths along the z-axis. For example, an MDCT with an adaptive array of 16 rows may be composed of two middle detectors of 1.0 mm each (2 mm total), followed

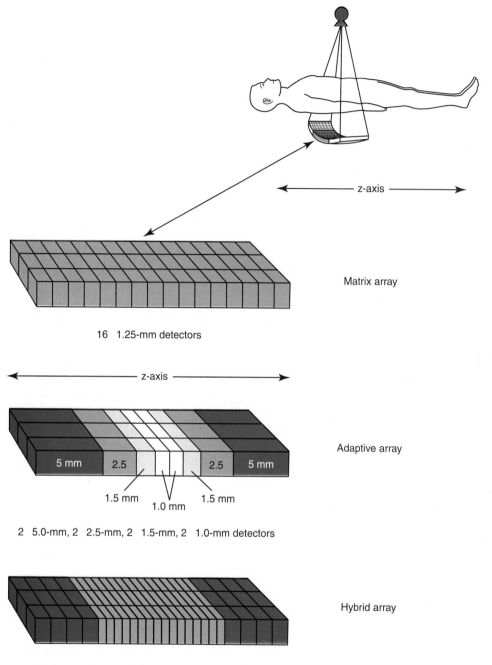

z-axis

Matrix array

16 1.25-mm detectors

z-axis

Adaptive array

5 mm 2.5 2.5 5 mm

1.5 mm 1.5 mm
1.0 mm

2 5.0-mm, 2 2.5-mm, 2 1.5-mm, 2 1.0-mm detectors

Hybrid array

4 1.25-mm, 16 0.625-mm, 4 1.25-mm detectors

FIG. 5.8 The predominant types of MDCT detector configurations: matrix, adaptive, and hybrid arrays.

by pairs of 1.5 mm (3 mm total), 2.5 mm (5 mm total), and 5.0 mm (10 mm total), moving outward from the center of the array. Added together, the detectors total 20 mm along the z-axis.

c. Hybrid array: Consists of two detector sizes. The narrower detectors are positioned midline, flanked by the wider detectors. For example, the central rows of a 16-channel MDCT system are 0.625 mm, with the remaining peripheral rows at 1.25 mm.

35. It is important to keep in mind the distinction between the number of data channels an MDCT system possesses and the quantity/size of its detectors:

a. The quantity of data channels controls the number of sections the scanner can simultaneously acquire with each gantry rotation. For example, what is commonly referred to as a 16-slice MDCT system has, in fact, 16 data channels at its disposal. The maximum number of sections that may be reconstructed from each gantry rotation is 16.

b. The number of detectors in the array is equal to or greater than the number of data channels. The 16-slice MDCT system may utilize an adaptive array of 24 detectors (Fig. 5.9A).

c. With 16 possible data channels, the maximum number of sections this system can simultaneously acquire is 16. Therefore when the beam collimation is set to a width of 20 mm, data from the middle 16 detectors (0.625 mm) are combined, or binned, to form eight sections, each 1.25 mm wide.

d. Data from the four 1.25-mm detectors from each side of the array contribute an additional eight sections per gantry rotation, each 1.25 mm thick.

e. The result is a total of 16 1.25-mm sections acquired for each rotation of the gantry (Fig. 5.9B).

f. *Binning* refers to the electronic combination of signal from adjacent detectors to form a reconstructed slice that is thicker than the individual detector width.

g. The effective section width for the preceding example is 1.25 mm. The minimum section width possible is 1.25 mm. However, it is possible to further apply the concept of binning to reconstruct thicker sections for the same data set.

h. The preceding examples illustrate the process of detector collimation. The width of the x-ray beam remains the same, but the signal emitted from each detector is manipulated to control section width.

i. In the example shown in Fig. 5.9C, signals from pairs of 1.25-mm detectors and quads of 0.625-mm detectors are electronically combined to form eight 2.5-mm-thick sections from data collected during each gantry rotation.

36. The relationship between beam collimation and section width in MDCT can be explored by modifying Fig. 5.9C as follows:

a. While utilizing the previously described 16-channel adaptive array MDCT system, the operator can choose to further collimate the primary beam to a width of 10 mm. After transmission through the patient, radiation is now incident upon only the central 16 detectors (0.625 mm × 16 = 10 mm).

b. In the example shown in Fig. 5.9D, the minimum effective section width is 0.625 mm. When clinically appropriate, the signal from each detector can be used to reconstruct images that represent 0.625 mm of tissue.

c. The user may also decide that the large quantity of 0.625-mm images required to cover a given volume of anatomy is not clinically indicated. In this case, signal from adjacent detectors can be electronically combined (binned) to form thicker (1.25-mm) images.

37. It is the combination of beam collimation and detector collimation that controls:

a. The number of sections that can be simultaneously acquired with each gantry rotation.

b. The minimum section width that can be reconstructed from the acquired volumetric data set.

38. The volumetric nature of MDCT data acquisition ensures that regardless of the section width chosen, images may be reconstructed at any point (increment) along the scanned volume.

39. Nonhelical, or axial, data acquisition is also possible with an MDCT system. Axial acquisition offers excellent image resolution and is often used during applications for which the accurate display of small anatomic details is vital.

40. During axial acquisition, the beam is collimated to the maximum desired section width and is incident upon a predetermined number of detectors.

41. For example, a four-channel MDCT system has an array of 16 detectors, each 1.25 mm wide. During axial acquisition mode, the user selects a beam collimation of 10 mm, exposing the middle eight detectors to transmitted radiation. For each complete rotation of the gantry around a fixed table location, a maximum of four images may be reconstructed from signal collected from the available four data channels in two ways:

a. Four 2.5-mm sections, each section combining data from two detectors.

b. Two 5.0-mm sections, each section combining data from four detectors.

42. Axial section width is therefore controlled by beam collimation and the summation of signal from a predetermined number of detector elements (Fig. 5.10).

43. *Cine CT acquisition* involves multiple axial scans obtained at a single anatomic level over a predetermined period. The primary clinical applications of cine CT acquisition involve dynamic imaging of physiologic processes such as respiration, swallowing, and the cardiac cycle as well as for CT perfusion studies.

44. Cine CT is also utilized during automated bolus tracking for optimal contrast enhancement. Multiple axial scans are acquired at a selected level—usually the vessel or organ of interest—and the helical acquisition is triggered once a predetermined level of contrast enhancement is reached.

45. Currently, the 64-slice MDCT system remains the most widely accepted, studied, and published standard for detector configuration.

46. Various other detector configurations remain available, including 256-slice and 320-slice volumetric acquisition MDCT systems.

47. Further advancement of multidetector technology continues in an effort to improve spatial and temporal resolution and to reduce patient radiation dose. Future directions for technologic improvements include smaller detectors, more detector rows, and better detector efficiency.

48. Flat-panel detector technology and its application for expansive volumetric data acquisition is another potential direction for CT.

49. Flat-panel detectors are essentially larger area detectors used in place of the segmented detector rows found in MDCT systems. The system uses a widely divergent cone beam of radiation to cover the expanded detector.

50. The detector itself consists of a film of scintillating crystals bonded to a matrix of silicon photosensors, similar to a digital radiography image receptor. The matrix array of photodiodes and transistors generates an electronic signal proportionate to the light emitted from the scintillating sheet.

51. A prototypical flat-panel detector has a dimension of 40 × 30 cm. For each gantry revolution, z-axis coverage up to 18 cm is possible.

52. The extensive volumetric scan coverage with each gantry rotation makes possible the acquisition of entire organs in a single axial scan.

53. Flat-panel detector systems also provide improved resolution through extremely thin reconstructed sections. Initial flat-panel CT detectors have achieved sections with sensitivity profiles as thin as 150 μm (0.15 mm).

54. The wide 2-D field of view made possible by a single, large area detector also allows such a system to operate as a conventional fluoroscopic device. This type of real-time CT fluoroscopy may have substantial applications for interventional CT and may offer a true dual-purpose radiographic imaging system.

55. C-arm systems with flat-panel CT capabilities have numerous applications during surgical procedures. A further application, termed an *O-arm*, incorporates a telescoping gantry that enables the acquisition of 3-D CT images in addition to standard fluoroscopy.

56. Additional clinical applications of flat-panel detector CT systems include:
    a. Ultra-high resolution of bony structures.
    b. Dynamic cardiac imaging.
    c. Whole-organ perfusion studies.

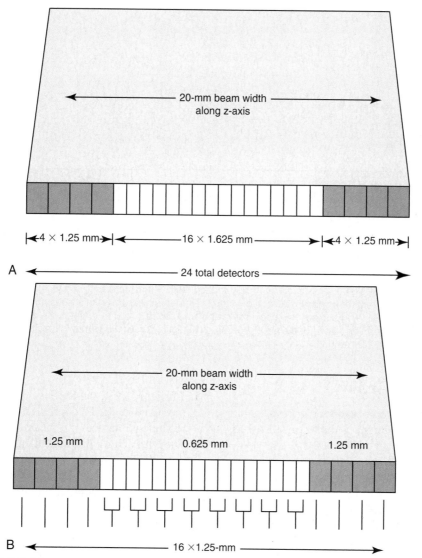

FIG. 5.9 (A) A diagrammatic representation of a 16-channel MDCT adaptive detector array. A total of 24 detectors; the central 16 are 0.625 mm wide, flanked by 8 detectors 1.25 mm wide. (B) With 16 available data channels, data from the 0.625-mm detectors are binned to form eight 1.25-mm sections. The maximum number of sections simultaneously acquired per gantry revolution is 16, each 1.25 mm in width.

Continued

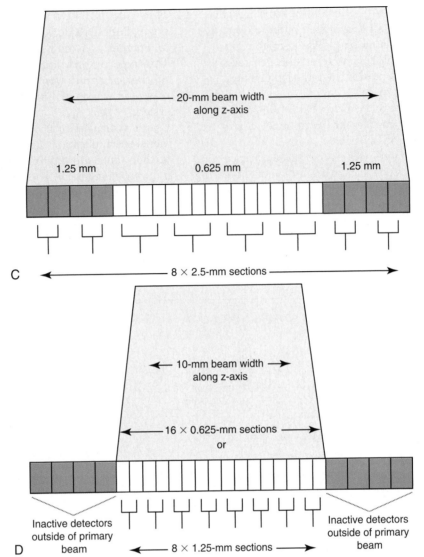

FIG. 5.9—cont'd (C) In this example, the signal measured by two adjacent 1.25-mm detectors is binned, and the signal measured from four adjacent 0.625-mm detectors is also electronically combined. The result is the reconstruction of eight 2.5-mm-thick sections from each gantry rotation. (D) In this example, the beam has been collimated to a width of 10 mm along the z-axis. The detector configuration allows for the reconstruction of 16 sections, each 0.625 mm thick; alternatively, binning can result in eight 1.25-mm-thick sections per gantry rotation.

F. Data Acquisition System

1. The DAS consists of electronic components responsible for measuring the transmitted x-radiation absorbed by the detectors.
2. Electronic amplifiers condition and boost the electronic signal that the detectors transmit in response to radiation absorption.
3. The analog-to-digital converter (ADC) is the component of the DAS responsible for converting the electronic signal into digital form. This digital data are then transmitted to the system computer for image reconstruction.
4. The vast range of tissue densities inherent in CT imaging results in extremely small fluctuations in attenuation. The ADC must be enormously sensitive to a vast range of signal intensities.

5. During MDCT, the DAS is responsible for controlling the signal emitted from the activated detectors exposed to the collimated x-ray beam.
6. The DAS of a MDCT system has a maximum number of data channels used to transmit data from the detectors to the computer system for image reconstruction.
7. The number of data channels controls the number of slices the system can acquire with each gantry rotation.
8. The following example may be used to illustrate the relationship between beam collimation, data channels, quantity of detectors, and the number of sections an MDCT system can acquire per gantry rotation:
   a. The DAS of a four-channel MDCT system has four z-axis data channels.

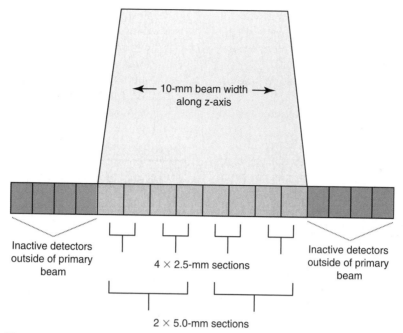

FIG. 5.10 In this example, axial acquisition may result in the reconstruction of four 2.5-mm sections or two 5.0-mm sections. The maximum number of sections acquired per gantry rotation is governed by the number of available data channels. The detectors that lie outside the collimated beam do not measure transmitted radiation or contribute signal to the reconstruction process.

b. The system's detector array contains 16 detectors, each measuring 1.25 mm along the z-axis (20 mm total).

c. When the beam collimation is set to 20 mm, all detectors measure transmitted radiation and produce proportional signal to be collected by the DAS.

d. Because only four z-axis data channels are available, the signal from four detectors may be combined, or binned, to form images that are 5 mm thick (4 × 1.25 mm = 5.0 mm).

e. Therefore with a beam collimation of 20 mm, this system is capable of producing four CT images per gantry rotation with a minimum thickness of 5.0 mm each (Fig. 5.11A).

f. If the beam is further collimated to 10 mm, the transmitted radiation exposes only the center 10 mm of the detector array, corresponding to the middle eight detectors out of the total of 16 (8 × 1.25 mm = 10 mm).

g. The four channels are now capable of producing four CT sections per gantry rotation, each 2.5 mm in thickness and representing the combined data from two detectors (2 × 1.25 mm = 2.5 mm) (Fig. 5.11B).

h. Beam collimation to 5 mm on this system would result in the possible reconstruction of four 1.25-mm-thick images for every gantry rotation (Fig. 5.11C).

G. Computer System

1. An in-depth analysis of the function of the CT computer system is beyond the scope of clinical practice and this review book.

2. However, the CT technologist should have a basic understanding of the fundamental operation of the CT computer system and should be able to identify the major technical components.

3. Fast and efficient data processing and extremely large data storage capacity are the most important characteristics of CT computer systems.

4. The central processing unit (CPU) is capable of performing multiple tasks simultaneously, a function called *parallel processing*.

5. *Pipelining* is an additional feature of CT computer systems that further improves the speed and efficiency with which it can perform multiple simultaneous functions, including detector signal preprocessing, convolution, postprocessing, and image manipulation.

6. The primary data processing component of the CT system is the array processor. A separate computer with its own CPU, the array processor is connected to the main host computer of the CT system.

7. The array processor is responsible for receiving scan data from the host computer, performing all of the major processing of the CT image, and returning the reconstructed image to the storage memory of the host computer.

8. The hard disk drive is the common choice for mass storage of CT computer system data.

9. The hard disk drive is a rewritable, nonremovable storage system that must be capable of storing a tremendous amount of data. It also must be able to transfer data quickly, in a manner quantified by the data transfer rate.

10. The operating system (OS) is the main software of the CT computer. It controls the utilization of the hardware resources, such as the available memory, CPU time, and disk space.

11. Common types of OS software include Windows, MS-DOS, OS/2, and UNIX.

12. The remaining software of the CT computer system may be organized as follows:

    a. Preprocessing software processes the signal data collected from the detectors and conditions it by applying appropriate correction factors for beam hardening, detector malfunction, and so on.

    b. Reconstruction software is responsible for mathematically constructing the raw data into image data using algorithms for the processes of convolution, back projection, data frequency filtering, and so on.

    c. Postprocessing software manipulates the image data for review and interpretation. This software controls the image visualization and analysis tools of the CT system, including applications such as windowing, image display filters, 3-D/MPR reformation, and analytic functions (ROI, distance).

IMAGE PROCESSING AND DISPLAY

A. Image Reconstruction

1. The data acquisition process can be outlined as follows:

    a. The x-ray tube rotates around the patient while emitting a constant beam of x-radiation. The quantity of radiation is controlled primarily by

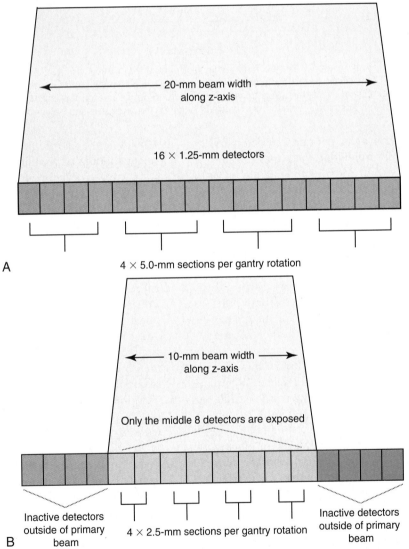

FIG. 5.11 (A) Four-channel MDCT acquisition with 20-mm beam width. For each gantry rotation at this selected beam width, the system is capable of reconstructing a maximum of four 5.0-mm CT sections. The data from four adjacent detector elements (1.25 mm each) are binned, or electronically combined. (B) Four-channel MDCT acquisition with 10-mm beam width. With only the central eight detectors exposed to transmitted radiation, a maximum of four 2.5-mm CT images may be reconstructed for each gantry rotation. The detectors that lie outside the collimated beam do not measure transmitted radiation and do not contribute signal to the reconstruction process.

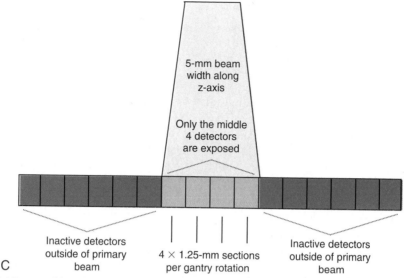

C

5-mm beam width along z-axis

Only the middle 4 detectors are exposed

Inactive detectors outside of primary beam

4 × 1.25-mm sections per gantry rotation

Inactive detectors outside of primary beam

FIG. 5.11—cont'd (C) Four-channel MDCT acquisition with 5.0-mm beam width. With only the central four detectors exposed to transmitted radiation, a maximum of four 1.25-mm CT images may be reconstructed for each gantry rotation. The detectors that lie outside the collimated beam do not measure transmitted radiation or contribute signal to the reconstruction process.

the mA setting, and the beam quality (penetrability) is controlled primarily by the kVp.

b. As the x-ray photons pass through the patient, some are absorbed completely and others lose a portion of their energy and change direction as scatter radiation. This process, termed *attenuation,* can be described as the reduction in intensity of the x-ray quantum as it travels along from tube to detector.

c. The extent of attenuation depends on multiple factors, including the x-ray energy and the atomic structure and density of the exposed tissue.

d. Attenuation values are calculated by mathematically comparing the radiation incident upon the patient (I_0) to the radiation transmitted through and measured by the detector (I).

e. The logarithmic relationship is mathematically described by the formula:

$$= \log \frac{\text{Intensity of x-ray at the source } (I_0)}{\text{Intensity of x-ray at the detector } (I)}$$

f. The portion of the x-ray beam transmitted through the patient and incident upon a single detector is termed a *ray*. Each ray undergoes a specific quantity of attenuation based on its particular path through the patient.

g. The measurement of transmitted radiation made by an individual detector is called a *ray sum*. It equals the total attenuation occurring along a straight-line path from tube to detector.

h. The ray sum, or transmission measurement, equals the total attenuation of all materials along the ray.

i. The detector emits an electronic analog signal in proportionate response to the transmitted radiation it absorbs. As the detector array rotates about the patient, the signal varies according to the measured x-ray energy flux.

j. During the process of data acquisition, ray sum measurements are made by the DAS hundreds of times per second. The term *view* is used to describe each data sample made by the DAS. A view contains transmission measurements made along multiple rays, each corresponding to a particular detector (ray sums).

k. The sampling rate may be quantified as *views per rotation* (VPR). The VPR determines the quantity of samples, and therefore transmission data, acquired during each gantry rotation.

2. The analog transmission values (signal) acquired by the DAS are digitized by the ADC and sent to the computer for processing as raw data.

3. From the thousands of ray sum measurements acquired, the computer system generates an attenuation map, spatially localizing the degree of attenuation that occurs across a given section of anatomy.

4. The large magnitude of data samples acquired during scanning allows for precise localization of attenuation values for each pinpoint area of tissue within a given section.

5. The ability of an object to attenuate the x-ray beam is assigned a value termed the *linear attenuation coefficient* (μ).

6. If the intensity of radiation incident upon an object is known, the magnitude of attenuation occurring as the x-ray beam passes through an object can be calculated by measuring the intensity of radiation transmitted.

7. The Lambert–Beer equation illustrates the relationship between radiation intensity and object density and

allows for the calculation of an object's linear attenuation coefficient (μ):

$$I = I_0 e^{-\mu x}$$

where e is Euler's constant (2.718) and x is object thickness.

8. The Lambert–Beer equation is valid only for homogeneous pencil-beam radiation sources, such as the first-generation CT system developed by Hounsfield.

9. The situation becomes much more complicated by the heterogeneous nature of the x-ray beam and the additional difficulties inherent in the cone beam geometry of modern MDCT systems. Nevertheless, the Lambert–Beer equation neatly demonstrates how the attenuation coefficients contained within a sample (section) of patient anatomy can be calculated.

10. The reconstructed CT image displays a 2-D map localizing the attenuation that occurs throughout each section of tissue.

11. The primary goal of CT image reconstruction is to spatially distribute the attenuation data recorded by the detector array.

12. The mathematical process primarily responsible for CT image reconstruction is called *back-projection*. During this reconstruction method, the ray sum data acquired from each projection (data sample) is projected back onto a matrix.

13. A *matrix* is a 2-D grid of numbers arranged in rows and columns.

14. The acquisition of an extremely large number of projections for each gantry rotation results in a detailed but relatively blurry digital representation of the object(s) in study.

15. An additional process called *convolution* is applied to reduce image unsharpness. An algorithm or convolution kernel acts as a mathematical filter, modifying the ray sum data and removing the unwanted burring effect of the back-projection.

16. The appearance of the CT image may be altered by the application of different algorithms to manipulate the signal during image reconstruction. For example, a soft tissue algorithm yields a smooth image, which is preferable for the evaluation of soft tissue structures. A bone algorithm sharpens edges and improves the demonstration of bony detail with high-resolution CT images.

17. This back-projection of ray sum data onto a matrix combined with mathematical filtration is the basis for what was historically the most common employed basic method of image reconstruction for the modern MDCT system—*the filtered back projection (FBP)*.

18. However, additional techniques are necessary to eliminate unwanted image degradation resulting from patient movement during helical data acquisition.

19. Conventional CT data acquisition consists of incremental, slice-by-slice scanning. For each 360-degree rotation of the gantry components, the patient/table remains stable and transmission data are recorded. The bed then moves to the next location, determined by the chosen section interval, and the process is repeated until the desired anatomic coverage is achieved.

20. Helical, or spiral, scanning refers to the volumetric data acquisition process whereby the gantry and bed undergo continuous motion. The acquired data are described as having a helical, or spiral, geometry.

21. During helical data acquisition, the patient bed is continuously feeding through the gantry as the tube and detector array rotate. Therefore no single slice of patient anatomy is ever exposed to a full 360 degrees of evaluation.

22. *Interpolation* is the mathematical process whereby data from tube rotations just above and just below a given slice position are used for image reconstruction.

23. Interpolation allows for the reconstruction of a thin, motion-free image from a volumetric data set acquired from a moving patient.

24. The technique known as *360-degree linear interpolation (360LI)* uses two sets of projection data acquired 360 degrees apart to form an image at a precise z-axis location.

25. More commonly used for current MDCT image reconstruction is the 180-degree linear interpolation technique (*180LI*).

26. The 180LI technique interpolates data acquired at a distance only 180 degrees away from the reconstructed slice location. For every one-half rotation of the gantry during scanning, a complementary ray is acquired, at the point where the x-ray tube and detectors are in exact opposite positions from those in the previous, complementary view.

27. Data acquired from the complementary ray are used to form an image at a precise z-axis location.

28. Interpolation of data from a shorter distance away along the z-axis reduces blurring and improves image quality.

29. Multidetector row CT systems utilize an additional process called *z-filtering* during image reconstruction. Z-filtering allows for thin sections to be reconstructed at any point along the acquired z-axis volume. This reconstruction method utilizes multiple complementary rays beyond those immediately above and below the particular slice plane.

30. Image reconstruction for MDCT helical acquisition is complicated further by the addition of cone beam geometry.

31. The widened 2-D detector array of MDCT systems requires a more divergent x-ray beam. The rays measured from a more divergent beam arrive at the detector at an oblique angle, which must be compensated for during the reconstruction process.

32. As the number of detector rows and subsequent beam divergence increase, the situation may arise in which not all of the rays measured by the detectors have

passed through a given section plane. Rays that are positioned at the periphery of the cone beam may never pass through a midline section as it relates to the total data acquired from a single gantry rotation.

33. Special cone beam reconstruction algorithms are used to overcome this issue. Examples are the Feldkamp–Davis–Kress (FDK) and advanced single-slice rebinning (ASSR) algorithms. The mathematical theory and function of these specialized algorithms are beyond the scope of both the clinical practice of CT and this review book.

34. Once the reconstruction process is completed, the raw data (ray sum or transmission measurements) is displayed as image data. The resultant images of this initial, or prospective, reconstruction are evaluated by a radiologist, further manipulated in 3-D or MPR, archived to long-term storage, and so on.

35. Multiple data reconstructions can be performed retrospectively, with adjustments to the section interval, display field of view (DFOV), image centering, or algorithm (kernel). MDCT systems also allow changes in section width through adjustment of the detector collimation.

36. The projection (raw) data must be available within the system to perform such retrospective reconstructions. Each CT system is capable of storing a finite amount of raw data for retrospective reconstruction.

37. *Iterative reconstruction* was historically used for image reconstruction in some of the earliest CT systems, dating back to Hounsfield's original work.

38. In modern MDCT systems, iterative techniques are commonly employed to reduce image noise and allow for significant reductions in technical factors, thus reducing patient dose.

39. This method of CT image reconstruction uses multiple image reconstruction passes (iterations) to arrive at a final image with reduced noise and artifacts, leading to improved overall quality.

40. Current computation power of CT computer systems allows for rapid reconstruction with iterative approaches.

41. Adaptive iterative reconstruction techniques are currently employed on CT systems from most major industry vendors. This technique begins with data analysis using standard FBP algorithms. This is followed by comparisons between the measured pixel values and those of an ideal data set. Through a repeated comparison process, new pixel values are calculated, resulting in a final image that approaches an ideal, noise-free version (iteration).

42. A second-generation type of iterative reconstruction technique known as *model-based iterative reconstruction* is also now available. This advanced technique considers the shape of the CT x-ray beam both prepatient and postpatient, and uses complex statistical analyses in both a forward and backward series of reconstructions to arrive at an improved image with reduced noise.

B. Image Display

1. *Digital image* is used to describe an image of an object that is numerically based. To review:
   a. The CT image is a digital image made up of numerical values acquired from a conversion of analog signal.
   b. The signal is generated by detectors that measure the attenuation of radiation by an object (patient).
   c. A numerical value called the *linear attenuation coefficient* (μ) is assigned to a sample of tissue quantifying its degree of attenuation.
   d. The digital CT image is therefore based on numerical values that quantify x-ray attenuation.

2. The digital CT image is displayed on an arrangement of numerical values called a *matrix*. The matrix is made up of a series of *picture* elements, arranged in rows and columns, called pixels (*pi-x-els*).

3. The number of pixels contained in a matrix varies throughout digital imaging but is 512 across and 512 down (512 × 512) in most CT systems.

4. As presented on a display screen, the CT image is two-dimensional. However, each pixel actually represents a volume of tissue. The volume data are referred to as a voxel, for *volume* element (*vo-x-el*) (Fig. 5.12).

5. The longitudinal dimension of the voxel corresponds to the z-axis of scanning, with a voxel depth equal to the reconstructed section width. For example, sections reconstructed at a 1.25-mm width have voxel lengths (z) of 1.25 mm.

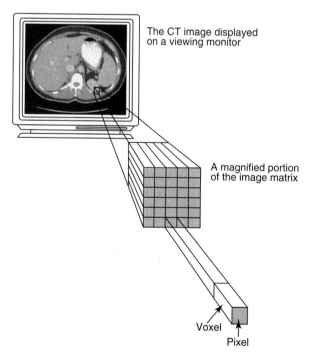

The CT image displayed on a viewing monitor

A magnified portion of the image matrix

Voxel

Pixel

FIG. 5.12 The digital CT image is displayed upon a matrix, which is composed of rows and columns of pixels. Each pixel represents a three-dimensional volume element called a voxel.

6. Each voxel digitally represents a quantity of scanned patient tissue. The tissue within the voxel has exhibited some measure of attenuation, and a corresponding linear attenuation coefficient (μ) is assigned to the pixel. The μ of each pixel represents the average attenuation exhibited by the tissue spatially localized within the voxel.

7. The calculated μ for each pixel is not an absolute value and can vary for an identical voxel scanned on a different CT system or at a different moment in time. This variation is because of naturally occurring fluctuations in the photon energy produced by the x-ray system.

8. The conversion of the linear attenuation value (μ) into a CT number normalizes the voxel attenuation and corrects for this potential variation in pixel number. The *CT number* is a relative value that standardizes the attenuation value (μ) of a tissue by comparing it with the attenuation of water for a particular CT system.

9. The mathematical relationship between linear attenuation coefficient (μ) and CT number is given as follows:

$$CT\ number = \frac{\mu_t - \mu_w}{\mu_w} \bullet K$$

where μ_t is the linear attenuation coefficient of the pixel/voxel in question, μ_w is the linear attenuation of water for a given CT system, and K is a constant value of 1000 termed the *contrast factor*.

10. The calculated CT number is given in Hounsfield units (HU), named for the inventor of CT technology, Sir Godfrey Hounsfield.

11. For example, during a body CT scan, a particular voxel of tissue has a total linear attenuation coefficient (μ) of 0.189. The μ of water for this scanner is known to be 0.181. The CT number for this pixel can be calculated as follows:

$$CT\ number = \frac{\mu_t - \mu_w}{\mu_w} \bullet K$$
$$= \frac{0.189 - 0.181}{0.181} \bullet 1000$$
$$= 0.044 \bullet 1000 = 44\ HU$$

12. This pixel value corresponds to a typical HU for soft tissue structures such as musculature and abdominal organ parenchyma.

13. Another voxel from the same section location has a total linear attenuation coefficient (μ) of 0.008. The CT number for this pixel can be calculated as follows:

$$CT\ number = \frac{\mu_t - \mu_w}{\mu_w} \bullet K$$
$$CT\ number = \frac{0.008 - 0.181}{0.181} \bullet 1000$$
$$CT\ number = -0.956 \bullet 1000 = -956\ HU$$

14. The HU for this pixel is a negative number because the tissue it represents has an attenuation value less than that of water. This pixel value corresponds to a typical HU for an air-filled structure such as the lungs or gastrointestinal tract.

15. This relationship also clearly illustrates why the CT number for a voxel containing water is at or around 0 HU:

$$CT\ number = \frac{\mu_t - \mu_w}{\mu_w} \bullet K$$
$$CT\ number = \frac{0.181 - 0.181}{0.181} \bullet 1000$$
$$CT\ number = 0 \bullet 1000 = 0\ HU$$

16. Table 5.1 lists approximate linear attenuation coefficients (μ) and relative Hounsfield values for assorted body tissues.

17. To review, the pixel value, given in Hounsfield units, is a numerical representation of the attenuation of a voxel of tissue as compared with that of water for an individual CT system.

18. The CT image is most accurate when a voxel represents only one tissue type. *Partial volume averaging* occurs when multiple types of tissue are represented by a single voxel. The attenuation coefficients for each tissue type are averaged, yielding a single pixel value whose HU attempts to represent the entire contents of the voxel.

19. Partial volume averaging can be reduced by minimizing the voxel dimension. Small voxels have a greater propensity to contain only one tissue type, thereby improving accuracy.

20. The simplest method of reducing voxel dimension is to reduce reconstructed section width. A thinner slice (section) is produced from voxels with shorter lengths along the z-axis. Thinner section widths reduce the partial volume effect.

21. The volume of a voxel may also be reduced by decreasing the pixel dimension. The pixel dimension, *d*, is given by the following formula, in relation to the DFOV:

$$d = \frac{DFOV\ (mm)}{matrix\ size}$$

22. The matrix size is relatively standard in CT imaging at 512^2, or 512 pixels across by 512 pixels down.

23. The SFOV is one of two fields of view described in CT imaging. SFOV is determined by the size (x- and y-axes) of the detector array. SFOV controls the diameter of the circular data acquisition field within the CT gantry:
    a. Most modern MDCT systems have an SFOV within the approximate range of 48 to 52 cm. Therefore the maximum circular field of data acquired is between 48 and 52 cm.
    b. A CT system allows for a reduction in SFOV for certain clinical applications by reducing the number of activated detectors during data acquisition.

TABLE 5.1	Computed Tomography Number for Various Tissues and X-Ray Linear Attenuation Coefficients at Four kVp Techniques				
Tissue	**CT Number**		**Linear Attenuation Coefficient (cm⁻¹)**		
		75 kVp	100 kVp	125 kVp	150 kVp
Dense bone	3000	0.604	0.528	0.460	0.410
Muscle	50	0.273	0.237	0.208	0.184
White matter	45	0.245	0.213	0.187	0.166
Gray matter	40	0.243	0.212	0.184	0.163
Blood	20	0.241	0.208	0.184	0.163
Cerebrospinal fluid	15	0.240	0.207	0.182	0.163
Water	0	0.239	0.207	0.181	0.160
Fat	−100	0.213	0.206	0.180	0.160
Lungs	−200	0.111	0.185	0.162	0.144
Air	−1000	0.0005	0.093	0.081	0.072
			0.0004	0.0003	0.0002

From Bushong SC: *Radiologic science for technologists,* ed 10, St Louis, 2013, Mosby.

c. Most CT systems have multiple SFOV choices. Common examples are large SFOV (50 cm) and small SFOV (25 cm).

d. Some modern CT systems may feature a larger bore with extended SFOV options to accommodate larger patients.

e. The selection of SFOV may also involve additional filtration and corrective algorithms for certain clinical applications. For example, CT systems typically offer some version of a specific SFOV for the head. It utilizes an acquisition diameter of 25 cm but also includes specific adaptations within the reconstruction process to improve the quality of CT images of the head.

24. The DFOV is chosen by the CT operator on the basis of the part size in question. The selected DFOV determines what portion of the acquired data will be displayed across the matrix:

a. For example, during a CT examination of the abdomen, the operator chooses a large SFOV (50 cm) to ensure that the entire patient circumference is included within the data acquisition field.

b. The DFOV for image reconstruction is selected on the basis of the dimension of the anatomic area the operator selects to display across the image matrix. The size of the DFOV equals the size of the part of interest.

c. Continuing with the example, a DFOV of 38 cm displays a reconstructed circle whose diameter equals 38 cm. A DFOV of 12 cm would display only 12 cm of the acquired 50 cm of scan data across the image matrix.

d. Choosing a smaller DFOV, or targeting:
- Limits the anatomic area displayed.
- Increases the size of the displayed anatomy and, most importantly, reduces the pixel dimension and the volume of each voxel (Fig. 5.13).

e. As a geometric cuboid, the volume of a voxel may be calculated as follows:

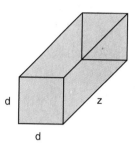

FIG. 5.13 Dimensions of a voxel. Pixel dimension (*d*) is controlled by the image matrix and the selected display field of view (DFOV). The voxel depth (*z*) is controlled by the section width.

$$\text{voxel volume (mm}^3) = d^2 \text{ (mm}^2) \bullet \text{section width (z, mm)}$$

25. To review, the pixel dimension and voxel volume are controlled by three technical parameters:
a. Matrix size.
b. DFOV.
c. Section width (z).

26. An important concept to keep in mind is that the actual size of the pixel does not change. A 512×512 matrix always has pixels of a consistent dimension. What changes is the amount of tissue spatially localized into each voxel and subsequently represented by each pixel's CT number.

27. Less tissue in each voxel reduces the partial volume effect and improves image quality (Fig. 5.14).

28. In addition to the size of a reconstructed image, the image centering may be altered with use of an application of the Cartesian coordinate system:
a. The x-y-axis is located within the rotational plane of the CT gantry.
b. The x-axis runs from right to left (or vice versa) when one is viewing an axial image.
c. The y-axis runs from anterior to posterior (or vice versa) when one is viewing an axial image.
d. The z-axis runs parallel to the movement of the CT table, in and out of the gantry. The z-axis corresponds to the plane running superior to inferior

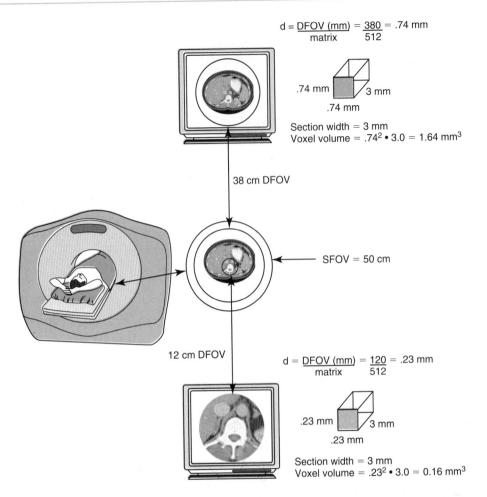

$$d = \frac{DFOV\ (mm)}{matrix} = \frac{380}{512} = .74\ mm$$

.74 mm
3 mm
.74 mm

Section width = 3 mm
Voxel volume = $.74^2 \cdot 3.0 = 1.64\ mm^3$

38 cm DFOV

SFOV = 50 cm

12 cm DFOV

$$d = \frac{DFOV\ (mm)}{matrix} = \frac{120}{512} = .23\ mm$$

.23 mm
3 mm
.23 mm

Section width = 3 mm
Voxel volume = $.23^2 \cdot 3.0 = 0.16\ mm^3$

FIG. 5.14 The combination of matrix, DFOV, and section width determines the amount of tissue that is spatially localized into each voxel. The pixel value (CT number) represents all of the tissue localized within a single pixel.

(or vice versa) when one is viewing sequential axial CT images of the head, neck, and trunk.

e. When one is imaging the upper or lower extremities, the z-axis runs parallel to the long axis of the part, from proximal to distal (or vice versa).

f. This coordinate system is sometimes referred to as *RAS* (for *r*ight, *a*nterior, and *s*uperior) coordinates.

g. The clinical images in Fig. 5.15 illustrate the display effects of DFOV reduction and targeting.

29. In contrast to targeting, the displayed CT image may also be electronically magnified.

30. Magnification is an electronic feature of the system software and display monitor. The process of image magnification results in a larger displayed image but has no effect on pixel/voxel dimension (Fig. 5.16).

31. Once image reconstruction is complete, the CT image exists as a digital matrix. Each pixel is assigned a Hounsfield value on the basis of the attenuation of the tissue localized in its corresponding voxel.

32. For visual display, the numerical data are converted into an image based on a gray scale. Each pixel is assigned a shade of gray according to its CT number.

33. *Windowing* is used to describe the process of grayscale mapping of the CT image. A basic understanding of computer language is helpful in comprehending how grayscale mapping of the CT image is accomplished.

34. Like any other computer system, the CT computer utilizes a binary system (0, 1) based on discrete units termed *bits*.

35. The bit depth of a digital imaging system defines the number of information bits contained within each pixel. The bit depth controls the maximum number of CT Hounsfield values that may be assigned to any one pixel, as illustrated by the following relationship:

$$\text{Pixel CT \#} = 2^k$$

where k is the bit number.

36. The CT computer system is typically capable of displaying 12 bits of data per pixel and is therefore able to display any of up to 4096 (or 2^{12}) Hounsfield values for each pixel.

37. The typical range of Hounsfield scale CT numbers is −1024 HU to +3071 HU. This range equals the 4096 different values possible with a 12-bit system ($2^{12} = 4096$).

DFOV = 48 cm   DFOV = 24 cm

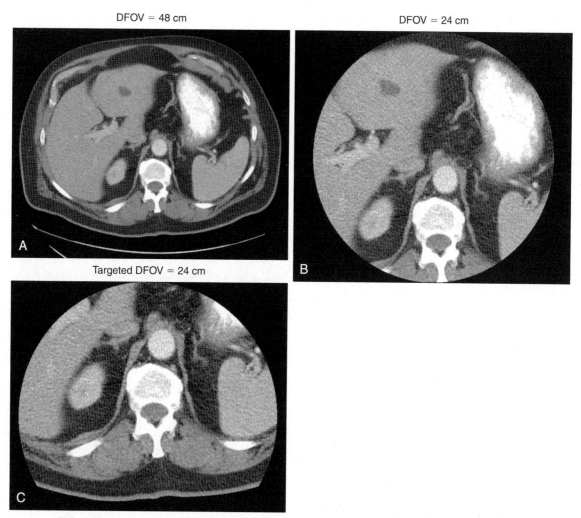

Targeted DFOV = 24 cm

FIG. 5.15 (A) A 5.0-mm axial CT section of the abdomen acquired with a large scan field of view (SFOV) of 50 cm. The display field of view (DFOV) is set at 48 cm, so almost all of the acquired data are displayed on the image matrix. The volume of each voxel equals (480/512)2 5 = 4.393 mm. (B) The same 50 cm of raw data retrospectively reconstructed with a DFOV of 24 cm. The volume of each voxel now equals (240/512)2 5 = 1.103 mm. Each voxel represents significantly less tissue in this targeted reconstruction. (C) An additional retrospective reconstruction with new RAS coordinates centering the targeted 24 cm DVOV over the spine.

38. During display of the CT image, each pixel is assigned a shade of gray on the basis of its CT number (HU). In theory, up to 4096 different shades of gray could be assigned to a given pixel.

39. Display monitors used for CT image evaluation possess a dynamic range of about 8 bits and can display 256 individual shades of gray.

40. Because the human eye is capable of differentiating only about 60 to 80 individual shades of gray, the 256 levels possible with an 8-bit system are more than sufficient.

41. Gray-scale mapping, or windowing, occurs when the display system assigns a shade of gray to an individual pixel on the basis of its CT number (HU).

42. The image window determines the range of pixel values that will be assigned a particular shade of gray.

Any pixel with a value outside the image window will not be assigned a shade of gray, but will appear either white or black.

43. The specifics of the displayed pixel range are determined by a user-selected *window level* (WL) and *window width* (WW).

44. The range of displayed pixels is controlled by the image WW. For example, for a WW of 150, a range of 150 pixel values are assigned individual shades of gray. Only pixels with Hounsfield values that fall within the set range are assigned one of the available 256 shades of gray.

45. Any pixel with a CT number lower than the set range appears black. Any pixel with a CT number higher than the set range appears white.

46. There are 256 shades of gray available to display 4096 possible pixel numbers. The selected WW determines

how many consecutive CT Hounsfield values will be displayed by a single shade of gray.

47. Narrow WW values assign fewer pixel values to each step along the gray scale. Wide WW values assign more pixel values to each shade of gray.

48. In the most basic example, a WW of 256 (WW/256) will display a single pixel value for each shade of gray. A WW of 2560 (WW/2560) assigns 10 consecutive pixel values for each step along the gray scale.

49. The WW is centered on a middle pixel value termed the *window level*.

50. The WL is the pixel value, given in HU, at the center of the WW. The WL is generally set at or near the Hounsfield value of the primary tissue of interest.

51. For example, if the previously cited WW of 150 (−25 to +125 HU) is centered at a CT number of +50 HU, the window may be graphically illustrated as shown in Fig. 5.17.

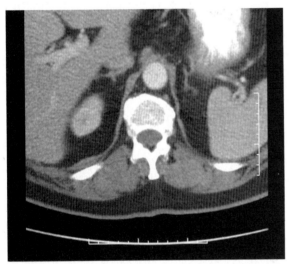

FIG. 5.16 The image from Fig. 5.15A is shown here magnified by a factor of 2. The DFOV remains at 50 cm, and the voxel volume is still 4.39 mm. The image has been electronically magnified on the display monitor and demonstrates a loss of sharpness in comparison with the targeted image in Fig. 5.15C.

52. In this example, only pixels with values between −25 HU and +125 HU will appear as some shade of gray. Any pixel with a Hounsfield value less than −25 HU will appear black. Any pixel with a Hounsfield value greater than +125 HU will appear white.

53. Fig. 5.18 provides an example of an axial CT image of the abdomen displayed with this window.

54. A window with a WL of −500 HU and a WW of 1000 may be graphically illustrated as shown in Fig. 5.19.

55. In this example, only pixels with values between −1000 HU and 0 HU will appear as some shade of gray. Any pixel with a Hounsfield value less than −1000 HU will appear black. Any pixel with a Hounsfield value greater than 0 HU will appear white.

56. Fig. 5.20 is an example of an axial CT image of the abdomen displayed with this window.

57. A window with a WL of +500 HU and a WW of 2000 may be graphically illustrated as shown in Fig. 5.21.

58. In this example, only pixels with values between −500 HU and +1500 HU will appear as some shade of gray. Any pixel with a Hounsfield value less than −500 HU will appear black. Any pixel with a Hounsfield value greater than +1500 HU will appear white.

59. Fig. 5.22 provides an example of an axial CT image of the abdomen displayed with this window.

60. Keep in mind that most CT imaging systems routinely have the ability to assign up to 4096 (2^{12}) Hounsfield values to any one pixel. With only 256 shades of gray available for display, pixels with similar Hounsfield values may be group-assigned a single shade of gray. The extent to which this grouping of pixel shade occurs depends on the WW.

61. For example, with a wider window setting, such as 4000, very few pixels if any will fall outside the display range and appear white or black. Groups of pixels whose CT numbers are similar will be assigned the same shade of gray (Fig. 5.23).

62. In general terms, the WW controls the contrast of a CT image, and the WL controls its brightness.

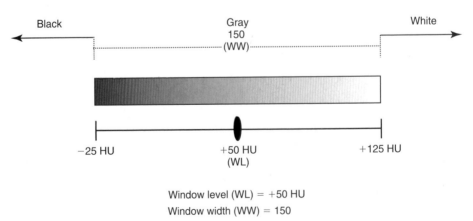

Window level (WL) = +50 HU

Window width (WW) = 150

FIG. 5.17 Pixels with values between −25 HU and +125 HU are each assigned a shade of gray. Pixels with values less than −25 HU are black, and those with values greater than +125 HU are white.

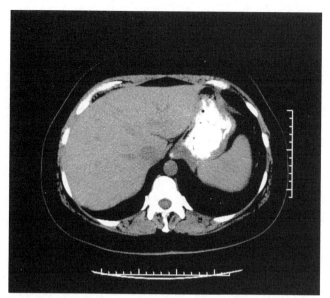

FIG. 5.18 An axial CT image of the abdomen displayed with a window level (WL) of +50 HU and a window width (WW) of 150. This narrow window setting results in a high-contrast image. There are many "black" and "white" pixels, with fewer pixels assigned shades of gray because of the narrow window setting.

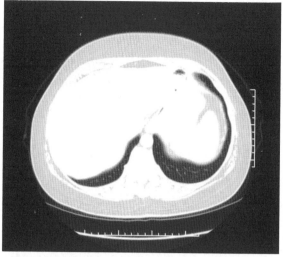

FIG. 5.20 The image from Fig. 4.20 is displayed here with a window level (WL) of −500 HU and a window width (WW) of 1000. This combination of settings would typically be referred to as a "lung window," because it offers good detail of the visualized lung parenchyma. Denser structures such as bone and soft tissue appear white because their pixel values are greater than 0 HU.

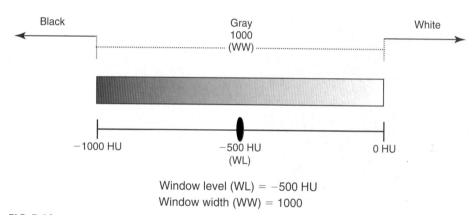

Window level (WL) = −500 HU
Window width (WW) = 1000

FIG. 5.19 Pixels with values between −1000 HU and 0 HU are each assigned a shade of gray. Pixels with values less than −1000 HU are black, and those with values greater than 0 HU are white.

63. Specific WW and level settings depend primarily on the visual preferences of the user. Some general guidelines to CT window settings can be found in Table 5.2.

64. The mathematical basis and digital display of the CT image may be summarized as follows:
   a. During data acquisition, a numerical value called the *linear attenuation coefficient* (μ) is assigned to a sample of tissue, quantifying its degree of attenuation.
   b. The pixel value, given in Hounsfield units, is a numerical representation of the attenuation of a voxel of tissue relative to that of water.
   c. During image display, each pixel is assigned a shade of gray on the basis of its CT number (Fig. 5.24).

65. Once the image is displayed on a computer monitor, CT software systems are capable of various analysis features including:

   a. *Image display filters*: Different from the algorithms utilized during image reconstruction, these display filters are used to visually enhance the CT image during certain clinical applications. Some are used to smooth the CT image for improved low-contrast resolution. Edge-enhancing filters sharpen the CT image during high-resolution imaging applications of the lungs and dense bones. Image filters do not affect the process of raw data reconstruction; rather, they alter the display characteristics of an image after the reconstruction process.

   b. Analytic functions: Quantitative software applications for evaluation of disease processes or other anatomic abnormalities:
   • *Region of interest* (ROI) provides a quantitative analysis of the Hounsfield values of a specific anatomic area. A graphic outline in the shape of a circle, square, freeform design, and so on is

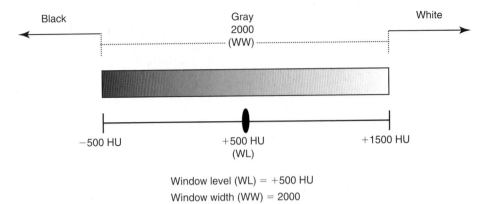

Window level (WL) = +500 HU

Window width (WW) = 2000

FIG. 5.21 Pixels with values between −500 HU and +1500 HU are each assigned a shade of gray. Pixels with values less than −500 HU are black, and those with values greater than +1500 HU are white.

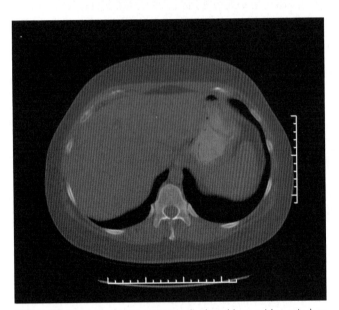

FIG. 5.22 The image in Fig. 4.20 is displayed here with a window level (WL) of +500 HU and a window width (WW) of 2000. This combination of settings would typically be referred to as a "bone window," because it offers good detail of the dense bony structures. The window is centered on a higher window level, resulting in pixels with greater Hounsfield values assigned shades of gray.

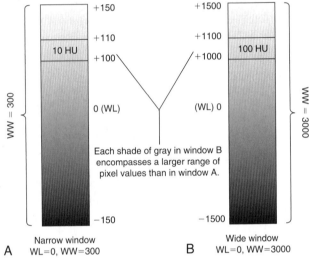

FIG. 5.23 The effects of window width (WW) settings on image contrast. Window A results in a narrow range of pixel values displayed as shades of gray. Small steps in pixel number are represented by large steps in gray shade. The image appears higher in contrast because of the predominance of white and black pixels with values that fall outside the WW. Window B offers a more gradual change in gray shade as pixel number changes. Larger steps in pixel number are required to elicit large steps in gray shade. The image appears lower in contrast because of the predominance of gray pixels with values that lie within the "wide" window.

TABLE 5.2	Sample Window Settings for Common Clinical Applications	
Window Name	**Window Level (WL)**	**Window Width (WW)**
Abdomen	+40 HU	350
Brain	+40 HU	100
Subdural	+50 HU	150
Stroke	+35 HU	35
Lung	−600 HU	1300
Vocal cords	−300 HU	1000
Liver	+50 HU	150
Trabecular bone	+250 HU	2000
Cortical bone	+350 HU	3000

placed over an area of the image. System software calculates the average CT number in HU within the defined ROI. The average ROI measurement provides information about tissue characteristics that may be helpful for clinical diagnosis.

- *Linear distance measurement* is a graphic used for precise size determination, distance for interventional procedures, and so on (Fig. 5.25).

c. *Cine viewing mode* allows the user to review large quantities of CT images at a high rate. The images are viewed in a motion loop, the speed of which can be controlled by the user. Cine viewing is particularly beneficial when one is reviewing the enormous image sets generated during MDCT studies.

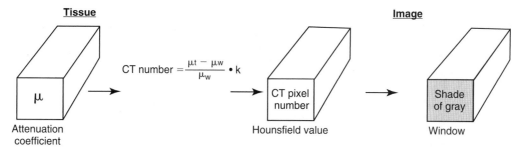

$$\text{CT number} = \frac{\mu t - \mu w}{\mu_w} \cdot k$$

Tissue

μ

Attenuation coefficient

Image

CT pixel number

Hounsfield value

Shade of gray

Window

FIG. 5.24 The numerical basis of the CT image. Linear attenuation coefficient (μ) is converted to CT pixel number (HU), which is then assigned a shade of gray for image display.

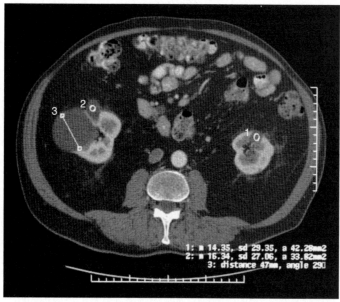

1: m 14.35, sd 29.35, a 42.28mm2
2: m 16.34, sd 27.06, a 33.82mm2
3: distance 47mm, angle 29⬚

FIG. 5.25 CT software systems are capable of various analysis features. ROI #1 calculates an average pixel value of 14.35 HU. ROI #2 calculates an average pixel value of 16.34 HU. Because of their relatively low (<20 HU) attenuation values, both renal masses most likely represent benign cystic masses. Each measurement also includes the statistical standard deviation (SD) of the pixel numbers within the ROI and the geometric area of the ROI. The linear distance indicated by graphic #3 can be utilized to measure size and/or angle.

C. Postprocessing

1. One of the major benefits of MDCT is the ability to produce superior MPR and 3-D images. This improvement is made possible by the acquisition of isotropic data sets.
2. *Isotropic* describes voxels with equal dimensions along the x-, y-, and z-axes. Isotropic resolution is approached by applying two key concepts:
   a. Choosing the thinnest detector collimation available to produce the thinnest slices available reduces voxel dimension in the z-axis.
   b. Reconstructing the acquired data with the smallest DFOV allowed on the basis of the part of interest reduces pixel dimension along the x- and y-axes.
3. For example, an abdominal CTA acquisition with a 64-slice MDCT system is made with a detector collimation of 0.6 mm. If images are reconstructed on a 512 matrix with a DFOV of 32 cm, the pixel dimension may be calculated as follows:

$$d = \frac{\text{DFOV}}{\text{matrix}}$$
$$= \frac{320}{512}$$
$$= 0.625 \, \text{mm}$$

4. In the example, the pixel dimension along the x- and y-axes is roughly equal to the z-axis dimension of the reconstructed section width (0.6 mm). This isotropic data set would result in high-quality MPR and 3-D images.
5. Reconstruction of such isotropic, overlapping, thin-section CT images greatly reduces the step artifact that can negatively affect the quality of MPR and 3-D CT images.

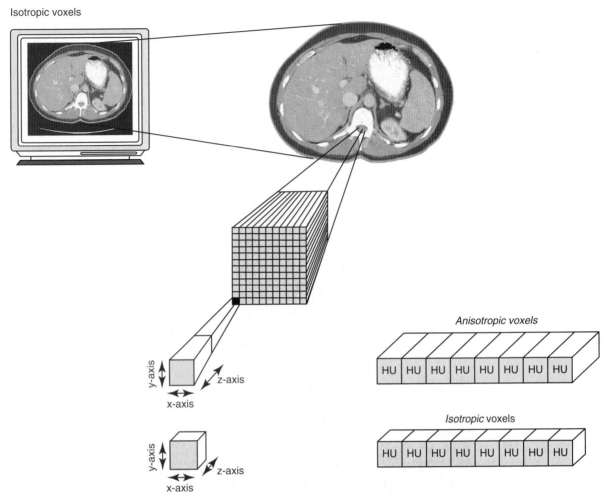

FIG. 5.26 Isotropic voxels. The x- and y-axis dimensions of the CT image pixel are determined by the selected display field of view (DFOV) value and reconstruction matrix. The width of the reconstructed section determines the voxel length along the z-axis. Isotropic resolution is achieved when the selected factors result in equal dimensions for the x-, y-, and z-axes.

6. An isotropic volumetric data set yields high-quality images with equal resolution in any reconstructed plane. It eliminates the need for data acquisition in two planes, as had been the norm for many applications, such as CT of the sinuses and small parts such as the wrist and ankle (Fig. 5.26).

7. *Multiplanar reformation* (MPR) describes the process of displaying CT images in a different orientation from the one used in the original reconstruction process.

8. Unlike retrospective reconstruction, reformation does not change the makeup of the image voxels. Reformation merely alters the viewing perspective of the images into a different anatomic plane.

9. The reformatted image is 1 voxel thick, with the pixels facing the viewer each representing the average attenuation occurring within the represented voxels.

10. MPR images are typically formed from a vertical stack of contiguous, helically acquired axial CT images. They are usually displayed in planes that are perpendicular, or orthogonal, to the original plane of data acquisition.

11. *Orthogonal planes* are at right angles to each other.

12. Because most CT examinations acquire data in the transverse, or axial plane, the most common orthogonal MPR planes are (Fig. 5.27):
    a. Coronal, the vertical plane that divides the part into anterior and posterior portions.
    b. Sagittal, the vertical plane that divides the part into right and left portions.

13. Reformats may also be constructed in a nonperpendicular or nonorthogonal plane, as follows:
    a. Oblique: Any plane that is tilted from the coronal, sagittal or axial plane
    b. Curved: Graphically designed reformation that samples an anatomic structure along points placed by the user. Curved reformations are common through areas such as blood vessels, pancreas, mandible, and spinal cord.

14. MPR images were historically displayed with a thickness equal to the acquired section width (i.e., one voxel thick). The truly volumetric acquisition made possible with MDCT allows for the display of MPR slabs of variable thickness, which average the attenuation values of multiple voxels.

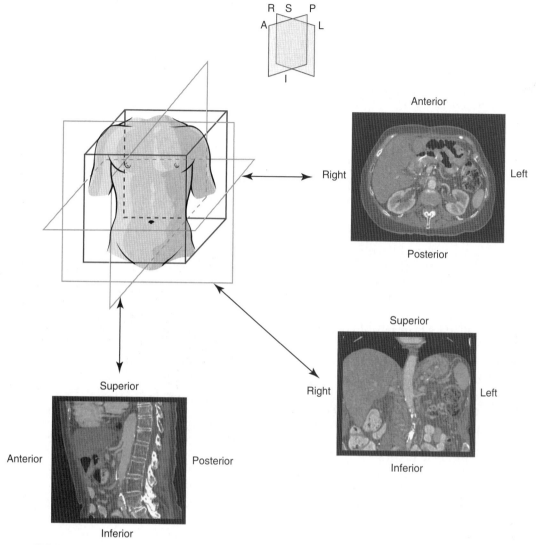

FIG. 5.27 Multiplanar reformation (MPR) and anatomic planes. *A,* Anterior; *R,* right; *S,* superior; *P,* posterior; *L,* left; and *I,* inferior.

15. MPRs may also be thickened to represent slabs of tissue with alternative techniques such as maximum intensity projection (MIP) and minimum intensity projection (min-IP).

16. MIP images display only the maximum pixel value along a ray traced through the object to the viewer's assumed perspective in front of the viewing monitor. Tissues with lower attenuation values are not displayed, leaving high-attenuation structures such as bone and contrast-enhanced soft tissue structures free of superimposition.

17. As the viewer faces a MIP image, each pixel represents the maximum attenuation that occurs in the associated voxel. The voxel length is determined by the user as the slab thickness.

18. For example, MIP images are valuable in demonstrating contrast-enhanced blood vessels during CTA and for the opacified urinary tract during CT urography.

19. Similar in principle, min-IP images display the minimum pixel value along each ray to the viewer.

Min-IP reformations are used primarily during the evaluation of the biliary tree, colon, lungs, and trachea.

20. *Three-dimensional (3-D) CT* describes the process of displaying volumetrically acquired CT data with a perception of 3-D depth on a computer monitor or recording film.

21. The CT system composes a 3-D model using the stack of acquired CT images displayed with definable shading, lighting, and rendering.

22. *Rendering* uses 3-D algorithms to provide a specific perspective to the construction of the 3-D model:

a. *Surface render*ing, also termed *shaded-surface display (SSD):* A technique that uses the concept of *thresholding* to limit the displayed volumetric data. The threshold allows the user to select the range of pixel values rendered in the 3-D model. For example a higher bone threshold (>300 HU) can be chosen to build a skeletal model of the patient's skull. Decreasing the threshold to include voxels with soft tissue attenuation values results in a 3-D model with the patient's skin intact.

b. *Volume rendering* (VR) adjusts the opacity of voxels included in the 3-D model according to their tissue characteristics. Unlike the thresholding concept used for SSD rendering, VR does not exclude voxels, but instead alters their appearance so that the 3-D model contains the entire volume dataset.

23. Rendering applications are also used to control the perspective of the viewer evaluating the 3-D model, as follows:

a. *Orthographic volume rendering* is the method of externally viewing a 3-D reconstructed object. The viewer's perspective is one of being outside the object and looking at its surface.

b. *Perspective volume rendering* provides a viewpoint of being within the lumen of the object, similar to an endoscopic view. Also referred to as *immersive rendering*, this type of 3-D reconstruction is commonly utilized during CT colonography and CT bronchography.

24. The quality of MPR and 3-D images can be improved by adhering to several basic principles:

a. Utilize the thinnest section width possible for the anatomical area, the clinical indication, and the need to keep patient radiation dose to a minimum. Thicker, anisotropic sections result in MPR images in which the separation of each axial section is apparent on the reformation. Commonly referred to as *step artifact,* this unwanted result can be avoided with an isotropic acquisition.

b. The section interval should be less than the reconstructed section width. Overlapping the reconstruction reduces the appearance of separate individual axial sections on the reformatted image. A 50% level of overlap is suggested for optimal reformatted image quality, for example, 1.0-mm sections reconstructed every 0.5 mm.

c. Optimize patient comfort to minimize motion. Movement during data acquisition severely degrades the quality of reformatted images. Patient motion can cause blurriness in the reformation and/or severe step artifact at the point of motion.

25. Quantitative analysis of CT data is available through various software applications including:

a. Linear distance and structure diameter from measurements made with the deposition of a cursor along the borders of a structure.

b. Calcium scoring during cardiac CT to measure the density of plaque deposits in the coronary arteries.

c. Ejection fraction measurement of the left ventricle during cardiac CT.

IMAGE QUALITY

1. The capacity to define, measure, and assess image quality is a primary responsibility of the CT technologist.

2. This responsibility includes, but is not limited to:

a. A thorough understanding of the parameters of CT image quality.

b. Prompt identification of the causes of CT image and study degradation.

c. The ability to implement appropriate technical solutions in response to image quality issues.

3. A distinct advantage of the digital nature of CT is that image quality can be easily defined and measured.

4. Several quantitative measurements are utilized to directly assess the image quality of a given CT system:

a. Spatial resolution.
b. Contrast resolution.
c. Temporal resolution.
d. Noise.
e. Uniformity.
f. Linearity.

5. These image quality criteria are affected not only by CT system efficacy, but also by the technical factors chosen during the performance of any CT examination.

6. The following section provides a definition of each image quality parameter, methods by which they can be quantitatively measured, and an outline of the controlling technical factors.

A. Spatial Resolution

1. The ability of a CT imaging system to display fine details separately is referred to as *spatial resolution* and sometimes as *high-contrast spatial resolution.*

2. The term describes a CT system's ability to resolve small, closely spaced objects when they are surrounded by material that is very different in density.

3. The measured spatial resolution of a CT system is given in units of line pairs per centimeter, or lp/cm.

4. There are two components of spatial resolution for helical CT systems:

a. In-plane spatial resolution.
b. Longitudinal spatial resolution.

5. *In-plane spatial resolution* can be demonstrated as a function of the actual object and the accuracy or fidelity with which the object is represented on the image.

6. During imaging of an object, signal is generated by the CT detectors in response to the transmitted radiation passing through the object.

7. The signal can be described as having a specific spatial frequency on the basis of the size and density of the object being imaged.

8. Larger objects of uniform density are represented by low spatial frequency signal.

9. Smaller dense objects and areas of sharp borders between varying densities are represented by high spatial frequency signal.

10. It is possible to quantify a CT system's response to these different spatial frequencies as a measure of spatial resolution. If the relationship of the generated signal to the actual object detail is plotted, a smooth

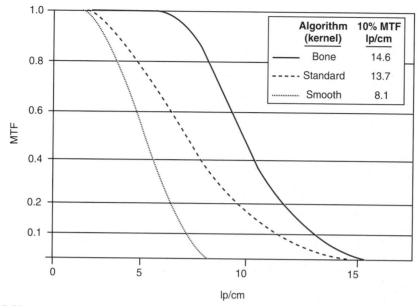

FIG. 5.28 Modulation transfer function (MTF) curves demonstrating the effects of algorithm selection on in-plane spatial resolution. Each curve represents CT image reconstruction utilizing three different algorithms. At an MTF of 0.1 (limiting resolution), the bone algorithm demonstrates the best in-plane spatial resolution, with an ability to resolve up to 14.6 lp/cm. *(Modified from Kalender WA:* Computed tomography, *ed 3, Erlangen, Germany, 2011, Publicis.)*

curve termed the *modulation transfer function* (MTF) is produced.

11. The MTF is a graphical representation of a CT system's response to a spatial frequency. The ability of a CT scanner to record a spatial frequency and thereby resolve an object can be shown graphically using an MTF curve.

12. The MTF of a CT system is an objective measurement of a system's in-plane spatial resolution. By evaluating an MTF curve of a particular image, the operator can assess the spatial resolution of a CT system and appraise changes in spatial resolution resulting from adjustments in technical factors.

13. At an MTF of 1.0, the image is a perfect reproduction of the object. At an MTF of 0.0, the object is not represented in the image (Fig. 5.28).

14. The MTF of a given scan is evaluated by observing the maximum signal frequency, in lp/cm, that the system can adequately display. The limiting resolution is read at a point on the graph where the signal frequency corresponding to a particular object has reached 10%; anything lower, and the object is no longer sufficiently imaged.

15. The details regarding the generation of MTF curves is beyond the scope of clinical CT practice and of this review book. However, the CT technologist should be familiar with MTF curves and should be able to utilize the information to compare and contrast the spatial resolution of different CT systems or when adjusting technical parameters.

16. The in-plane spatial resolution of a modern MDCT system can reach levels of 25 lp/cm or more, with

the ability to resolve objects smaller than 1-mm in size.

17. Practical measurement of MTF and in-plane spatial resolution is achieved by scanning a quality control (QC) device called a *phantom*.

18. The construction of CT phantoms vary, but they are primarily composed of a radiolucent plastic material and contain specialized inserts used to measure specific image quality criteria.

19. One high-resolution insert consists of metal bars arranged in patterns of increasing line pairs per centimeter. The phantom is scanned with use of a variety of technical factors, and the in-plane spatial resolution is measured by determining the maximum lp/cm that can be visually separated (Fig. 5.29).

20. The in-plane spatial resolution can also be measured by evaluating the *point spread function* (PSF) of a CT system. The PSF is used to quantify the amount of blurring that occurs within an image of an object.

21. To measure the PSF, a phantom containing a small wire is scanned. MTF curves for the image of the wire are generated, and the amount of blur is measured.

22. Alternatively, a pattern of decreasingly sized holes is scanned, and the evaluator measures the smallest range of closely spaced holes than can be discerned as separate.

23. The technical factors affecting in-plane spatial resolution include the following:
    a. *Focal spot size:* Small focal spot size improves in-plane spatial resolution. Larger focal spots increase geometric unsharpness because of penumbra. The selection of focal spot size is usually

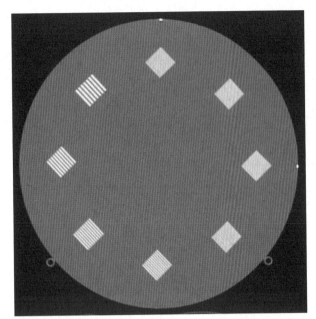

FIG. 5.29 A high-contrast spatial resolution phantom containing eight bar resolution patterns ranging from 4 to 12 lp/cm. The phantom insert is scanned with use of a specific set of technical parameters, (section width, DFOV and so on). The reconstructed phantom image is evaluated for the maximum number of individual line-pairs that may be resolved as separate, yielding the spatial resolution of the CT system at the specified technical parameters.

tied to the mA setting for an acquisition. Each CT system has an mA cutoff point, at which the focal spot switches from small to large according to the associated filament size.

b. *Detector size*: Smaller, more closely spaced detectors improve spatial resolution. Referred to as *detector aperture* and *detector spacing*, respectively, these attributes of the detector configuration have a direct effect on the sensitivity of a CT system to small changes in spatial frequency. There are geometric limits to the number of detectors an array may contain. An array with smaller, more closely spaced detectors can simply have more of them. More detectors increase the signal recording capability of a detector array, improving its sensitivity to the wide range of encountered spatial frequencies and increasing the in-plane spatial resolution.

c. *Reconstruction algorithm*: Also referred to as a *convolution kernel*, the reconstruction algorithm shapes the spatial frequencies used during the image reconstruction process. High spatial frequency algorithms, such as those for edge or bone, emphasize high spatial frequency signal during image reconstruction. The resulting image demonstrates superior spatial resolution. Lower spatial frequency algorithms, such as those termed *standard or soft tissue*, emphasize low spatial frequency signal and yield images lower in spatial resolution. The selection of algorithm (kernel) is made on the basis of the clinical application and the existing trade-off

between spatial resolution and image noise (see the later section on noise).

d. *Pixel dimension*: The combination of large matrix and small DFOV (large zoom factor) results in a smaller pixel dimension and an increase in the in-plane spatial resolution. This relationship of matrix with DFOV directly controls the size of the smallest detail a CT system is able to resolve. In general terms, smaller pixels, responsible for representing less tissue, will represent the tissues more accurately.

e. *Sampling frequency*: The number of views obtained by the CT system during the data acquisition of an image. This sampling rate may also be referred to as *VPR*. The VPR determines the quantity of samples, and therefore transmission data, acquired during each gantry rotation. Inherent to the system design and not adjustable by the user, a higher sampling frequency is obtained by increasing the temporal data sampling rate or by the number of detectors. For example, a very small object (detail) exhibits a very high spatial frequency. The *Nyquist theorem* dictates that the data sampling frequency must be at least twice the object's spatial frequency in order for the object to be resolved by the CT system.

24. *Longitudinal spatial resolution* is a relatively new term in CT image quality. It is introduced as way of describing how patient movement during volumetric acquisition can affect image detail.

25. The longitudinal spatial resolution is usually qualified by the degree of broadening that occurs to the *slice sensitivity profile* (SSP) during volumetric acquisition.

26. The SSP represents the amount of broadening that occurs along the z-axis during volumetric data acquisition.

27. The section width (slice) for a volumetric acquisition may be graphically displayed as an SSP (Fig. 5.30).

28. The SSP of a conventional nonhelical CT image is rectangular. The section represents a known thickness of tissue centered at a specific location along the patient's longitudinal (z-) axis.

29. As a result of the patient/bed translation during scanning, the SSP of a volumetrically acquired image is curved. The increase in partial volume averaging that occurs during helical acquisition slightly widens the slice profile for each image.

30. Effective section width corresponds to the SSP of the reconstructed section in consideration of the widening that occurs during helical data acquisition.

31. The effective section width is defined as the *full width at half maximum* (FWHM) of the SSP. It is measured by examining the SSP at half of its maximum height.

32. SSP broadening may also be evaluated by measuring the illustrated slice profile at a value termed full width at tenth maximum (FWTM).

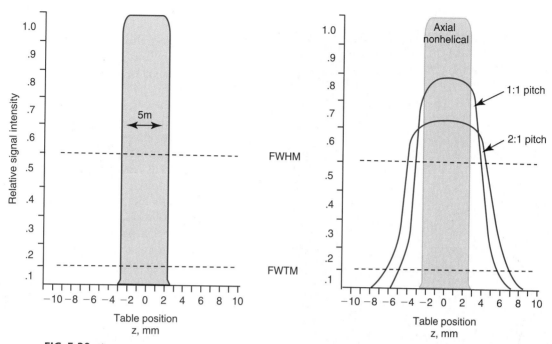

FIG. 5.30 Slice sensitivity profiles (SSPs) with measurement of section thickness at full width at half maximum (FWHM) and full width at tenth maximum (FWTM). The SSP of a conventional nonhelical CT acquisition is rectangular. SSP broadening effects are inherent in helical acquisition and worsen with increasing beam pitch.

33. Some CT systems display the effective section width for an acquisition as a function of other selected scan parameters.
34. The factors that affect longitudinal spatial resolution and the SSP are as follows:
    a. *Spiral interpolation algorithm:* This is an inherent component of the reconstruction process that is not influenced by the operator. This additional algorithm is applied to the image reconstruction of helically acquired images to reduce SSP-broadening effects. The 180LI interpolation algorithm is most commonly used. It provides thinner SSP than the 360LI algorithm at the cost of increased image noise.
    b. *Pitch:* For SSCT scanners, increases in detector pitch cause a substantial widening of the SSP and subsequent loss of longitudinal spatial resolution. For MDCT systems, the greater spatial resolution made possible by detector collimation along the z-axis compensates for the negative effects of pitch.
35. Excessive widening of the SSP and a loss of spatial resolution along the z-axis during MDCT examinations may be avoided by using the following general guidelines:
    a. Choose the thinnest beam collimation possible in consideration of patient radiation dose ramifications and the clinical needs of the study (i.e., breathholds, contrast enhancement patterns, and so on).
    b. Limit pitch by selecting the slowest table translation speed possible. Again, this step must be taken in consideration of patient radiation dose ramifications and the clinical requirements of the study.
    c. Reconstruct images using the thinnest detector collimation possible. Thin-section reconstruction reduces the partial volume effect, reduces or completely eliminates broadening of the SSP, and improves longitudinal spatial resolution.

B. Contrast Resolution

1. The ability of the CT system to detect an object with a small difference in linear attenuation coefficient as compared with the surrounding tissue is called *contrast resolution.*
2. It describes the CT system's ability to differentiate between two adjacent tissues of similar attenuation values and may also be referred to as *low-contrast detectability* or the *sensitivity* of the CT system.
3. Excellent low-contrast resolution remains one of the most important advantages of CT over other radiographic imaging modalities.
4. MDCT systems are typically capable of differentiating adjacent objects with attenuation differences as small as 3 HU.
5. Contrast resolution is measured by scanning the low-contrast detectability portion of a CT phantom

The average pixel values (HU) should demonstrate a difference comparable to the known difference in the densities of each material.

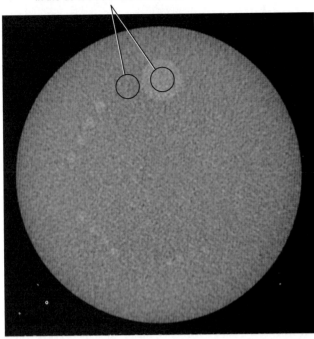

FIG. 5.31 Low-contrast resolution insert of the American College of Radiology (ACR) phantom, consisting of a series of cylinders of gradually decreasing diameter. Each cylinder is slightly different in density from the background material. The image is visually evaluated to assess the low-contrast sensitivity of the CT system utilizing a range of technical parameters (section width, mA, and so on). ROI measurements can be made to quantify the contrast exhibited between the two slightly different substances.

(Fig. 5.31). This insert typically consists of several series of discs or spheres arranged in size order. The discs or spheres exhibit varying contrast from the surrounding material, ranging between 0.3% and 1.0%.

6. Each 1.0% in contrast between adjacent objects amounts to a difference in pixel value of approximately 10 HU.

7. Scans through the insert are performed with various technical factors. Assessment of low-contrast resolution is made by determining the smallest, lowest contrast circles demonstrated in the image.

8. The technical factors affecting contrast resolution include:

   a. *Inherent subject contrast*: The thickness and atomic density of an object largely determine its image contrast as compared with surrounding tissue. The inherent contrast of an anatomic area can be augmented with the administration of oral and/or IV contrast media. Both negative and positive contrast agents work to alter the inherent contrast of certain tissues.

   b. *Beam collimation*: Scatter radiation reduces contrast resolution. Increasing beam collimation reduces scatter radiation and improves contrast resolution.

   c. *Algorithm selection*: Low spatial frequency algorithms (kernels), such as those used to display soft tissue structures, offer improved contrast resolution.

   d. *Window setting*: A narrow WW can improve contrast resolution by exaggerating the difference in gray shade assignment to pixels with only small differences in attenuation value.

   e. *Detector collimation*: Increased detector collimation results in the reconstruction of thinner sections. As section width decreases, the photon flux for each pixel also decreases. Unless the mA setting is raised to compensate, an increase in noise occurs. Any increase in noise results in a decrease in contrast resolution. In fact, the major limiting factor for contrast resolution is noise.

   f. *Noise:* Any change in technical factor resulting in a decrease in noise also results in an improvement to contrast resolution. The factors affecting noise, and therefore contrast resolution, are further discussed later.

C. Temporal Resolution

1. The stop-motion capability of a CT system is referred to as *temporal resolution*. Temporal resolution quantifies the CT system's ability to freeze motion and provide an image free of blurring.

2. The advent of cardiac MDCT has greatly increased the importance of temporal resolution as a CT image quality factor.

3. Historically, the temporal resolution of a CT scanner could be simply equated to the time needed for a complete 360-degree rotation of the gantry. For example, a 1-second scan consisted of a complete gantry revolution in 1 second, yielding a temporal resolution of 1 second.

4. The controlling factors of the temporal resolution of a CT system are the gantry rotation speed and reconstruction method.

5. Current MDCT systems allow complete 360-degree gantry rotations in as little as a quarter of a second (250 msec).

6. Temporal resolution can be improved by segmenting the data acquisition process into separate components of smaller rotation angles. For example, as described in Chapter 4 in the section on cardiac CT, single-segment or half-scan acquisitions reconstruct data obtained from half of the rotation time. This segmentation results in a 250-msec temporal resolution from a 0.5-sec gantry rotation time.

7. Further improvements in temporal resolution are possible with multisegment reconstructions. At time of publication, state-of-the art temporal resolution has been reduced to well under 200 msec, with dual-slice CT systems reaching as low as 75 msec.

D. Noise

1. In general terms, *noise* in a digital imaging system is any portion of the signal that contains no useful information.
2. Noise can also be described as random (*stochastic*) statistical variations in the signal. Occurring during the computations for each pixel value, these variations interfere with the imaging system's ability to display an accurate image.
3. Noise in the CT image, similar in appearance to the quantum mottle of radiography, manifests as an overall graininess on the reconstructed image.
4. There are three general types of noise in the CT image:
   a. *Quantum* noise: The result of an insufficient x-ray photon flux per voxel. When the CT system attempts to calculate the Hounsfield value for a pixel, but has failed to expose the coinciding voxel to a sufficient amount of x-ray interaction, noise appears on the reconstructed image. The amount of quantum noise is inversely related to the amount of radiation exposed to each voxel. Altering either the voxel dimension or the x-ray flux affects the noise level.
   b. *Electronic system* noise: Signal may be lost and noise introduced to the reconstruction process by the various electronic components of the CT system.
   c. *Artifactual* nose: Artifacts may be viewed as a type of noise. Artifacts can represent a portion of the signal that contains no useful information and may obscure the information present in the image. Please refer to the next section for a detailed review of artifacts.
5. *Signal-to-noise ratio* (SNR) is a descriptive term used to quantify the amount of noise in a displayed CT image. The goal is to produce images with an acceptable noise level—one in which the SNR is high—while maintaining dose and spatial resolution at appropriate levels.
6. As previously mentioned, image noise is the major quality factor affecting low-contrast resolution in the CT image.
7. There are many adjustments to technical factors that improve SNR and contrast resolution while simultaneously decreasing spatial resolution. The inverse of this relationship is also true: technical factor adjustments that positively affect spatial resolution may negatively affect SNR and contrast resolution.
8. When one is choosing technical parameters for CT protocol design, a compromise must be established between the two. This relationship may be further illustrated by the following formula:

$$D = \frac{SNR^2}{\Delta^3 T}$$

where D is radiation dose, Δ is pixel dimension, and T is section width

9. This formula mathematically illustrates the following principle: Adjustments made to voxel dimension in an effort to improve spatial resolution must be compensated for with an appropriate increase in dose to maintain SNR and contrast resolution (Fig. 5.32).
10. Noise is most commonly measured by scanning a water-filled phantom with a standardized set of technical factors. The image noise is equal to the standard deviation of pixel values within an ROI measurement of the image (Fig. 5.33).
11. According to relative scale of pixel values, an ROI of a water-filled phantom should measure near 0 HU. However, within the measured ROI, pixel values range above and below 0 HU. The degree to which this variation occurs is dictated by noise.

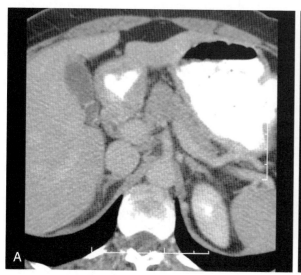
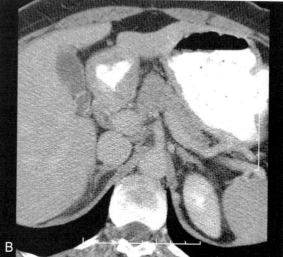

FIG. 5.32 The effects of noise on the CT image. Note the "grainy" or "mottled" appearance of B as compared with A. A was reconstructed with a low-spatial frequency algorithm, whereas B is the product of a high-spatial frequency algorithm.

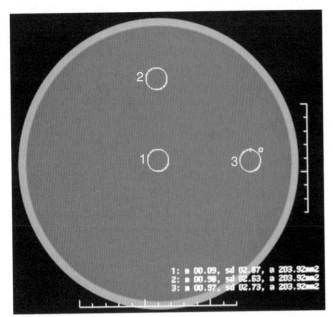

FIG. 5.33 Water-filled phantom used to measure the noise and uniformity of a CT system. The average CT value of ROI #1 accurately demonstrates a water density of 0.09 HU with an acceptable standard deviation (noise) of 2.87. As a measure of the uniformity of the CT system, the values for ROI #2 and ROI #3 are within acceptable range in comparison with ROI #1.

12. Noise as standard deviation (σ) can be defined by the following equation:

$$\text{Noise} (\sigma) = \frac{\sqrt{\sum(X_i - X)^2}}{n - 1}$$

where x_i is each CT value, x is the average of at least 100 values, n is the total number of CT values in the ROI.

13. This formula is used solely as a guide for understanding the principle of standard deviation as it relates to image noise. The CT system software automatically calculates the standard deviation within a given ROI to be used as a measure of noise for a given set of technical factors.

14. The technical parameters that most directly affect noise include:

a. *X-ray photon flux:* This equals the rate at which x-ray photons pass through a given unit of tissue over a given unit of time. Any decrease in photon flux causes an increase in image noise. Photon flux is largely determined by the operator-controlled settings of mA and time. Voxel dimension, which also directly affects photon flux, is covered separately later. An increase in either mA setting or scan time increases photon flux, SNR, and patient radiation dose. Raising the kVp value can also increase photon flux, but at an overall cost to contrast resolution resulting from changes in beam quality. In general, the amount of noise present in the CT image may be reduced by a factor of two (halved) with any setting change that increases the photon flux by a factor of four (4×).

Quadruple # of photons → image noise is halved

b. *Voxel dimension:* Noise can be decreased by increasing the dimensions of the voxel. A larger voxel has a greater photon flux and is subject to less noise. Voxel dimension may be increased by increasing the DFOV (decreasing zoom factor), decreasing the matrix size, or increasing the section width. Remember that DFOV and matrix size determine the amount of tissue represented by each pixel. As the pixel dimension increases, it is representative of a greater quantity of photon flux and exhibits less noise. Increases in section width also increase pixel/voxel dimension, with one additional drawback: Any improvement in noise is overshadowed by an overall loss of detail resulting from the partial volume effect.

c. *Pitch/table speed:* As pitch increases, the speed at which the patient travels through the gantry also increases. For each gantry rotation, scans acquired at a higher pitch expose each voxel to less photon flux. Unless dose is increased, a higher pitch results in greater image noise.

d. *Detector sensitivity and efficiency:* Improvements in these factors decrease noise and allow for an overall reduction in patient exposure. Beyond the control of the operator, CT detector array sensitivity and efficiency are areas of continuing technical advancement for manufacturers.

e. *Patient factors:* With patient radiation dose constant, acquisitions of larger patients and of denser parts result in noisier CT images. As a method of balancing SNR and patient radiation dose, ATCM systems adjusts dose according to a predetermined SNR. The acceptable image noise level is predetermined by the user. The CT system automatically adjusts dose to a minimum, while not exceeding the set noise level.

f. *Algorithm/kernel:* The use of low spatial frequency algorithms (kernels), such as smooth or soft tissue algorithms, reduce noise. High spatial frequency algorithms increase noise on the reconstructed CT image.

E. Uniformity

1. When imaged, a phantom of uniform material such as water should demonstrate consistent CT values regardless of a pixel's position on the image matrix. Pixels at the center of the image should measure as water density (~0 HU), as should pixels at various other points in the image.

2. Beam hardening occurs as the x-ray beam passes through the object (phantom, patient). The beam exposing the center of the object has a higher average photon energy than the beam exposing the periphery of the object. This beam-hardening effect may slightly alter the pixel values at different points across an image of an object of uniform inherent density.

3. The *spatial uniformity* of a CT system describes its ability to maintain relatively consistent CT values across the entire image of an object of equal density.
4. Uniformity may be evaluated by positioning several ROI measurements at different locations along the center and periphery of an image. The CT values should not differ by more than 2 HU from one location to another (Fig. 5.33).

F. Linearity

1. The relative accuracy between calculated CT numbers and their respective linear attenuation coefficients is termed *linearity*.
2. The CT number for water is 0 HU. According to the formula for the calculation of CT number relative to water discussed previously (see "Image Display"), the CT number for air is −1000 HU, and the CT number for water is 0 HU.
3. The CT system is calibrated according to these two known values. Daily calibration procedures should be performed using a water-filled phantom or a gantry cleared of all objects and exposing only room air.
4. Calibration and routine vendor maintenance procedures work to establish and maintain CT system linearity.

5. Linearity may be periodically evaluated by scanning of a specialized phantom insert containing an assortment of materials—acrylic, polyethylene, water, air, artificial bone, and so on (Fig. 5.34). Known ranges of CT values are compared with those obtained by CT acquisition to ensure system accuracy and linearity.

G. Quality Assurance and Accreditation

1. A quality control (QC) program monitors the overall technical performance of the CT system by measuring specific aspects of its function and comparing the measurements with a set standard.
2. Any QC program consists of two main parts:
   a. *Quality assurance,* the measurement of the scanner's performance through quality testing procedures and evaluation of the test results.
   b. *Quality control,* the implementation of corrective actions to improve any identified performance inadequacies of the CT system.
3. Each facility maintains a CT QC program that involves daily, weekly, monthly, and annual tests to ensure optimal performance in the following areas:
   a. Accuracy and linearity of CT numbers.
   b. Spatial resolution.
   c. Contrast resolution/low-contrast detectability.

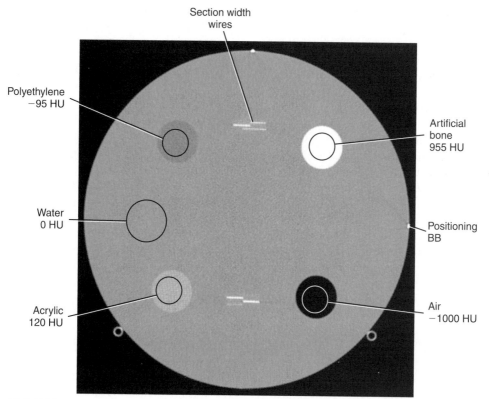

FIG. 5.34 A linearity phantom containing four inserts of various materials surrounded by water. This American College of Radiology (ACR) phantom also contains two ramps consisting of a series of wires spaced 0.5 mm apart along the phantom's z-axis. The accuracy of the selected section width is evaluated by counting the number of wires visible in cross section. The phantom image in this figure was acquired at a section width of 1.25 mm. The BBs are used to ensure that the phantom is positioned correctly for true axial sections.

d. Noise.
e. Uniformity.
f. Section width/SSP.
g. Accuracy of laser light alignment.
h. Table indexing and section localization.
i. Patient radiation dose.
j. Scatter radiation.

4. The frequency of the tests is determined by the radiology department's overall QC program and by the requirements of specified accrediting agencies.

5. Consistency in the technical factors utilized for QC testing is imperative. Tests should be performed with the same settings for mA, kVp, section width, DFOV, and so on, to ensure accuracy of results.

6. The hallmarks of a superior QC program are routine frequency of testing, prompt taking of corrective actions as needed, and accurate recordkeeping.

7. The QC program in CT is usually a component of a larger, department-wide program in total quality improvement (TQI).

8. The responsibilities for implementing the facility-specific QC tests and procedures vary among technologists, physicists, and QC officers.

9. In 2002 the American College of Radiology (ACR) implemented an accreditation process for CT departments to become ACR-accredited.

10. ACR accreditation in CT involves the submission of acquired clinical and phantom images, dose measurements, and scanning protocols.

11. Details regarding the process for ACR accreditation in CT are beyond the scope of this review book; they are available on the ACR's website (www.acr.org).

ARTIFACT RECOGNITION AND REDUCTION

1. Errors during the measurement of transmitted radiation by the detectors can result in a form of noise on the image termed an *artifact*.

2. An artifact contains no useful information and can severely disrupt the quality of an image by interfering with anatomic detail contained on the CT image.

3. CT image artifacts can take many forms and shapes, including streaks, bands, rings, and shading errors.

4. It is a primary responsibility of the CT technologist to identify artifacts, diagnose their origins, and implement appropriate corrective actions when possible.

A. Beam Hardening

1. As previously described, the average photon energy of the beam increases as it traverses an object (patient). Lower-energy photons are absorbed along the path of each measured ray.

2. The beam that interacts with the center of an object (patient) has a higher average photon energy than the beam that exposed the periphery of the object (patient).

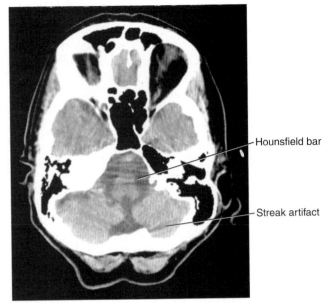

Hounsfield bar

Streak artifact

FIG. 5.35 Beam-hardening artifact in the posterior fossa of the skull. Extremely dense regions at the temporal bone and the internal occipital protuberance cause beam-hardening artifact in the form of "streaking" and the Hounsfield bar.

3. An artifact appears when the degree of beam hardening exceeds the CT system's ability to correct during the reconstruction process.

4. Beam-hardening artifacts typically manifest as areas of light and dark streaking bands across portions of the image.

5. The dense bony areas of the posterior fossa of the skull are especially prone to beam-hardening artifacts. The term *Hounsfield bar* is commonly used to describe this particular artifact (Fig. 5.35).

6. Unfortunately, beyond the mathematical corrections included in the image reconstruction process, there is little that can be done technically to resolve beam-hardening artifacts.

7. The use of higher kVp techniques (120 to 140 kVp) may help to slightly reduce this phenomenon, particularly in the area of the brain's posterior fossa.

8. Some current CT systems may offer reconstruction filters that smooth (reduce) the appearance of beam hardening artifacts on the image.

B. Partial Volume Averaging

1. The *partial volume effect* is an unavoidable phenomenon in CT imaging. The complex anatomic structures under examination do not easily lend themselves to representation by series of cubes arranged in matrix form.

2. The attenuation values for an object are often spread over large numbers of voxels. Each voxel also contains values for multiple tissue types. The values are averaged together to yield a single pixel value attempting to represent an assortment of different materials.

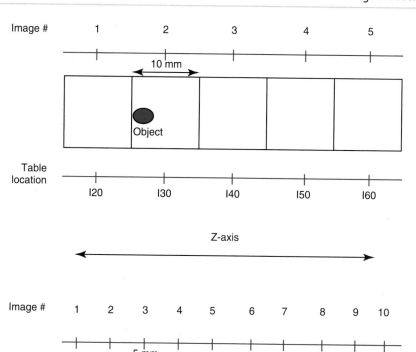

The attenuation values for the object in image #2 are averaged for the calculation of a single pixel CT # (HU). Partial volume artifact results, as the object is not well demonstrated on the 10-mm-thick image.

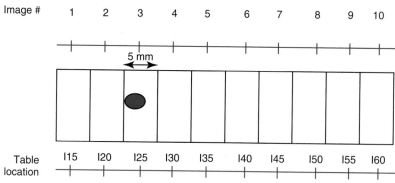

A second 5-mm-thick acquisition improves the slice sensitivity profile and helps to eliminate the partial volume artifact. MSCT technology allows for this change in section width to occur via retrospective reconstruction of the original data-set, eliminating the need for a second acquisition.

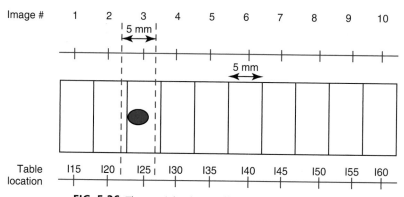

The volumetric acquisitions of helical SSCT and MDCT also allow for retrospective adjustments to the section interval. Overlapping reconstructions further reduce partial volume artifact as in this example, where the object of interest is better positioned within an individual section obtained at a new location along the z-axis.

FIG. 5.36 The partial volume effect that occurs when an object is only partly positioned within a voxel or is much smaller than the overall voxel volume. The object's attenuation is not accurately represented by the pixel value.

3. *Partial volume artifact* occurs when a structure is only partly positioned within a voxel and the attenuation for the object is not accurately represented by a pixel value (Fig. 5.36).
4. Partial volume artifact typically appears as a generalized unsharpness or haziness of the borders of objects. Contrast of the object from its surroundings is compromised.

5. The posterior fossa and the interface between the diaphragm and the abdominal contents are common locations for the appearance of partial volume artifact.
6. The cupping artifact that occurs at the superior portion of the skull is another form of partial volume artifact, which is also heavily influenced by the phenomenon of beam hardening. Here the dense skull table averages

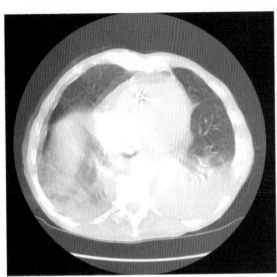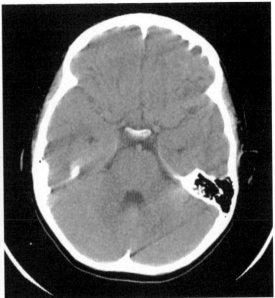

FIG. 5.37 Patient motion during data acquisition, resulting in noticeable image degradation referred to as motion artifact. The images shown are examples of image degradation resulting from voluntary patient movement.

with the low-attenuating brain tissue, causing an artifact in which the brain parenchyma may appear abnormally dense.

7. Also, areas of potential pathology, such as small masses, nodules, and fractures, may not be sharply demonstrated because of the partial volume effect.

8. The use of thin sections is the main method of reducing or eliminating partial volume artifact. Thin sections improve accuracy in the calculation of the pixel's CT number by reducing the voxel volume and limiting the contents of the voxel to fewer varying tissue types.

9. Use of overlapping sections may also improve the reconstructed voxel's position with respect to an object of interest. If the object is well-centered within a single voxel, its attenuation is better represented in the calculation of the pixel's Hounsfield value.

C. Motion

1. Any significant motion on the part of the patient during data acquisition causes noticeable image degradation in the form of a motion artifact.

2. Blurring and streaking are common manifestations of motion artifact on the CT image. Patient motion during volumetric data acquisition may also appear as a step artifact on 3-D and MPR images.

3. Patient motion may be involuntary, as with peristalsis, cardiac contraction, and tremors.

4. Technical adjustments to improve the temporal resolution of the CT system may help reduce involuntary motion artifacts. Reductions in scan time (gantry rotation), image segmentation, and physiologic gating can be used to diminish the effects of involuntary motion.

5. Voluntary patient motion, including breathing and swallowing, cause substantial motion artifact on the CT image (Fig. 5.37).

6. There are two basic methods of reducing CT image artifact from voluntary motion:
   a. Communication: Clear and thorough explanation of the patient's responsibilities with regard to suspension or respiration, swallowing, and remaining still.
   b. Immobilization: Appropriate use of positioning and immobilization straps, cushions, holders, and so on.

D. Metallic Artifacts

1. Highly dense metallic objects in and around the patient cause significant image streaking (Fig. 5.38).

2. Objects such as surgical clips, prosthetic devices, guidewires, electrodes, dental fillings, jewelry, zippers, foreign bodies, and dense barium may cause streaking artifacts on the image.

3. Metallic artifacts occur as a result of a combination of errors involving the beam hardening from the metal and the partial volume averaging of the extremely dense object with the less dense surrounding material.

4. In addition, the metallic object may cause severe discrepancies in the obtained projection profiles because of its abnormally high attenuation.

5. Methods of reducing metallic artifact from CT images include:
   a. Removing the metal object from the acquisition whenever possible.
   b. Decreasing the section width to reduce partial volume averaging.
   c. Increasing the kVp value to improve the beam's penetrability through the object.

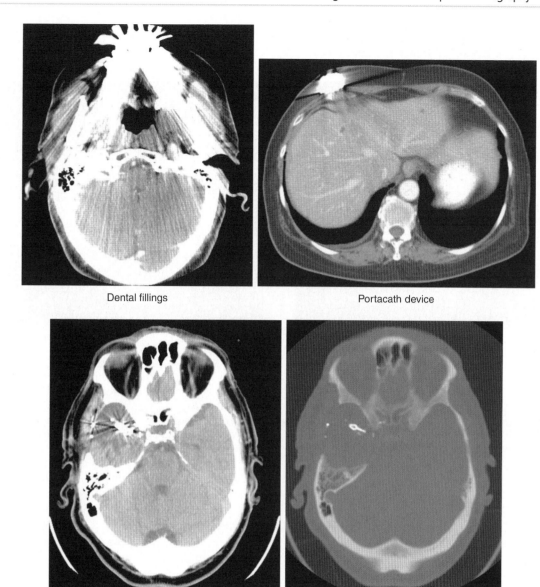

Dental fillings

Portacath device

Intracranial aneurysm clip
displayed in a soft tissue window.

Identical axial brain image
displaying an intracranial aneurysm
displayed in a bone window.

FIG. 5.38 Examples of metallic streaking artifacts.

d. Adjusting the WW and WL settings, which may slightly reduce the degrading effect of the streak artifact.

e. Reorienting data acquisition to avoid having the metal object in the scanned field. For example, axially acquired sections through the sinuses avoid the streak artifact caused by dental fillings. Volumetric MDCT axial acquisition through the sinuses allows for high-quality coronal MPR images through the sinuses without metal artifact.

f. CT manufactures may offer metallic artifact reduction (MAR) software in an effort to reduce streaking artifact from metal substances. This continues to be an area of further development in CT image quality.

E. Edge Gradient

1. Streak artifact occurs at the interface between a high-density object surrounded by lower-attenuation material.

2. Edge gradient artifacts are caused by the system's inability to process the high spatial frequency signal that represents the interface between two substances with widely different attenuation values (Fig. 5.39).

3. Common sites for edge gradient artifacts to occur include:

   a. The interface between dense bone and surrounding tissue.

   b. Bowel loops that are densely opacified with oral or rectal contrast media.

   c. Bowel loops distended with air.

Streaking artifact caused by severe edge gradients between air-filled bowel, with walls coated by dense barium, surrounded by low-density fat in the abdominal cavity.

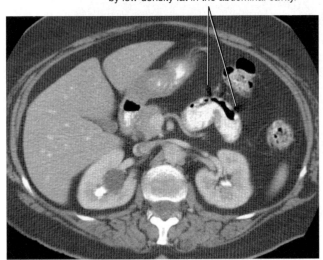

FIG. 5.39 Edge gradient artifact occurs at the interface between two objects with a great difference in density.

d. Blood vessels that are densely opacified with IV iodinated contrast media.
e. Areas surrounding biopsy needles during invasive CT procedures.

F. Patient Positioning

1. An *out-of-field artifact* occurs when a portion of the patient has been positioned outside of the SFOV.
2. Hyperdense streaking occurs in the anatomic region that lies outside the scan field (Fig. 5.40).
3. Adjusting patient position from right to left or adjusting the table height relative to the center of the gantry may eliminate the artifact by moving the entire anatomic area into the SFOV.
4. Out-of-field artifacts may be unavoidable when the patient's dimension exceeds the maximum SFOV.
5. The shoulders, abdomen, and lower pelvis are the most common regions where out-of-field artifacts occur.

G. Step Artifact

1. A primary advantage of the volumetric acquisitions of helical SSCT and MDCT is the ability to produce high-quality 3-D and MPR images.
2. The step artifact was especially common to older, nonhelically acquired reformations. With step artifact, the image demonstrates the individual sections used to build the reformatted model, and the MPR or 3-D image suffers from a lack of overall sharpness and detail (Fig. 5.41).
3. In modern MDCT systems, the highest quality 3-D and MPR images are obtained with the acquisition of an isotropic or near-isotropic data set.

Patient anatomy lies outside of the scan field of view (SFOV), causing a hyperdense streaking artifact.

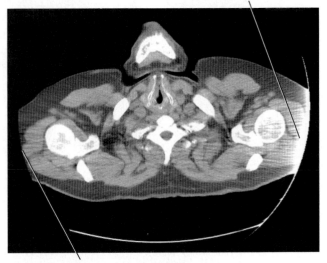

Patient anatomy lies outside of the display field of view (DFOV) but within the scan field of view (SFOV). Anatomy is cut off, but no artifact occurs.

FIG. 5.40 When a portion of the patient is positioned outside the scan field of view, the out-of-field artifact occurs. This dense streaking may occur because of improper positioning or when the patient's body extends beyond the limits of the scan field.

4. Near-isotropic acquisitions are attained when the section width (z-axis) is minimized as much as clinically and technically possible to approach a dimension equal to that of the pixel in the x- and y-axes.
5. True *isotropic acquisitions* occur when the section width equals the pixel dimension and the voxel is cube-shaped. Isotropic data sets have become more commonplace with the greater availability of 64-slice technology.
6. Isotropic data are only one component of high-quality 3-D and MPR images. The other equally important piece is an overlapping data set.
7. As previously discussed, overlapping images are those in which the reconstruction interval is less than the section width.
8. Step artifact may still occur in an MDCT system unless thin, overlapping sections are used to build the 3-D and MPR images.

H. Equipment-Induced Artifacts

1. Numerous artifacts result from the improper performance of the CT system.
2. Equipment-induced artifacts may be unavoidable and seldom depend on technical selections made by the system operator.
3. The CT technologist must readily identify these types of artifacts and implement appropriate corrective actions to assure their resolution.
4. These types of artifacts include:

Stair-step artifact

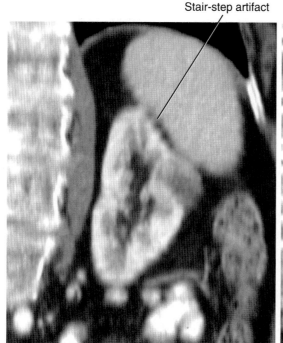
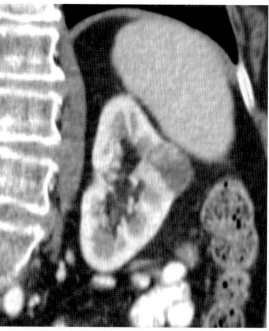

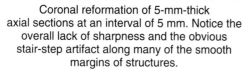

Coronal reformation of 5-mm-thick axial sections at an interval of 5 mm. Notice the overall lack of sharpness and the obvious stair-step artifact along many of the smooth margins of structures.

Coronal reformation of 2.5-mm-thick axial sections at an interval of 1.25 mm. The stair-step artifact is effectively eliminated, and the reformat exhibits improved anatomic detail and sharpness.

FIG. 5.41 Step artifact present on a coronal multiplanar reformation (MPR) image of the left kidney.

a. *Rings:* These are usually caused by faulty detectors. An error in a detector results in the back-projection of an incorrect ring of density on the reconstructed CT image.

b. *Streaks:* Detector malfunction and/or misalignment of the tube and detectors may cause the appearance of streak artifact on the CT image.

c. *Aliasing:* This is another form of streak artifact caused by an insufficient number of views (data samples) obtained during data acquisition.

d. *Tube arcing:* This refers to short-circuiting within the x-ray tube during data acquisition that results in severe streak artifacts in the CT image.

e. *Cone beam artifacts:* These are unique to the cone beam geometry of MDCT systems. Cone beam artifacts typically appear similar to partial volume artifacts. In theory, cone beam artifacts worsen as the number of detector rows increases. However, manufacturers address the issue by employing specialized cone beam reconstruction algorithms to compensate for potential errors.

f. *Windmill:* Also referred to as *z-spacing* or *interpolation artifact,* this artifact may occur from the use of increased pitch during a volumetric acquisition. The term *windmill artifacts* comes from the spiraling appearance of shading artifact that appears as a large number of volumetrically acquired images are paged through for review.

INFORMATICS

1. Once reconstructed, the CT image is displayed on a computer display for further manipulation, review, and evaluation. The images are stored locally on the hard drive of the CT system.

2. The CT system has limited short-term storage capabilities, and the images must then be transferred for long-term safekeeping as part of the patient's medical record.

3. Each CT image reconstructed on a 512^2 matrix is approximately 0.5 megabytes (MB) in digital size. Each CT examination can contain thousands of individual CT images. The long-term archival of CT data requires substantial physical and financial resources.

4. *Image compression* is a complex computer technique that reduces the size of digital CT image data. Compression of CT images reduces the storage requirements and increases the speed at which CT images may be transmitted among computer systems.

5. The technical details of digital image compression are well beyond the scope of clinical CT practice and of this review book. However, the CT technologist should at least be familiar with the two main types of digital image compression:

   a. Lossless (reversible) compression, in which the image is digitally compressed without loss of data and is identical to the original.

b. Lossy (irreversible) compression, in which data are lost during the compression process and the image does not exactly match the original. Lossy compression results in the loss of data but is capable of much higher compression rates than lossless compression.

6. All CT images are networked and stored in accordance with a standard protocol known as the *Digital Imaging and Communications in Medicine (DICOM) standard*. The DICOM standard confirms the process of recording, storing, printing, and transmitting medical image data.

7. The DICOM standard was cooperatively developed in 1985 by the ACR and the National Electrical Manufacturers Association (NEMA). The DICOM standard is continuously updated and augmented to meet the changing needs of medical imaging and CT.

8. The purpose of DICOM conformance is to ensure that all medical image files can be conveniently archived and transmitted along various systems and networks, regardless of the manufacturing vendor.

9. Medical images must exist in DICOM file format and must be transferred along networks conforming to a DICOM communications protocol.

10. Archival or storage of the CT image data can be divided into two main options:
    a. *Hard copy*, which is storage of CT image data on digital image film. Laser imager systems record CT images on light-sensitive film in multiple formats (12:1, 6:1, and so on). Hard copy films allow for convenient viewing on view boxes but are limited by physical space-occupying demands for long-term storage.
    b. *Soft copy*, by which CT image data are stored in digital file format. Mass storage devices, such as hard drives, magnetic tape drives, and magnetic optical disks (MODs), can be used to archive the CT image data for long-term storage.

11. Common digital media such as CD-ROM and DVD are actually optical disks and may also be utilized for CT image storage and transfer. These storage devices have become particularly important because of the dramatic increase in volume of image data with the advent of MDCT and advanced CT procedures. As an alternative to laser film, entire CT examinations can be stored on such media for long-term storage and for communication to patients, referring physicians, surgeons, and so on.

12. Optical discs can be characterized according to their storage capabilities:
    a. *Read-only* discs contain image data for review only; the data cannot be modified or added to.
    b. *Write-once, read-many times* (WORM) discs, which allow the initial storage of large quantities of digital image data and subsequent unlimited viewing, without the ability to reuse the discs. Writable

CDs (CD-R) and DVDs (DVD-R) are common examples of WORM media.
    c. *Rewritable discs* allow data to be recorded multiple times. MODs and rewritable CDs (CD-RW) and DVDs (DVD-RW) are examples of rewritable media.

13. *Picture archival and communications system* (PACS) are computerized networks charged with the responsibility of storing, retrieving, distributing, and displaying CT and other digital medical images.

14. A PACS consists of several key components:
    a. An interface to the CT system and other imaging modalities for transfer of image data from the scanner(s) to the PACS.
    b. Large, expandable digital archive for long-term image storage.
    c. Display workstations for image review and manipulation.
    d. Digital links to the facilities radiology information system and/or hospital information system for retrieval and archival of demographic information and other pertinent aspects of the patient's electronic medical record.
    e. Additional elements of a PACS may include film digitizers for the archival of hard copy images, dictation/transcription components, CD/DVD burners, printers, and so on.

15. A PACS communicates with the CT system(s) and other modalities and peripherals via a computerized communication system, or *network*.

16. When the network is of sufficient size to support the PACS over limited geographical distance, such as within a radiology department, it is termed a *local area network* (LAN).

17. A wired version of a LAN, commonly known by the proprietary name Ethernet, is routinely used for PACS. Wireless LANs are also available; they are commonly known by the name *Wi-Fi* (a trademark of the Wi-Fi Alliance that can be used for certified products).

18. *Wide area networks* (WANs) are used to connect multiple LANs over a larger distances, such as entire medical centers. The Internet or World Wide Web is the largest WAN.

19. *Teleradiology* refers to the ability of a PACS to transmit image data across a LAN or WAN from the imaging facility to an off-site location.

20. Web-based teleradiology systems use the geographically unlimited WAN of the World Wide Web to transmit images for physician review.

21. In accordance with federal requirements regarding the confidentiality of patient information, networks transferring medical record and image data are subject to strict security measures.

22. Safeguards used to secure networked medical image data include:

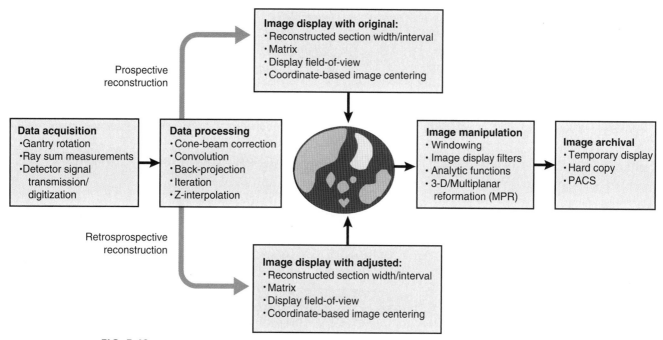

FIG. 5.42 CT process flow chart illustrating the imaging chain through data acquisition, image reconstruction (prospective and retrospective), image display, image manipulation and image archival.

a. The use of security software programs and hardware devices such as secure network routers and firewalls.

b. Digital encryption designed to code the transmitted data in a form decipherable only by software at the destination location.

c. Privacy and authentication procedures that require the use of log-in and password combinations to access patient information.

23. Fig. 5.42 outlines the processes of image display, data acquisition, data processing, image manipulation, and image archival.

PART II

Simulated Examination One

QUESTIONS

PATIENT CARE

1. An average range for activated partial thromboplastin time (PTT) is:
   a. 10–12 seconds
   b. 17–21 seconds
   c. 25–35 seconds
   d. 43–55 seconds

2. Which of the following is the correct angle of insertion for placing a butterfly needle into a vein for intravenous administration of a contrast agent?
   a. 5 degrees
   b. 15 degrees
   c. 45 degrees
   d. 60 degrees

3. A total volume of 125 mL of an iodinated contrast agent is administered intravenously via automatic injector in 50 seconds. The flow rate for this injection is:
   a. 0.75 mL/sec
   b. 1.25 mL/sec
   c. 1.75 mL/sec
   d. 2.5 mL/sec

4. The condition whereby the patient suffers from a low concentration of oxygen in the blood is called:
   a. hypoxemia
   b. hypotension
   c. hypoxia
   d. hyponatremia

5. While one is obtaining a thorough history from a patient before the intravenous injection of an iodinated contrast material, which of the following topics should be included?
   1. any prior allergic reactions to contrast media
   2. presence of HIV or hepatitis infection
   3. history of asthma
   a. 1 only
   b. 1 and 2 only
   c. 1 and 3 only
   d. 1, 2, and 3

6. Which of the following factors may affect a patient's calculated glomerular filtration rate (GFR)?
   1. age
   2. sex
   3. race
   a. 1 and 2 only
   b. 2 and 3 only
   c. 1 and 3 only
   d. 1, 2, and 3

7. Which of the following intravenous contrast agent administration methods provides the greatest overall plasma iodine concentration?
   a. drip infusion
   b. bolus technique
   c. biphasic technique
   d. CT portography

8. A patient in shock may exhibit which of the following symptoms?
   1. tachycardia
   2. rapid, shallow breathing
   3. cyanosis
   a. 1 only
   b. 1 and 2 only
   c. 1 and 3 only
   d. 1, 2, and 3

9. The drug SOLU-CORTEF may be classified as which of the following?
   a. anticholinergic
   b. bronchodilator
   c. antihistamine
   d. corticosteroid

10. Which of the following is a nonionic contrast material?
    a. iodamide
    b. iothalamate
    c. iohexol
    d. diatrizoate

11. Which of the following terms is used to describe a patient who is having difficulty breathing?
    a. dyslexia
    b. dyspnea
    c. dysphagia
    d. dysphasia

12. Which of the following describes the situation in which an assumption is made that an unconscious or otherwise physically unable patient consents to medical treatment?
    a. informed consent
    b. witnessed consent
    c. patient proxy
    d. implied consent

13. Complete cardiac diastole corresponds to which portion of the cardiac cycle on an electrocardiogram (ECG)?
    a. P wave
    b. QRS complex
    c. alpha wave
    d. T wave

14. During CT arthrography, iodinated contrast media is injected directly into the:
    a. joint space
    b. intrathecal space
    c. subarachnoid space
    d. venous bloodstream

15. Which of the following is considered one of the iso-osmolar contrast media (IOCM)?
    a. iodixanol
    b. iopamidol
    c. iohexol
    d. ioversol

16. A common site for the IV administration of iodinated contrast media is the anterior recess of the elbow, otherwise known as the:
    a. brachial fossa
    b. olecranon fossa
    c. retroulnar space
    d. antecubital space

17. The potentially serious decline in renal function after the IV administration of contrast material is called:
    a. anaphylaxis
    b. bronchospasm
    c. contrast-induced nephrotoxicity (CIN)
    d. urticaria

18. Advantages of a saline flush immediately after the IV administration of iodinated contrast material include:
    1. reduction in required contrast agent dose
    2. reduction in the incidence of contrast-induced nephrotoxicity (CIN)
    3. reduction of streaking artifact from dense contrast agent in the vasculature
    a. 1 only
    b. 3 only
    c. 2 and 3 only
    d. 1, 2, and 3

19. Which of the following medications may be administered to dilate the coronary vasculature prior to a cardiac CT examination?
    a. sublingual nitroglycerine
    b. a β-adrenergic receptor blocking agent (β-blocker)
    c. atropine
    d. albuterol

20. A normal range for diastolic blood pressure in an adult is:
    a. 40–60 mm Hg
    b. 60–90 mm Hg
    c. 80–120 mm Hg
    d. 95–140 mm Hg

21. Which of the following is a parenteral route of medication administration?
    a. sublingual
    b. intramuscular
    c. transdermal
    d. oral

22. Which of the following types of isolation techniques protects against infection transmitted through fecal material?
    a. acid-fast bacillus isolation
    b. contact isolation
    c. enteric precautions
    d. drainage-secretion precautions

23. Which of the following is considered one of the ionic radiopaque contrast media (RCM)?
    a. iohexol
    b. iothalamate meglumine
    c. iopamidol
    d. ioversol

24. A patient who appears drowsy but can be aroused is said to be:
    a. comatose
    b. lethargic
    c. obtunded
    d. semicomatose

25. Direct contraindications to the administration of iodinated contrast material include:
    1. prior life-threatening reaction to iodinated contrast material
    2. multiple myeloma
    3. diabetes
    a. 1 only
    b. 1 and 2 only
    c. 1 and 3 only
    d. 1, 2, and 3

SAFETY

26. The acronym CTDI is used to describe which of the following?
    a. a specialized CT imaging technique used to measure bone mineral density
    b. a quality control test that measures the accuracy of the laser lighting system
    c. the radiation dose to the patient during a CT scan
    d. a high-speed CT scanner used for cardiac imaging

27. Contact shields made of _____ may be used to selectively protect radiosensitive organs that lie within the scanned region during a CT acquisition.
    a. bismuth
    b. aluminum
    c. lead
    d. molybdenum

28. Which of the following technical factors has a direct effect on patient dose?
    a. matrix size
    b. algorithm
    c. mAs
    d. window level

29. Which of the following devices is used to measure the patient dose from a CT examination?
    a. Geiger counter
    b. proportional counter
    c. ionization chamber
    d. film badge

30. To meet current industry standards for required dose reduction measures, a CT system must employ which of the following:
    1. automatic exposure control (AEC)
    2. adult and pediatric protocols
    3. Digital Imaging and Communications in Medicine (DICOM) radiation dose structured reporting (RDSR)
    a. 1 only
    b. 1 and 2 only
    c. 2 and 3 only
    d. 1, 2, and 3

31. When implementing a scan protocol for a CT of the abdomen without contrast on a pediatric patient (40 lb/18 kg), which technical factor should be primarily adjusted?
    a. detector configuration
    b. tube milliamperage (mAs)
    c. scan field of view (SFOV)
    d. reconstruction algorithm

32. Whole-body risk based upon the radiosensitivity of exposed tissues may be estimated using the unit:
    a. stochastic dose
    b. kerma
    c. effective dose
    d. CT dose index (CTDI)

33. The use of iterative reconstruction techniques for CT data processing results in:
    1. decreased noise on the reconstructed image
    2. decreased radiation dose to the patient
    3. decreased image reconstruction time
    a. 3 only
    b. 1 and 2 only
    c. 1 and 3 only
    d. 1, 2, and 3

34. Which of the following methods may be employed to reduce the radiation dose to the pediatric patient undergoing CT?
    1. reduce mA
    2. limit phases of acquisition
    3. increase pitch
    a. 1 only
    b. 1 and 2 only
    c. 1 and 3 only
    d. 1, 2, and 3

35. A decrease in the focus-to-detector distance of a multidetector CT (MDCT) system would result in:
    a. increased patient dose
    b. decreased patient dose
    c. magnification of the image
    d. loss of contrast resolution

36. The radiation dose index calculation that takes into account the variations in absorption across the field of view due to beam hardening is termed:
    a. $CTDI_W$
    b. $CTDI_{100}$
    c. $CTDI_{vol}$
    d. MSAD

37. The radiation dose structured report (RDSR) must include which of the following details regarding a CT acquisition:
    1. tube current (mA)
    2. display field of view (DFOV)
    3. tube voltage (kVp)
    4. acquisition time (seconds)
    5. acquisition length (millimeters)
    a. 1 only
    b. 1, 2, and 4
    c. 1, 3, 4, and 5
    d. All (1–5)

38. The reduction in intensity of the CT x-ray beam as it passes through patient issue may be generally termed:
    a. isotropy
    b. photodisintegration
    c. attenuation
    d. absorption

39. Which of the following clinical scenarios could result in an unnecessary increase in radiation dose to the patient?
    1. using in-plane bismuth shielding with longitudinal and angular tube current modulation (ATCM)
    2. increasing the tube potential (kVp) without a compensatory decrease in tube current (mA)
    3. increasing technical parameters to produce a noise-free image
    a. 3 only
    b. 1 and 2 only
    c. 2 and 3 only
    d. 1, 2, and 3

40. The dose length product (DLP) of a given CT acquisition may be calculated according to which of the following?
    1. MSAD × slice width (cm) × number of slices in scan volume
    2. $CTDI_{vol}$ × scan length (cm)
    3. pitch × $CTDI_W$
    a. 3 only
    b. 1 and 2 only
    c. 1 and 3 only
    d. 1, 2, and 3

41. A modern CT system may employ complex collimation along the z-axis to reduce patient radiation exposure due to:
    a. binning
    b. beam hardening
    c. overbeaming
    d. interpolation

42. Which of the following units is used to express the total patient dose from a helically acquired CT examination?
    a. roentgen (R)
    b. curie (Ci)
    c. R-cm (roentgens per centimeter)
    d. mGy-cm (milligrays per centimeter)

PROCEDURES

43. Components of a comprehensive CT stroke management protocol typically include:
    1. precontrast sequence of the brain
    2. CT angiogram (CTA) of the brain and carotids
    3. CT perfusion (CTP) of the brain
    a. 2 only
    b. 1 and 2 only
    c. 2 and 3 only
    d. 1, 2, and 3

Use Fig. 6.1 to answer questions 44–46.

44. Number 1 on the figure corresponds to which of the following?
    a. left pulmonary artery
    b. ascending aorta
    c. inferior vena cava
    d. descending aorta

45. Which number on the figure corresponds to the superior vena cava?
    a. 2
    b. 3
    c. 4
    d. 5

46. The abnormal density located in the posterior portion of the left lung field on the figure has an average attenuation value of +5.0 Hounsfield units. This density most likely represents:
    a. pneumothorax
    b. hemothorax
    c. atelectasis
    d. pleural effusion

47. Simple cysts of the kidney have average attenuation values in the range of:
    a. −40 to 0 Hounsfield units
    b. 0 to +20 Hounsfield units
    c. +30 to +50 Hounsfield units
    d. above +60 Hounsfield units

48. After initiation of rapid bolus administration of an iodinated contrast agent, the arterial phase of hepatic contrast enhancement occurs at approximately:
    a. 15–20 seconds
    b. 25–35 seconds
    c. 60–70 seconds
    d. 120–180 seconds

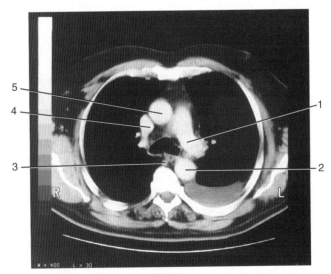

FIG. 6.1

Use Fig. 6.2 to answer questions 49–51.

49. Number 2 on the figure corresponds to which of the following?
    a. left internal jugular vein
    b. left external carotid artery
    c. left internal carotid artery
    d. left external jugular vein

50. Number 5 on the figure corresponds to which of the following?
    a. right internal jugular vein
    b. right external carotid artery
    c. right internal carotid artery
    d. right external jugular vein

51. Number 1 on the figure corresponds to which of the following?
    a. vocal cords
    b. uvula
    c. aryepiglottic fold
    d. epiglottis

52. The abdominal aorta bifurcates at the level of:
    a. T10
    b. T12
    c. L2
    d. L4

53. The accumulation of gas within a degenerating intervertebral disc is called the:
    a. aeration effect
    b. vacuum phenomenon
    c. oxygen saturation point
    d. carbonization sign

54. Which of the following CT studies of the head is typically performed without a contrast agent?
    a. CT angiogram for circle of Willis
    b. coronal scan to rule out (R/O) pituitary tumor
    c. CT of brain to R/O subdural hematoma
    d. CT of brain to R/O metastatic disease

55. Which of the following phases of renal contrast enhancement best demonstrates transitional cell carcinoma (TCC) of the bladder?
    a. early arterial
    b. corticomedullary
    c. nephrographic
    d. excretory

Use Fig. 6.3 to answer questions 56–59.

56. Number 5 on the figure corresponds to which of the following?
    a. transverse colon
    b. stomach
    c. duodenum
    d. hepatic flexure

57. Which of the following most likely describes the patient position during the formation of the image in the figure?
    a. supine
    b. prone
    c. left lateral decubitus
    d. right lateral decubitus

58. CT examinations of the abdomen are often performed in the position on the figure to demonstrate the relationship between the:
    a. ureters and renal collecting systems
    b. duodenum and pancreatic head
    c. large and small colon
    d. liver and gallbladder

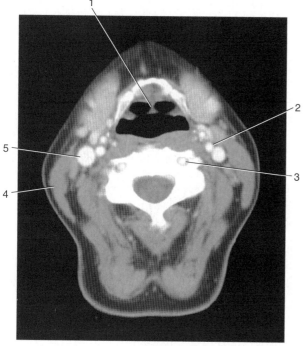

FIG. 6.2

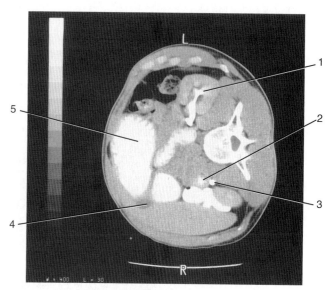

FIG. 6.3

59. Number 3 on the figure corresponds to which of the following?
    a. right ureter
    b. inferior vena cava
    c. renal calculi
    d. right renal artery
60. The still-viable ischemic cerebral tissue that surrounds the infarct core in a patient with an acute stroke is termed the:
    a. thrombolytic zone
    b. hemorrhage focus
    c. ischemic penumbra
    d. stroke volume
61. Complex fractures of the wrist are most common in which of the following carpal bones?
    a. hamate
    b. scaphoid
    c. capitate
    d. triquetrum
62. A complete CT study of the orbits should include:
    a. Thick section (5–10 mm) axial images only
    b. Thick section (5–10 mm) axial and coronal images
    c. Thin section (1–3 mm) coronal sections only
    d. Thin section (1–3 mm) axial and coronal sections
63. High-resolution computed tomography (HRCT) is most commonly used for the evaluation of the:
    a. pancreas
    b. brain
    c. lungs
    d. pelvis
64. During a general CT examination of the abdomen, an intravenous contrast agent is indicated and is administered with the aid of an automatic injector. Which of the following ranges of flow rate should be used?
    a. 0.2–1.0 mL/sec
    b. 1.0–3.0 mL/sec
    c. 4.0–6.0 mL/sec
    d. 7.0–10.0 mL/sec

65. Diffuse fatty infiltration of the hepatic parenchyma may be referred to as:
    a. chromatosis
    b. steatosis
    c. cirrhosis
    d. lipomatosis

Use Fig. 6.4 to answer questions 66–69.

66. Which of the following corresponds to the low-attenuation area indicated by number 3 on the figure?
    a. renal cortex
    b. renal pelvis
    c. renal calyx
    d. renal pyramid
67. The data for this reformatted image of the abdomen was most likely acquired in which of the following renal enhancement phases?
    a. precontrast
    b. corticomedullary
    c. nephrographic
    d. excretory
68. Number 2 on the figure corresponds to which of the following?
    a. hepatic vein
    b. suprarenal lymph node
    c. adrenal gland
    d. common bile duct
69. Number 6 on the figure corresponds to which of the following?
    a. psoas muscle
    b. omentum
    c. piriformis muscle
    d. erector spinae muscle
70. CT images of the chest should be acquired with the patient:
    a. at full inspiration
    b. breathing quietly
    c. at full expiration
    d. breathing normally

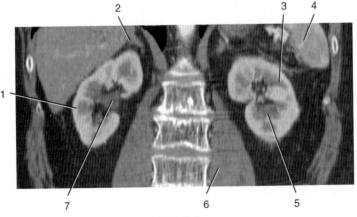

FIG. 6.4

71. During CT scanning of the head, the gantry should be angled:
    a. 15 degrees above the infraorbital-meatal line (IOML)
    b. 10 degrees below the IOML
    c. 0 degrees
    d. 20 degrees above the skull base
72. During CT examination of the larynx, the patient is often instructed to phonate the letter "E" in order to properly evaluate the:
    a. epiglottis
    b. uvula
    c. trachea
    d. vocal cords

Use Fig. 6.5 to answer questions 73–76.

73. Number 2 corresponds to which of the following?
    a. carotid canal
    b. incus
    c. cochlea
    d. vestibule
74. Number 4 corresponds to which of the following?
    a. external auditory meatus
    b. internal auditory canal
    c. vestibule
    d. carotid canal
75. Which of the following display field of view (DFOV) values was most likely used to display the image?
    a. 9.6 cm
    b. 18.0 cm
    c. 25.6 cm
    d. 51.2 cm

76. Number 3 on the figure corresponds to which of the following?
    a. vestibule
    b. semicircular canal
    c. cochlea
    d. incus
77. During a CT examination of a female pelvis for a suspected malignancy, ascites may be present in an area posterior to the uterus and ovaries known as:
    a. the cul-de-sac
    b. Morison pouch
    c. the space of Retzius
    d. the prevesical compartment
78. Which of the following pathologic processes may be considered an interstitial disease of the lungs?
    a. bronchiectasis
    b. mediastinal lymphadenopathy
    c. pulmonary metastasis
    d. bronchogenic carcinoma
79. An enterovesical fistula is an abnormal communication between the bowel and the:
    a. uterus
    b. bladder
    c. vagina
    d. umbilicus
80. Positioning the patient with the knees flexed over a foam cushion during a CT examination of the lumbar spine assists in:
    1. decreasing the kyphotic curvature of the lumbar spine
    2. making the patient more comfortable throughout the examination
    3. decreasing the lordotic curvature of the lumbar spine
    a. 1 only
    b. 2 only
    c. 3 only
    d. 2 and 3 only
81. The imaging plane that is parallel to the foot's plantar surface is called the:
    a. coronal plane
    b. sagittal plane
    c. axial plane
    d. oblique axial plane
82. The condition of intermittent cramping pain in the legs due to poor circulation is called:
    a. varices
    b. claudication
    c. stenosis
    d. thrombosis

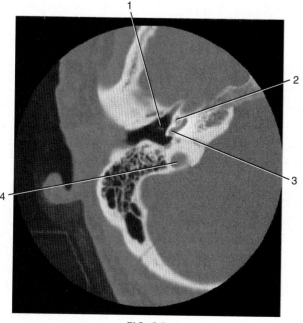

FIG. 6.5

Use Fig. 6.6 to answer questions 83–86.

83. The pathologic process indicated by number 3 on the figure most likely corresponds to:
    a. atelectasis
    b. lymphadenopathy
    c. pleural effusion
    d. ground-glass opacity

84. Number 1 on the figure corresponds to which of the following?
    a. right atrium
    b. pulmonary trunk
    c. ascending aorta
    d. right ventricle

85. This high-resolution computed tomography (HRCT) image of the chest was most likely acquired with a section width of:
    a. 1 mm
    b. 5 mm
    c. 7 mm
    d. 10 mm

86. Number 2 on the figure corresponds to which of the following?
    a. left mainstem bronchus
    b. anterior segment of left upper lobe bronchus
    c. posterior segment of left upper lobe bronchus
    d. anterior segment of left lower lobe bronchus

87. The pituitary gland is best demonstrated during CT in which of the following imaging planes?
    a. axial
    b. coronal
    c. sagittal
    d. transaxial

88. The most common site of organ injury due to blunt abdominal trauma is the:
    a. liver
    b. kidney
    c. spleen
    d. pancreas

Use Fig. 6.7 to answer questions 93–91.

89. Number 7 on the figure corresponds to which of the following?
    a. duodenum
    b. pancreatic head
    c. jejunum
    d. gallbladder

90. Number 2 on the figure corresponds to which of the following?
    a. superior mesenteric vein
    b. superior mesenteric artery
    c. renal artery
    d. portal vein

91. Number 8 on the figure corresponds to which of the following?
    a. duodenum
    b. descending colon
    c. jejunum
    d. ascending colon

92. The adult spinal cord ends at what vertebral level?
    a. T11–T12
    b. L1–L2
    c. L3–L4
    d. superior portion of the coccyx

93. Which of the following terms is used to describe a fibroid tumor of the uterus?
    a. leiomyoma
    b. cystic teratoma
    c. endometriosis
    d. corpus luteum

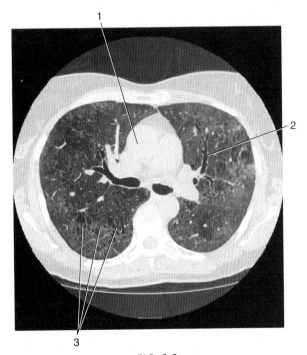

FIG. 6.6

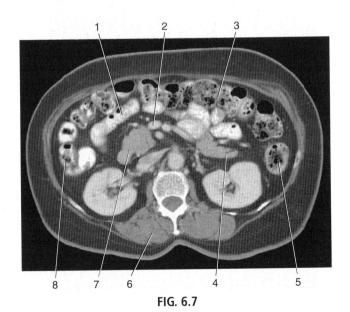

FIG. 6.7

Use Fig. 6.8 to answer questions 94–96.

94. Number 1 on the figure corresponds to which of the following?
   a. sphenoid sinus
   b. ethmoid sinus
   c. frontal sinus
   d. maxillary sinus

95. The section thickness that would demonstrate the greatest detail of the paranasal sinuses is:
   a. 3 mm
   b. 5 mm
   c. 7 mm
   d. 10 mm

96. Which number on the figure corresponds to the zygomatic bone?
   a. 3
   b. 1
   c. 2
   d. 6

97. Which of the following anatomic organs is located within the peritoneal cavity?
   a. pancreas
   b. kidneys
   c. uterus
   d. liver

98. Which of the following may be included as part of a routine preparation for a general contrast-enhanced CT examination of the abdomen and pelvis?
   1. instructing the patient to take nothing by mouth (NPO) for 4 hours before the examination
   2. 1200 mL of oral contrast agent administered 90 minutes before the examination
   3. having the patient drink 4 liters of polyethylene glycol (PEG) 24 hours before the examination
   a. 1 only
   b. 2 only
   c. 1 and 2 only
   d. 1 and 3 only

99. During a complete CT scan of the pelvis, sections should be obtained from the:
   a. iliac crests to the pubic symphysis
   b. kidneys through the bladder
   c. bottom of the kidneys to the pubic symphysis
   d. iliac crests to the lesser trochanter

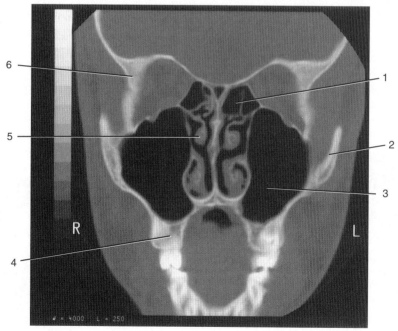

FIG. 6.8

Use Fig. 6.9 to answer questions 100–103.

100. Number 4 on the figure corresponds to which of the following?
    a. navicular
    b. cuboid
    c. calcaneus
    d. talus

101. Which of the following best describes the type of image displayed in the figure?
    a. sagittal maximum intensity projection (MIP)
    b. direct sagittal acquisition
    c. sagittal multiplanar reformation (MPR)
    d. volume-rendered 3-D

102. Number 6 on the figure corresponds to which of the following?
    a. navicular
    b. cuboid
    c. calcaneus
    d. talus

103. Number 1 on the figure corresponds to which of the following?
    a. navicular
    b. cuboid
    c. calcaneus
    d. talus

104. Because of its inherent iodine concentration, the thyroid gland appears _____ on CT images.
    a. hypodense
    b. isodense
    c. hyperdense
    d. mottled

105. Air trapping within the trachea and bronchial tree may be optimally demonstrated with multiplanar volume reconstructions (MPVRs) of the thorax known as:
    a. maximum intensity projections (MIPs)
    b. 3-D volume renderings
    c. shaded-surface displays (SSDs)
    d. minimum intensity projections (min-IPs)

Use Fig. 6.10 to answer questions 106–108.

106. Which number on the figure corresponds to the anterior horn of the lateral ventricle?
    a. 1
    b. 5
    c. 3
    d. 2

107. Number 3 on the figure corresponds to which of the following?
    a. caudate nucleus
    b. thalamus
    c. third ventricle
    d. pineal gland

108. Which number on the figure corresponds to the septum pellucidum?
    a. 2
    b. 3
    c. 4
    d. 5

109. Which of the following is *not* a portion of the small bowel?
    a. duodenum
    b. jejunum
    c. ileum
    d. cecum

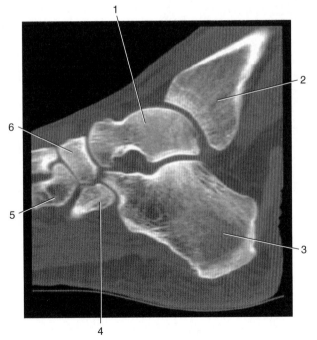

FIG. 6.9

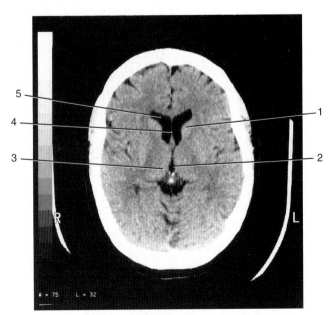

FIG. 6.10

110. The specialized CT examination of the bladder in which an iodinated contrast agent is directly administered under gravity into the bladder via Foley catheter is termed:
   a. CT intravenous pyelogram (IVP)
   b. CT urogram
   c. CT enteroclysis
   d. CT cystography

IMAGE PRODUCTION

111. Which of the following best describes the shape of the x-ray beam utilized in multidetector CT (MDCT)?
   a. pencil beam
   b. fan-shaped
   c. electron beam
   d. cone-shaped
112. Collimation of the CT x-ray beam occurs:
   1. at the x-ray tube, regulating slice thickness
   2. just beyond the patient, focusing off-axis transmitted radiation
   3. before the detectors, limiting the amount of scatter radiation absorbed
   a. 1 only
   b. 1 and 2 only
   c. 1 and 3 only
   d. 1, 2, and 3
113. CT numbers are usually provided in the form of:
   a. Hounsfield units
   b. EMI numbers
   c. Cormacks
   d. μ
114. The mathematical technique allowing the reconstruction of motion-free images from helically acquired CT data is called:
   a. convolution
   b. radon transformation
   c. interpolation
   d. Fourier reconstruction
115. The full width at half maximum (FWHM) of a CT scanner is used to describe:
   a. spatial resolution
   b. contrast resolution
   c. noise
   d. calibration accuracy
116. A first-generation CT scanner consists of an x-ray tube and two detectors that translate across the patient's head while rotating in 1-degree increments for a total of:
   a. 45 degrees
   b. 90 degrees
   c. 180 degrees
   d. 360 degrees

117. Which of the following abbreviations is used to identify a computerized network that stores, retrieves, communicates, and displays digital medical images?
   a. WORM
   b. PACS
   c. DICOM
   d. HIPAA
118. The CT "window" controls the _____ of the CT image as it appears to the viewer.
   a. density and detail
   b. spatial and contrast resolution
   c. contrast and brightness
   d. attenuation coefficient and Hounsfield value
119. Voxels with equal dimensions along the x-, y-, and z-axes are referred to as:
   a. prospective
   b. isotropic
   c. retrospective
   d. anisotropic
120. Which of the following artifacts is not affected by the CT technologist?
   a. motion
   b. partial volume
   c. edge gradient
   d. ring
121. When one is viewing a multiplanar reformation (MPR) image, each pixel represents:
   a. the maximum attenuation occurring within the voxel
   b. the average attenuation occurring within the voxel
   c. the minimum attenuation occurring within the voxel
   d. all attenuation occurring within the voxel above a set threshold value
122. Statistical noise appears as _____ on a CT image.
   a. decreased contrast
   b. increased brightness
   c. concentric circles
   d. graininess
123. An acquisition is made on a 64-slice multidetector CT (MDCT) system in which each detector element has a z-axis dimension of 0.625 mm. With a selected beam width of 40 mm and the beam pitch set at 1.50, how much will the table move with each rotation of the gantry?
   a. 20 mm
   b. 40 mm
   c. 60 mm
   d. 80 mm
124. The component of the CT computer system responsible for the data processing of image reconstruction is the:
   a. pipeline memory
   b. array processor
   c. hard disk drive
   d. RAM microprocessor

125. The loss of anatomic information between contiguous sections due to inconsistent patient breathing is called:
    a. cupping artifact
    b. misregistration
    c. overshoot artifact
    d. out-of-field artifact

126. Before a CT image can be reconstructed by a computer, the transmission signal produced by the detectors must be converted into numerical information by a(n):
    a. kernel
    b. analog-to-digital converter (ADC)
    c. array processor
    d. digital-to-analog converter (DAC)

127. A CT image is formed in part by projecting back all of the attenuation values recorded during data acquisition onto a:
    a. pixel
    b. voxel
    c. matrix
    d. reformat

128. Areas of a CT image that contain abrupt changes in tissue density are electronically represented by which of the following?
    a. positive CT numbers
    b. high spatial frequencies
    c. negative CT numbers
    d. low spatial frequencies

Use Fig. 6.11 to answer questions 129–131.

129. Which of the following components of CT image quality are being evaluated in the figure?
    1. low-contrast detectability
    2. noise
    3. uniformity
    a. 2 only
    b. 1 and 2 only
    c. 1 and 3 only
    d. 2 and 3 only

130. The differences in Hounsfield value exhibited in the regions of interest (ROIs) measured on this CT image of a water-filled phantom are most likely due to the phenomenon referred to as:
    a. partial volume averaging
    b. noise
    c. beam hardening
    d. detector drift

131. Which region of interest (ROI) on the figure demonstrates the greatest amount of image noise?
    a. 1
    b. 2
    c. 3
    d. impossible to determine from the information provided

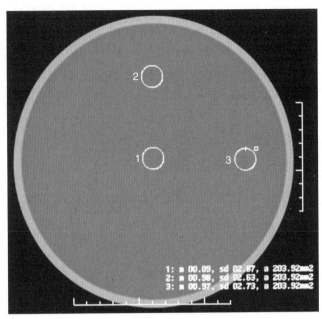

FIG. 6.11

132. Which of the following terms is used to describe a set of rules for solving a mathematical problem?
    a. reconstruction
    b. algorithm
    c. function
    d. array

133. Which of the following factors does not affect the dimensions of a voxel?
    a. slice thickness
    b. matrix size
    c. kernel
    d. display field of view

134. The size of the CT image displayed on a computer monitor can be enlarged by increasing the:
    1. display field of view (DFOV)
    2. scan field of view (SFOV)
    3. image magnification
    a. 1 only
    b. 3 only
    c. 1 and 2 only
    d. 1 and 3 only

135. The average photon energy of the primary beam of a CT scanner operating at a tube potential of 120 kVp is approximately:
    a. 50 keV
    b. 70 keV
    c. 100 keV
    d. 120 keV

136. Multidetector CT (MDCT) systems typically employ which of the following detector geometries?
    a. first-generation
    b. second-generation
    c. third-generation
    d. fourth-generation

137. The acquisition of a series of CT images at a single anatomic location over a set period is referred to as:
    a. ultrafast CT
    b. cine CT
    c. conventional CT
    d. temporal CT

138. The rate at which a quantity of x-radiation emitted from a CT tube passes through a unit area over a unit of time is called the:
    a. effective mAs
    b. photon flux
    c. constant mAs
    d. photon fluence

139. An average CT number value for bone is:
    a. +100 HU
    b. +500 HU
    c. +1000 HU
    d. +3000 HU

140. A standard CT image reconstructed on a 512^2 matrix has a digital size of approximately:
    a. 0.5 MB
    b. 3.0 MB
    c. 5.0 MB
    d. 10.0 MB

141. The term used to describe the relationship between the linear attenuation coefficient of an object and the calculated CT number is:
    a. linearity
    b. mottle
    c. quantum noise
    d. spatial resolution

142. Quality control measurements to test the accuracy of the CT scanner's calibration should be performed:
    a. daily
    b. weekly
    c. monthly
    d. annually

143. The 3-D CT technique that includes all of the acquired voxel information in the reconstructed model with adjustments to its opacity is termed:
    a. surface rendering
    b. maximum intensity projection (MIP)
    c. curved multiplanar reformation
    d. volume rendering

144. Where is the high-frequency generator often located in a modern CT scanner?
    a. inside the gantry
    b. just outside the scan room
    c. beneath the CT table
    d. inside the operator's console

145. The smallest unit of information used in the binary language of computers is the:
    a. bit
    b. chip
    c. base
    d. byte

146. The continuous gantry rotation required by helical CT acquisition is made possible by the application of:
    a. electromagnetic bushings
    b. titanium bearings
    c. slip-rings
    d. oil-cooled couplings

147. The process of applying a mathematical filter to remove blurring from the reconstructed CT image is termed:
    a. convolution
    b. interpolation
    c. iteration
    d. z-filtration

148. Which of the following acquisitions may be characterized as contiguous?
    a. 2.5-mm sections reconstructed every 1.25 mm
    b. 5.0-mm sections reconstructed every 7.5 mm
    c. 3.75-mm sections reconstructed every 3.75 mm
    d. 20-second cine acquisition with 1.25-mm sections

149. Pixels representing tissues with average attenuation coefficients greater than that of water have which of the following types of values?
    a. extremely small
    b. positive
    c. negative
    d. low contrast

150. Digital CT images are networked and archived in accordance with a standardized computer protocol identified by which of the following abbreviations?
    a. HIPAA
    b. HTTP
    c. TCP/IP
    d. DICOM

151. The contrast resolution of a CT scanner is *not* related to which of the following?
    a. focal spot size
    b. section width
    c. reconstruction algorithm
    d. signal-to-noise ratio

Use Fig. 6.12 to answer questions 152–153.

152. The artifact present on the lateral borders of the image in the figure most likely represents which of the following?
    a. edge gradient
    b. out-of-field artifact
    c. tube arcing
    d. beam hardening

153. The image in the figure was produced using the following parameters: large (full) scan field of view (SFOV); maximum display field of view (DFOV) (48 cm); 200 mA, 120 kVp; soft tissue algorithm. Which of the following technical adjustments would serve to reduce the artifact present?
    a. switching to a detail or bone algorithm
    b. using a smaller SFOV
    c. increasing the mA to 240 and the kVp to 140
    d. centering the patient within the SFOV

154. The average photon energy of the CT x-ray beam can be increased by:
    a. increasing mAs
    b. increasing filtration
    c. increasing collimation
    d. all of the above

155. Which of the following is a solid-state device used to record the light flashes given off by a scintillation crystal?
    a. photomultiplier tube
    b. anode
    c. photodiode
    d. input phosphor

156. Automatic tube current modulation (ATCM) software is used in current multidetector CT (MDCT) systems to control:
    a. patient radiation dose
    b. cardiac motion
    c. timing of the contrast agent bolus
    d. tissue perfusion assessment

157. The type of multidetector CT (MDCT) detector array that contains multiple rows of detector elements, each of the same length, is called a(n):
    a. uniform matrix array
    b. adaptive array
    c. hybrid array
    d. stationary array

158. A CT image is displayed in a window with a level of 0 and a width of 500. Which of the following statements is correct?
    a. Pixels with values between 0 HU and 500 HU will appear white.
    b. Pixels with values between –250 HU and +250 HU will be assigned shades of gray.
    c. Pixels with values greater than +500 HU will be black.
    d. Pixels with values less than 0 HU will appear white.

159. Reformatted CT image planes that lie perpendicular to the original plane of acquisition may be described as:
    a. oblique
    b. orthogonal
    c. obtuse
    d. orthographic

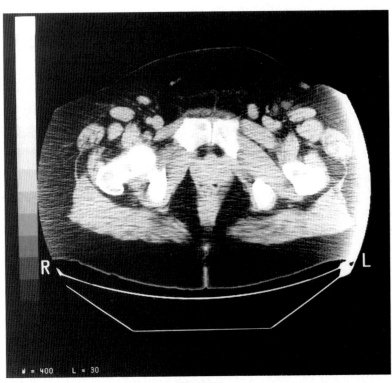

FIG. 6.12

160. Segmenting the data acquisition process into separate components of smaller rotation angles may improve which of the following components of CT image quality?
    a. temporal resolution
    b. longitudinal spatial resolution
    c. contrast resolution
    d. in-plane spatial resolution

161. Which of the following image artifacts is unique to multidetector CT (MDCT) systems?
    a. step artifact
    b. aliasing artifact
    c. out-of-field artifact
    d. cone beam artifact

162. Which of the following is considered an analytic form of image reconstruction?
    1. iterative technique
    2. Fourier reconstruction
    3. filtered back-projection
    a. 1 only
    b. 1 and 2 only
    c. 2 and 3 only
    d. 1, 2, and 3

163. A 16-slice MDCT system utilizes an adaptive array of 24 detectors, each ranging in size from 0.625 to 1.25 mm. What is the maximum number of sections the system can acquire with each rotation of the gantry?
    a. 8
    b. 16
    c. 32
    d. 64

164. The measurement of transmitted radiation made by an individual detector is called a(n):
    a. attenuation coefficient
    b. Hounsfield value
    c. CT number
    d. ray sum

165. The information included during the 3-D reconstruction of a CT scan is controlled by the:
    a. algorithm
    b. window setting
    c. threshold setting
    d. grayscale map

Simulated Examination Two

PATIENT CARE

1. As related to the cardiac cycle, the term _____ refers to the relaxation of heart muscle.
   a. diastole
   b. equilibrium
   c. systole
   d. a-fib

2. Which of the following may be considered one of the high-osmolar contrast media (HOCM)?
   1. iothalamate meglumine
   2. diatrizoate sodium
   3. iohexol
   a. 1 only
   b. 3 only
   c. 1 and 2 only
   d. 1, 2, and 3

3. Which of the following medications may be administered to a patient who is having a severe anaphylactoid reaction to iodinated contrast material?
   1. epinephrine
   2. atropine
   3. diphenhydramine
   a. 1 only
   b. 1 and 2 only
   c. 1 and 3 only
   d. 1, 2, and 3

4. The escape of contrast material from a needle or blood vessel into the subcutaneous tissues is called:
   a. infusion
   b. extraversion
   c. influxation
   d. extravasation

5. Thorough explanation of the CT procedure and proper communication with the patient are vital in ensuring that:
   1. breathing instructions are properly followed
   2. motion artifact does not occur
   3. patient anxiety is kept at a minimum
   a. 1 and 2 only
   b. 1 and 3 only
   c. 2 and 3 only
   d. 1, 2, and 3

6. Risk factors for contrast-induced nephrotoxicity (CIN) include:
   1. pheochromocytoma
   2. allergy to shellfish
   3. dehydration
   a. 2 only
   b. 3 only
   c. 1 and 2 only
   d. 1, 2, and 3

7. Normal range for oxygen (O_2) saturation is:
   a. 20%–25%
   b. 50%–60%
   c. 80%–85%
   d. 95%–100%

8. Which of the following laboratory measurements can be used to evaluate the renal function of a patient?
   1. blood urea nitrogen (BUN)
   2. partial thromboplastin time (PTT)
   3. creatinine
   a. 1 only
   b. 1 and 2 only
   c. 1 and 3 only
   d. 1, 2, and 3

9. Which of the following would be best suited for intravenous injection of contrast material with a power injector?
   a. butterfly needle
   b. central venous line
   c. 23-gauge spinal needle
   d. angiocatheter

10. Before the intravenous injection of iodinated contrast material, patients should be questioned regarding their:
    1. renal function
    2. allergic history
    3. cardiac history
    a. 1 only
    b. 2 only
    c. 3 only
    d. 1, 2, and 3

11. A(n) _____ infection is one that a patient acquires during a stay in a health care institution.
    a. blood-borne
    b. nosocomial
    c. iatrogenic
    d. staphylococcal

12. Which of the following sets of values would be considered normal levels for creatinine and blood urea nitrogen (BUN), respectively?
    a. 3.1 mg/dL; 1.2 mg/dL
    b. 1.2 mg/dL; 14 mg/dL
    c. 0.7 mg/dL; 39 mg/dL
    d. 5.2 mg/dL; 12 mg/dL

13. Which of the following sizes of butterfly needles allows for the most rapid administration of iodinated intravenous contrast media?
    a. 19 gauge
    b. 21 gauge
    c. 23 gauge
    d. 25 gauge

14. The choice between ionic and nonionic contrast media should be based on:
    1. the allergic history of the patient
    2. the cost of the contrast material
    3. the age and physical condition of the patient
    a. 1 only
    b. 1 and 2 only
    c. 1 and 3 only
    d. 1, 2, and 3

15. Which of the following is an example of a mild reaction to iodinated intravenous contrast media?
    a. dyspnea
    b. shock
    c. pulmonary edema
    d. vomiting

16. During which of the following CT procedures is the patient required to give informed consent?
    a. noncontrast CT of the chest
    b. renal stone survey
    c. 3-D reconstruction of the hip
    d. abdomen scan after IV contrast agent administration

17. The international normalized ratio (INR) is calculated to standardize which of the following laboratory values?
    a. prothrombin time (PT)
    b. partial thromboplastin time (PTT)
    c. blood urea nitrogen (BUN)
    d. glomerular filtration rate (GFR)

18. Which of the following infection control techniques is required at the site of an intravenous injection of iodinated contrast media?
    a. contact isolation
    b. surgical asepsis
    c. medical asepsis
    d. enteric precautions

19. Which of the following is a common site for the intravenous injection of iodinated contrast media?
    1. cephalic vein
    2. antecubital vein
    3. basilic vein
    a. 1 only
    b. 3 only
    c. 2 and 3 only
    d. 1, 2, and 3

20. An intrathecal injection before a CT examination of the lumber spine administers iodinated contrast material directly into the:
    a. subarachnoid space
    b. dura mater
    c. vertebral foramen
    d. subdural space

21. The range of serum iodine concentration for adequate tissue opacification during contrast-enhanced CT examinations is:
    a. 2–8 mg/mL
    b. 12–20 mg/mL
    c. 30–42 mg/mL
    d. 75–105 mg/mL

22. Components of the aseptic technique utilized for the IV administration of contrast agents include:
    1. thorough hand washing between patients
    2. wearing of disposable gloves
    3. establishment of a sterile field around the site
    a. 1 and 2 only
    b. 1 and 3 only
    c. 2 and 3 only
    d. 1, 2, and 3

SAFETY

23. During data acquisition, a CT system may continuously adjust the mA relative to the measured image noise for a method of dose reduction referred to as:
    a. iterative reconstruction
    b. automatic tube current modulation
    c. attenuation correction
    d. Nyquist sampling

24. The amount of x-ray energy absorbed in a quantity of air is termed:
    a. dose profile
    b. kerma
    c. becquerel
    d. multiple scan average dose (MSAD)

25. Which of the following technical changes would serve to decrease patient radiation dose during a CT examination?
    a. increase in matrix size
    b. change from soft tissue to bone algorithm
    c. decrease of tube rotation from 360 to 180 degrees
    d. decrease in display field of view (DFOV)

26. In an effort to reduce patient radiation dose, the technical factors of the applied CT protocol should be optimized on the basis of:
    a. age
    b. sex
    c. size or weight
    d. physical condition

27. Which of the following is considered in the calculation of the multiple scan average dose (MSAD) for an axial (step-and-shoot) CT examination?
    a. bed index
    b. gantry rotation time
    c. mA setting
    d. pitch

28. During CT examinations, the patient's body should be shielded above and below because of:
    a. the rotational nature of the x-ray tube
    b. extremely high kVp techniques
    c. lack of filtration of the CT beam
    d. reduced collimation of the CT beam

29. $CTDI_w$ is a weighted index that approximates radiation dose on the basis of the variations that occur across the field of view because of:
    1. beam hardening
    2. detector configuration
    3. pitch
    a. 1 only
    b. 1 and 2 only
    c. 2 and 3 only
    d. 1, 2, and 3

30. The embryo or fetus is most sensitive to ionizing radiation during which portion of gestation?
    a. first trimester
    b. second trimester
    c. third trimester
    d. the fetus is equally radiosensitive during all trimesters

31. To uniformly expose the entire detector array in a multidetector CT (MDCT) system, the primary beam must be expanded beyond the physical extent of the array in a process known as:
    a. interpolation
    b. overbeaming
    c. photon flux
    d. back-projection

32. Automatic tube current modulation (ATCM) is employed by a multidetector CT (MDCT) system for the purpose of:
    a. z-axis interpolation
    b. improving 3-D and multiplanar reformation (MPR) image quality
    c. reducing patient radiation dose
    d. freezing heart motion during cardiac CT

33. In an effort to avoid excessive radiation exposure to the patient, a CT system may be equipped with a(n) _____ system that automatically notifies the technologist about improper technical factors before data acquisition.
    a. dose alert
    b. electrocardiogram (ECG) trigger
    c. multiple scan average dose (MSAD)
    d. interpolation

34. The distance between the x-ray source (CT tube) and the center of the gantry may be referred to as the:
    a. focus-to-detector distance
    b. focus-to-isocenter distance
    c. source-to-object distance
    d. source-to-image receptor distance

35. The interaction between radiation and matter that results in the complete attenuation of an x-ray photon due to ionization of a target atom's inner shell electron is termed:
    a. photodisintegration
    b. Compton scatter
    c. Bremsstrahlung
    d. photoelectric effect

36. The inherent filtration of the x-ray tube used in a CT system typically amounts to an equivalent thickness of:
    a. 0.5 mm Al
    b. 3.0 mm Al
    c. 10.0 mm Al
    d. 15.0 mm Al

37. Adaptive collimation may be utilized to reduce the unnecessary radiation exposure at the start and end of a helical acquisition that may be referred to as:
    a. overbeaming
    b. interpolation
    c. overranging
    d. binning

38. Which of the following pitch settings would result in the largest radiation dose to the patient?
    a. 1.0
    b. 1.2
    c. 1.7
    d. 2.0

39. Optimization of CT techniques and procedures for the purpose of radiation dose reduction for patients and personnel should include:
    1. restricting the acquired acquisition volume to the area of clinical interest
    2. controlling access to the CT imaging room to essential personnel only
    3. adjusting technical parameters (e.g., mA, kVp) to the size of the patient
    a. 2 only
    b. 1 and 3 only
    c. 2 and 3 only
    d. 1, 2, and 3

40. When employing bismuth shielding, which of the following techniques will reduce streaking artifact while still offering radiation dose savings to sensitive tissues?
    a. Placing a foam spacer between the patient surface and the bismuth shield.
    b. Placing the bismuth shielding outside of the scan acquisition range.
    c. Placing the bismuth shielding after the acquisition of the localizer image.
    d. Placing a foam spacer on top of the bismuth shield to intercept the incoming beam.

41. The weighted computed tomography dose index ($CTDI_W$) can be converted into a volumetric CT dose index ($CTDI_{vol}$) that is useful for estimating patient dose during helical acquisitions by dividing the $CTDI_W$ by the scan's:
    a. milliamperage (mA)
    b. pitch
    c. multiple scan average dose (MSAD)
    d. section width

42. During the use of CT fluoroscopy for guided interventional procedures, which of the following technical considerations may be used to reduce occupational radiation exposure?
    1. increased kVp
    2. lead shielding
    3. use of a needle holder
    a. 2 only
    b. 1 and 2 only
    c. 1 and 3 only
    d. 2 and 3 only

PROCEDURES

Use Fig. 7.1 to answer questions 43–47.

43. Number 4 in the figure corresponds to which of the following?
    a. spleen
    b. duodenum
    c. left adrenal gland
    d. large colon

44. Number 2 in the figure corresponds to which of the following?
    a. inferior vena cava
    b. common bile duct
    c. portal vein
    d. superior mesenteric vein

45. The abdominal space indicated by number 7 in the figure is commonly referred to as:
    a. Morison pouch
    b. cul-de-sac
    c. splenorenal recess
    d. subphrenic space

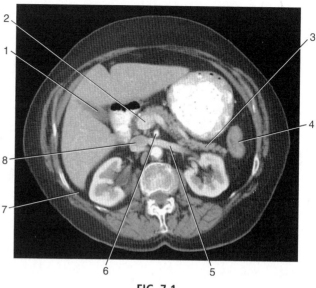

FIG. 7.1

46. Number 6 in the figure corresponds to which of the following?
    a. superior mesenteric vein
    b. superior mesenteric artery
    c. gastric artery
    d. right renal vein

47. Number 3 in the figure corresponds to which of the following?
    a. duodenum
    b. splenic vein
    c. jejunum
    d. pancreas

48. Abnormalities of the middle and inner ear may be best demonstrated with CT utilizing _____ sections.
    a. 1- to 2-mm
    b. 3- to 4-mm
    c. 5-mm
    d. 10-mm

49. The Lisfranc joint is the articulation between the:
    a. tarsals and metatarsals
    b. tarsals and lower leg
    c. metatarsals and phalanges
    d. proximal and middle phalanges

50. The volume and density of calcium measured in the coronary arteries on multidetector CT (MDCT) examination are quantified with use of a value called the:
    a. Euler constant
    b. Hounsfield number
    c. Agatston score
    d. Lambert–Beer value

51. Which of the following is/are (a) component(s) of the adnexal area of the uterus?
    1. ovaries
    2. fallopian tubes
    3. vagina
    a. 1 only
    b. 1 and 2 only
    c. 2 and 3 only
    d. 1, 2, and 3

52. Which of the following contrast media may be utilized during the CT evaluation of the gastrointestinal tract?
    1. diatrizoate meglumine (Gastrografin)
    2. effervescent agents
    3. iopamidol (Isovue)
    a. 1 only
    b. 1 and 3 only
    c. 2 and 3 only
    d. 1, 2, and 3

53. The liver has a dual blood supply and receives 75% of its blood from the:
    a. hepatic artery
    b. superior mesenteric artery
    c. portal vein
    d. superior mesenteric vein

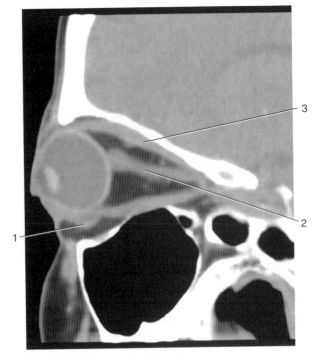

FIG. 7.2

Use Fig. 7.2 to answer questions 54–57.

54. Number 3 on the figure corresponds to which of the following?
    a. superior rectus muscle
    b. lateral rectus muscle
    c. medial rectus muscle
    d. inferior rectus muscle

55. Number 2 on the figure corresponds to which of the following?
    a. medial rectus muscle
    b. optic nerve
    c. lateral rectus muscle
    d. superior oblique muscle

56. Which of the following best describes the type of image featured in the figure?
    a. direct coronal acquisition
    b. sagittal maximum intensity projection (MIP)
    c. coronal multiplanar reformation (MPR)
    d. oblique sagittal MPR

57. Number 1 on the figure corresponds to which of the following?
    a. inferior rectus muscle
    b. optic chiasm
    c. inferior oblique muscle
    d. levator palpebrae superioris

Use Figure 7.3 to answer questions 58–61.

58. Number 6 on the figure corresponds to which of the following?
    a. descending aorta
    b. azygos vein
    c. inferior vena cava
    d. brachiocephalic artery

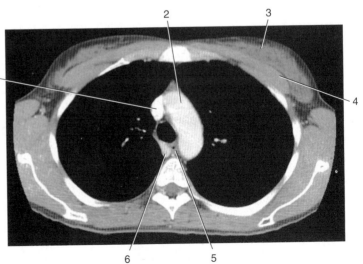

FIG. 7.3

59. Number 4 on the figure corresponds to which of the following muscles?
    a. pectoralis major
    b. pectoralis minor
    c. intercostal
    d. serratus posterior superior
60. Which of the following window settings was used to display the image in the figure?
    a. WL −400, WW 1500
    b. WL 0, WW 150
    c. WL +50, WW 400
    d. WL +275, WW 2500
61. Number 1 on the figure corresponds to which of the following?
    a. superior vena cava
    b. ascending aorta
    c. right brachiocephalic vein
    d. right brachiocephalic artery
62. At what percentage of overlap should CT sections be reconstructed to improve the quality of multiplanar reformation (MPR) images?
    a. 10%
    b. 25%
    c. 50%
    d. 100%
63. A primary responsibility of computed tomography in combined PET-CT is to:
    1. provide precise anatomic location of tumor activity
    2. reduce patient radiation dose
    3. provide attenuation correction information
    a. 1 only
    b. 1 and 3 only
    c. 2 and 3 only
    d. 1, 2, and 3
64. The degenerative pathologic process involving the forward slipping of an upper vertebral body over a lower vertebral body is called:
    a. spondylolisthesis
    b. spondylolysis
    c. herniated nucleus pulposus
    d. spinal stenosis

Use Fig. 7.4 to answer questions 65–68.

65. Number 2 on the figure corresponds to which of the following?
    a. jejunum
    b. sigmoid colon
    c. ileum
    d. cecum

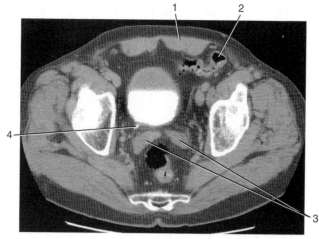

FIG. 7.4

66. Number 3 on the figure corresponds to which of the following?
    a. ureters
    b. cervix
    c. seminal vesicles
    d. vaginal cuff
67. Number 1 on the figure corresponds to which of the following?
    a. rectus abdominis muscle
    b. external oblique muscle
    c. transverse abdominis muscle
    d. internal oblique muscle
68. Number 4 on the figure corresponds to which of the following?
    a. ureteropelvic junction
    b. phlebolith
    c. ureterovesical junction
    d. appendicolith
69. Accurate demonstration of _____ would most likely require the intravenous injection of an iodinated contrast agent during a CT study of the chest.
    a. bronchiectasis
    b. pneumonia
    c. mediastinal lymphadenopathy
    d. pulmonary nodule
70. A focused, thin-section axial CT acquisition through just the region of the vocal cords should extend:
    a. from the external auditory meatus inferiorly to the mandible
    b. from the hard palate inferiorly to the hyoid bone
    c. from just above the hyoid bone inferiorly through the cricoid cartilage
    d. from the cricoid cartilage inferiorly through sternoclavicular joint

Use Fig. 7.5 to answer questions 71–73.

71. Number 3 on the figure corresponds to which of the following?
    a. coracoid process
    b. acromion
    c. glenoid process
    d. clavicle

72. The anatomic plane of the image in the figure can be best described as the:
    a. coronal plane
    b. sagittal plane
    c. axial plane
    d. oblique axial plane

73. Number 2 in the figure corresponds to which of the following?
    a. coracoid process
    b. acromion
    c. glenoid process
    d. clavicle

74. Which of the following contrast agent administration techniques should be used for a general CT survey of the abdomen?
    1. 400–600 mL oral contrast agent 45–90 minutes before the examination
    2. 250 mL oral contrast agent immediately before the examination
    3. 700–900 mL contrast agent administered as an enema immediately before the examination
    a. 1 only
    b. 1 and 2 only
    c. 1 and 3 only
    d. 1, 2, and 3

75. During CT perfusion studies, the quantity of blood (in mL) that moves through 100 g of tissue each minute is termed the:
    a. mean transit time (MTT)
    b. cerebral blood flow (CBF)
    c. cerebral blood volume (CBV)
    d. percentage washout value (PWV)

Use Fig. 7.6 to answer questions 76–79.

76. Which number in the figure corresponds to the trapezius muscle?
    a. 4
    b. 3
    c. 6
    d. 5

77. An adequate volume of intravenous contrast agent for the single-slice CT (SSCT) examination of the neck in this figure would be:
    a. 25 mL
    b. 50 mL
    c. 125 mL
    d. 225 mL

78. Number 1 on the figure corresponds to which of the following?
    a. common carotid artery
    b. external jugular vein
    c. internal jugular vein
    d. brachiocephalic artery

79. Number 4 on the figure corresponds to which of the following?
    a. erector spinae muscle
    b. rhomboid major muscle
    c. deltoid muscle
    d. levator scapulae muscle

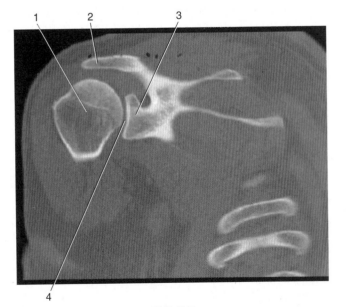

FIG. 7.5

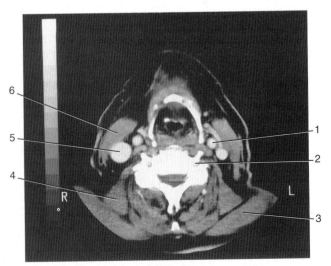

FIG. 7.6

80. The enhancement washout technique for CT characterization of adrenal masses includes:
    1. thin-section precontrast acquisition through the adrenals
    2. arterial phase postcontrast acquisition through the adrenals
    3. 10- to 15-minute delayed postcontrast acquisition through the adrenals
    a. 1 and 2 only
    b. 1 and 3 only
    c. 2 and 3 only
    d. 1, 2, and 3

81. Bowel obstruction due to loss of normal contractile motion in an area of intestine is termed:
    a. dyspepsia
    b. intussusception
    c. ileus
    d. adhesion

Use Fig. 7.7 to answer questions 82–85.

82. Number 5 on the figure corresponds to which of the following?
    a. ascending colon
    b. descending colon
    c. sigmoid colon
    d. cecum

83. Number 3 on the figure corresponds to which of the following?
    a. inferior vena cava
    b. common iliac artery
    c. abdominal aorta
    d. superior mesenteric artery

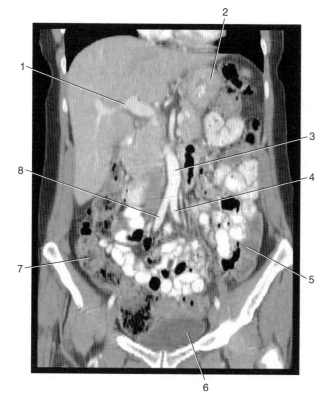

FIG. 7.7

84. Which of the following reformation techniques best describes the image in the figure?
    a. Multiplanar reformation (MPR)
    b. Volume-rendered 3-D
    c. Maximum intensity projection (MIP)
    d. Minimum intensity projection (min-IP)

85. Number 6 on the figure corresponds to which of the following?
    a. uterus
    b. rectum
    c. bladder
    d. sigmoid colon

86. The third ventricle of the brain communicates with the fourth ventricle through the:
    a. anterior commissure
    b. septum pellucidum
    c. cerebral aqueduct
    d. fornix

87. Complete CT examinations of the chest for investigation of bronchogenic carcinoma should include sections from the:
    a. mandible through the liver
    b. apices to the diaphragm
    c. top of the apices through the liver
    d. clavicles through the adrenals

88. The mediastinum includes which of the following anatomic structures?
    1. superior vena cava
    2. stomach
    3. ascending aorta
    a. 1 only
    b. 1 and 2 only
    c. 1 and 3 only
    d. 1, 2, and 3

89. The proper scan field of view (SFOV) for a CT of the abdomen of a patient who measures 42 cm is:
    a. head (25 cm)
    b. small (25 cm)
    c. medium (35 cm)
    d. large (48 cm)

90. The kidneys are located in the retroperitoneum and are bound by a band of fibrous connective tissue called:
    a. Cooper ligament
    b. Camper fascia
    c. linea alba
    d. Gerota's fascia

91. After initiation of rapid bolus administration of an iodinated contrast agent, the portal venous phase of hepatic contrast enhancement occurs at approximately:
    a. 15–20 seconds
    b. 25–35 seconds
    c. 60–70 seconds
    d. 120–180 seconds

Use Fig. 7.8 to answer questions 92–95.

92. Number 1 on the figure corresponds to which of the following?
    a. splenium of the corpus callosum
    b. internal capsule
    c. body of the corpus callosum
    d. genu of the corpus callosum

93. Number 6 on the figure corresponds to which of the following?
    a. anterior cerebral artery
    b. falx cerebri
    c. callosal marginal artery
    d. middle cerebral artery

94. Which number on the figure corresponds to the internal capsule?
    a. 1
    b. 2
    c. 4
    d. 5

95. Number 3 on the figure corresponds to which of the following?
    a. pineal gland
    b. middle cerebral artery
    c. fourth ventricle
    d. aqueduct of Sylvius

96. The prone position may be used for a postmyelogram CT examination of the lumbar spine in an effort to:
    a. reduce the lordotic curve
    b. decrease patient gonadal radiation dose
    c. reduce metrizamide pooling
    d. increase the lordotic curve

97. The bolus duration of any IV contrast agent administration can be calculated as the product of injection flow rate and:
    a. scan time
    b. osmolality
    c. cardiac output
    d. contrast agent volume

Use Figure 7.9 to answer questions 98–101.

98. Number 4 on the figure corresponds to which of the following?
    a. spinous process
    b. lamina
    c. transverse process
    d. pedicle

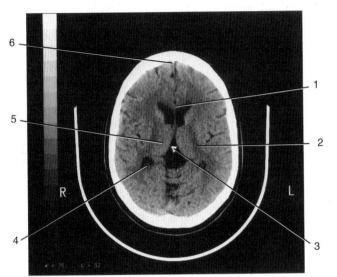

FIG. 7.8

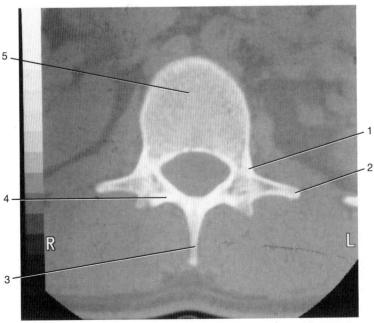

FIG. 7.9

99. Which number on the figure corresponds to the pedicle?
  a. 1
  b. 4
  c. 2
  d. 3

100. The intrathecal administration of an iodinated contrast agent in the patient in the figure would allow for greater visualization of the:
  1. spinal cord
  2. nerve roots
  3. anulus fibrosis
  a. 1 only
  b. 1 and 2 only
  c. 1 and 3 only
  d. 1, 2, and 3

101. Number 3 on the figure corresponds to which of the following?
  a. pedicle
  b. transverse process
  c. lamina
  d. spinous process

102. After initiation of rapid bolus administration of iodinated contrast material, the pancreatic phase of contrast enhancement occurs at approximately:
  a. 15–25 seconds
  b. 35–45 seconds
  c. 60–70 seconds
  d. 120–180 seconds

103. Following the IV administration of iodinated contrast media, a tumor that exhibits a greater density than the surrounding parenchyma is characterized as:
  a. hypervascular
  b. isovascular
  c. hypovascular
  d. cavernous

104. Which of the following is *not* a component of the "triple rule-out" multidetector CT (MDCT) protocol for patients complaining of chest pain?
  a. computed tomography angiogram (CTA) of the pulmonary arteries
  b. prone high-resolution CT (HRCT) of the lungs
  c. CTA of the aorta
  d. coronary CTA

105. During contrast-enhanced CT examinations of the chest, streaking artifact may obscure portions of the superior mediastinum because of dense concentrations of iodine in the:
  a. descending aorta
  b. superior vena cava
  c. ascending aorta
  d. pulmonary arteries

Use Fig. 7.10 to answer questions 106–109.

106. Number 3 on the figure corresponds to which of the following?
  a. esophagus
  b. left pulmonary vein
  c. trachea
  d. left primary bronchus

107. The image in the figure was most likely acquired during which of the following phases of contrast enhancement?
  a. precontrast
  b. arterial phase
  c. venous phase
  d. delayed phase

108. Number 2 on the figure corresponds to which of the following?
  a. left pulmonary artery
  b. descending aorta
  c. left brachiocephalic artery
  d. left subclavian artery

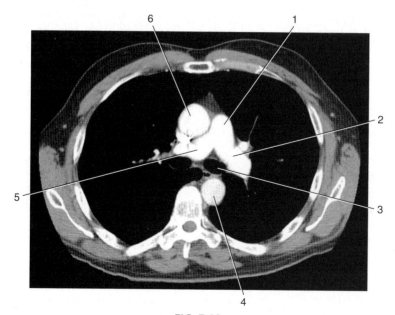

FIG. 7.10

109. Number 6 on the figure corresponds to which of the following?
    a. right atrium
    b. pulmonary trunk
    c. ascending aorta
    d. descending aorta
110. The average density of a mass within the kidney measures −75 Hounsfield units (HU). The mass is most likely a:
    a. cyst
    b. lipoma
    c. stone
    d. hydrocele

IMAGE PRODUCTION

111. The component of the CT scanner responsible for the mathematical calculations of the image reconstruction process is the:
    a. data acquisition system (DAS)
    b. analog-to-digital converter (ADC)
    c. digital-to-analog converter (DAC)
    d. array processor
112. Filament sizes for modern CT x-ray tubes range between:
    a. 0.5 and 1.2 mm
    b. 2.0 and 3.0 mm
    c. 5.5 and 7.8 mm
    d. 25.0 and 31.5 mm
113. Which of the following would serve to increase spatial resolution of a CT examinations using a large focal spot size, 5-mm sections, and a 512^2 matrix?
    1. change to small focal spot size
    2. acquire 2.5-mm sections
    3. reconstruct images in a 320^2 matrix
    a. 1 only
    b. 1 and 2 only
    c. 1 and 3 only
    d. 1, 2, and 3
114. A CT image is formed in part by projecting back all of the attenuation values recorded during data acquisition onto a:
    a. pixel
    b. voxel
    c. matrix
    d. reformat
115. The mathematical process that allows multidetector CT (MDCT) images to be reconstructed at any point along the acquired volume is commonly referred to as:
    a. iteration
    b. filtered back-projection
    c. Fourier reconstruction
    d. z-filtering

116. Fourth-generation CT scanners use a _____ tube-detector configuration.
    a. rotate–translate
    b. electron beam–stationary
    c. rotate–stationary
    d. rotate–rotate
117. Which of the following is considered an equipment-induced CT image artifact?
    a. step artifact
    b. metallic artifact
    c. cupping artifact
    d. aliasing artifact
118. The measurement of CT system performance through quality testing procedures and evaluation of the test results is referred to as:
    a. calibration
    b. uniformity
    c. quality assurance
    d. linearity
119. During CT x-ray exposure, the product of the selected mA setting and the scan time is called the:
    a. effective mAs
    b. peak mAs
    c. absorbed mAs
    d. constant mAs
120. Which of the following mathematical reconstruction methods may be used by a CT system to decrease image noise and offer patient dose savings?
    a. convolution
    b. iterative reconstruction
    c. Fourier transform
    d. back-projection
121. What matrix size was used to reconstruct an image with a display field of view (DFOV) of 25 cm and a pixel area 0.25 mm²?
    a. 80 × 80 pixels
    b. 256 × 256 pixels
    c. 320 × 320 pixels
    d. 512 × 512 pixels
122. When one is viewing a minimum intensity projection (min-IP) image, each pixel represents:
    a. the maximum attenuation occurring within the voxel
    b. the average attenuation occurring within the voxel
    c. the minimum attenuation occurring within the voxel
    d. all attenuation occurring within the voxel above a set threshold value
123. Which of the following statements regarding predetector collimation of the CT x-ray beam is true?
    a. Predetector collimation reduces patient radiation dose.
    b. Predetector collimation reduces the production of scatter radiation.
    c. Predetector collimation determines the scan field of view (SFOV).
    d. Predetector collimation removes scatter radiation before it reaches the detectors.

124. Which of the following equations shows the Lambert–Beer law, which describes the relationship between matter and attenuation?

  a. $\text{Attenuation} = \dfrac{I_0}{I}$

  b. $\text{CT number} = \dfrac{\mu_t - \mu_w}{\mu_w \times K}$

  c. $I_0 = Ix^{-e\mu}$
  d. $I = I_0 e^{-\mu x}$

Use Fig. 7.11 to answer questions 125 and 126.

125. The graph in the figure is used to evaluate which of the following components of CT image quality?
  a. in-plane spatial resolution
  b. longitudinal spatial resolution
  c. temporal resolution
  d. contrast resolution

126. On the basis of the information provided on the graph in the figure, which of the following statements is true?
  a. The limiting resolution in section A is less than that in section B.
  b. The signal-to-noise ratio (SNR) of section A is greater than that of section B.
  c. The effective width of section B is greater than that of section A.
  d. Section B is isotropic in dimension.

127. Which of the following would be considered the best method to reduce respiratory motion on the CT image?
  a. good patient–technologist communication
  b. reduced scan times
  c. immobilization devices
  d. glucagon administration

128. Power output for a modern multidetector CT (MDCT) x-ray tube has an approximate range of:
  a. 3–5 kilowatts (kW)
  b. 15–20 kilowatts (kW)
  c. 40–48 kilowatts (kW)
  d. 60–100 kilowatts (kW)

129. The mathematical manipulations required during the reconstruction of a CT image are accomplished using a(n):
  1. algorithm
  2. kernel
  3. mathematical filter function
  a. 1 only
  b. 1 and 2 only
  c. 1 and 3 only
  d. 1, 2, and 3

130. When an operator reduces the scan field of view for a particular body part, which of the following technical changes occurs?
  1. The displayed image appears larger.
  2. Spatial resolution increases.
  3. A smaller number of detectors are activated.
  4. The displayed image appears smaller.

131. An average CT number value for blood is:
  a. –20 HU
  b. +10 HU
  c. +45 HU
  d. +100 HU

132. The electronic combination of signals from adjacent detectors to form a CT image is called:
  a. binning
  b. interpolation
  c. z-filtering
  d. partial volume averaging

133. Which of the following technical adjustments may be employed to improve the temporal resolution of a multidetector CT (MDCT) system?
  1. decrease in section width
  2. image segmentation
  3. physiologic gating
  a. 1 only
  b. 3 only
  c. 1 and 2 only
  d. 2 and 3 only

134. The streaking artifact that occurs in the area of the posterior fossa during a CT examination of the brain may be referred to as:
  a. cupping
  b. the "boiled egg" artifact
  c. stairstep
  d. the Hounsfield bar

135. The relative accuracy between calculated CT numbers and their respective linear attenuation coefficients is referred to as:
  a. linearity
  b. calibration
  c. uniformity
  d. contrast resolution

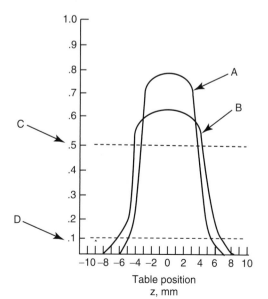

Table position
z, mm

FIG. 7.11

136. To maintain security and patient privacy when medical images are transmitted across a network, the images may be coded in a form decipherable only by software at the destination location. This process is referred to as:
    a. write-once, read-many (WORM)
    b. Hypertext Transfer Protocol (HTTP)
    c. teleradiology
    d. encryption

137. Which of the following 3-D imaging techniques is utilized to provide "fly-through" images during CT colonography?
    a. orthographic volume rendering
    b. shaded surface display (SSD)
    c. perspective volume rendering
    d. minimum intensity projection (min-IP)

138. Which of the following sets of technical factors would yield an isotropic data set when a multidetector CT (MDCT) image is reconstructed using a 512^2 matrix?
    a. 5.0-mm sections, 17-cm DFOV
    b. 3.0-mm sections, 25-cm DFOV
    c. 1.25-mm sections, 48-cm DFOV
    d. 0.625-mm sections, 32-cm DFOV

139. Which of the following is *not* commonly used as a CT scintillation detector material?
    a. ceramic rare earth
    b. silver halide
    c. bismuth germanate
    d. cadmium tungstate

140. The mathematical technique that involves the estimation of an unknown value from values on either side of it is known as:
    a. filtering
    b. interpolation
    c. convolution
    d. summation

141. During which of the following CT examinations is a misregistration artifact most likely to occur?
    a. brain
    b. pelvis
    c. neck
    d. abdomen

142. In a single-slice CT (SSCT) system, which of the following technical parameters may be adjusted retrospectively?
    1. section width
    2. section increment
    3. reconstruction algorithm
    a. 2 only
    b. 1 and 2 only
    c. 2 and 3 only
    d. 1, 2, and 3

143. Bow-tie filters are employed in a CT x-ray system to reduce:
    a. image noise
    b. low spatial frequency signal
    c. patient radiation dose
    d. high spatial frequency signal

144. Which of the following technical factors is/are involved in the determination of section width for multidetector CT (MDCT) images?
    1. scan field of view (SFOV)
    2. beam collimation
    3. detector configuration
    a. 2 only
    b. 1 and 2 only
    c. 1 and 3 only
    d. 2 and 3 only

145. The fluctuation of CT numbers in an image of uniform, homogeneous material may occur because of:
    a. linearity
    b. noise
    c. aliasing
    d. partial volume effect

146. A region of interest (ROI) measurement placed over a portion of a CT image provides which of the following?
    a. distance (mm)
    b. diameter (mm)
    c. linear attenuation coefficient (μ)
    d. average CT number (HU)

147. A multidetector CT (MDCT) image is reconstructed using a 512^2 matrix and a display field of view (DFOV) of 38 cm. If the detector collimation is set to a section width of 1.25 mm, what is the volume of each voxel?
    a. 0.69 mm^3
    b. 0.93 mm^3
    c. 1.26 mm^3
    d. 1.68 mm^3

Use Fig. 7.12 to answer questions 148–150.

148. Which of the following is the common term for the artifact present on the image in the figure?
     a. aliasing
     b. streaking
     c. edge gradient
     d. tube arcing

149. Which of the following would be the most common cause of the artifact in the figure?
     a. metallic dental fillings
     b. partial volume averaging
     c. beam hardening
     d. detector malfunction

150. Reduction of the type of artifact seen in the figure on a coronal multidetector CT (MDCT) view of the sinuses may be accomplished through:
     a. an increase in the mA
     b. a decrease in the kVp
     c. coronal multiplanar reformation (MPR) images built from an axial acquisition
     d. a reduction in the scan field of view (SFOV)

151. First-generation CT scanners used a method of data acquisition based on a _____ principle.
     a. multiplanar
     b. rotation-only
     c. translate–rotate
     d. transaxial

152. The maximum beam collimation for a multidetector CT (MDCT) system with a detector array of 64 detectors, each 0.625 mm wide, is:
     a. 1.25 mm
     b. 5.00 mm
     c. 10.00 mm
     d. 40.00 mm

153. Compared with conventional radiography, computed tomography produces diagnostic images with better:
     a. low-contrast resolution
     b. spatial resolution
     c. minute detail
     d. patient radiation dose reduction

154. Writable CD and DVD media are optical disks that may be described as:
     a. read-only
     b. lossy
     c. write-once, read-many (WORM)
     d. lossless

155. A CT system measures the average linear attenuation coefficient of a voxel of tissue to be 0.008. The linear attenuation coefficient of water for this scanner equals 0.181. The CT number assigned to the pixel representing this voxel of tissue equals:
     a. −956 HU
     b. −173 HU
     c. +44 HU
     d. +1044 HU

156. Which of the following statements comparing the efficiency of scintillation and gas ionization detectors is correct?
     a. Both have approximately the same capture efficiency.
     b. The scintillation detector has a higher capture efficiency.
     c. Unlike the scintillation detector, the gas ionization detector has a problem with afterglow.
     d. Gas ionization detectors have a higher conversion efficiency.

157. The data acquisition system (DAS) of a CT scanner is responsible for:
     1. measuring transmitted intensity
     2. converting the transmission data into a digital signal
     3. sending the digital information to the computer for processing
     a. 1 only
     b. 2 only
     c. 1 and 3 only
     d. 1, 2, and 3

158. Which of the following is used to remove image blurring during the back-projection method of CT image reconstruction?
     1. z-filtering
     2. convolution kernel
     3. Feldkamp–Davis–Kress (FDK) algorithm
     a. 2 only
     b. 3 only
     c. 1 and 2 only
     d. 2 and 3 only

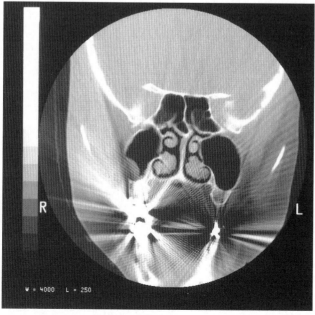

FIG. 7.12

159. During CT x-ray production, the electromagnetic steering of the electron beam from the cathode to two alternating targets is referred to as:
   a. prospective gating
   b. ultrafast CT
   c. twin CAT
   d. flying focal spot

Use Fig. 7.13 to answer questions 160–162.

160. The region of interest (ROI) measurement in the figure provides an average density of +1.9 HU. This material is most likely:
   a. fat
   b. blood
   c. tumor
   d. water

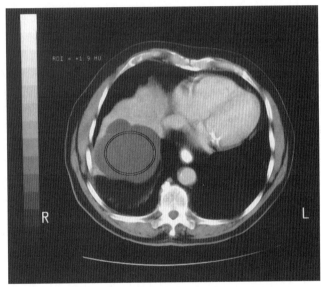

FIG. 7.13

161. The material within the region of interest (ROI) measurement in the figure has a linear attenuation coefficient of:
   a. 0.0007
   b. 0.185
   c. 0.206
   d. 0.530

162. The image in the figure was most likely displayed with the use of which of the following window widths?
   a. 70
   b. 400
   c. 1300
   d. 3800

163. Areas of a CT image that contain minimal changes in tissue density are electronically represented by:
   a. positive CT numbers
   b. high spatial frequencies
   c. negative CT numbers
   d. low spatial frequencies

164. A CT image is displayed in a window with a level of +200 and a width of 1000. Which of the following statements is correct?
   a. Pixels with values between +200 HU and −1000 HU will appear white.
   b. Pixels with values greater than +200 HU will appear black.
   c. Pixels with values between −300 HU and +700 HU will be assigned shades of gray.
   d. Pixels with values between −1200 HU and +1200 HU will be assigned shades of gray.

165. In the binary number system, a byte is a series of _____ bits of information.
   a. two
   b. four
   c. eight
   d. sixteen

8

Simulated Examination Three

QUESTIONS

PATIENT CARE

1. The use of water as an oral contrast material for CT of the abdomen and/or pelvis has several potential advantages, including:
   1. increased palatability and improved patient comfort
   2. better demonstration of enhancing bowel wall
   3. no interference with 3-D applications
   a. 1 only
   b. 1 and 2 only
   c. 1 and 3 only
   d. 1, 2, and 3

2. A patient's blood pressure is measured as 140/70 mm Hg. The number 140 represents:
   a. the pressure within the arterial vessels during contraction of the heart
   b. the pressure exerted on the chambers of the heart while it is relaxed
   c. the pressure within the arterial vessels while the heart is relaxed
   d. the pressure exerted on the chambers of the heart during a contraction

3. A(n) _____ contrast material may be described as one that does not dissociate into charged particles in solution.
   a. neutral
   b. nonionic
   c. osmolar
   d. ionic

4. Proper immobilization during a CT procedure may involve the use of:
   1. soft, hook-and-loop (e.g., Velcro) immobilization straps
   2. adhesive medical tape
   3. good patient communication
   a. 1 only
   b. 1 and 2 only
   c. 1 and 3 only
   d. 1, 2, and 3

5. The normal range of glomerular filtration rate (GFR) for men is:
   a. 50 ± 14 mL/min/m^2
   b. 60 ± 10 mL/min/m^2
   c. 70 ± 14 mL/min/m^2
   d. 80 ± 10 mL/min/m^2

6. Risk factors for contrast-induced nephrotoxicity (CIN) include:
   1. diabetes
   2. advanced age
   3. hematuria
   a. 1 only
   b. 3 only
   c. 1 and 2 only
   d. 1, 2, and 3

7. The reduction in number of infectious organisms without a complete elimination is termed:
   a. medical asepsis
   b. sterilization
   c. surgical asepsis
   d. immunization

8. Which of the following is the preferred range for patient heart rate for optimal cardiac CT studies?
   a. 65–75 bpm
   b. 75–85 bpm
   c. 85–95 bpm
   d. >100 bpm

9. *Urticaria* is which of the following?
   a. severe nausea with associated vomiting
   b. urinary tract infection
   c. hives
   d. bronchospasm

10. Which of the following type(s) of oral contrast material could cause peritonitis if leakage from the digestive tract occurs from perforation?
    a. iopamidol (Gastrografin)
    b. barium sulfate
    c. diatrizoate (Hypaque)
    d. effervescent granules

11. Which of the following is not an advantage of an automatic power injector over the manual bolus method of intravenous contrast agent administration?
    a. uniform contrast enhancement throughout the examination
    b. consistent contrast agent administration for all patients
    c. decreased risk of contrast-induced nephrotoxicity (CIN)
    d. shorter injection times

12. Which of the following is/are severe adverse reaction(s) to iodinated intravenous contrast media?
    1. anaphylaxis
    2. urticaria
    3. vomiting
    a. 1 only
    b. 1 and 2 only
    c. 1 and 3 only
    d. 1, 2, and 3

13. Which of the following laboratory values is the most dependable measure of renal function?
    a. Blood urea nitrogen (BUN)
    b. creatinine
    c. Prothrombin time (PT)
    d. Partial thromboplastin time (PTT)

14. Which of the following angiocatheter sizes may be safely used for the automated power injection of iodinated contrast agents at flow rates higher than 3 mL/sec?
    1. 18-gauge
    2. 20-gauge
    3. 22-gauge
    a. 1 only
    b. 3 only
    c. 1 and 2 only
    d. 1, 2, and 3

15. Which of the following portions of the electrocardiogram (ECG) corresponds to the period of atrial systole?
    a. P wave
    b. QRS complex
    c. alpha wave
    d. T wave

16. Which of the following terms is used to describe the intravenous injection of medication or contrast agent in one complete dose over a short time?
    a. infusion
    b. bolus
    c. IV drip
    d. Infus-A-Port

17. Used in determining the biologic effect of iodinated contrast media, the term _____ refers to the number of ions formed when a substance dissociates in solution.
    a. solubility
    b. osmolality
    c. concentration
    d. iodination

18. The injection rate of an automatic injector is set at 1.5 mL/sec. What is the injection time for a contrast agent volume of 150 mL?
    a. 60 seconds
    b. 90 seconds
    c. 100 seconds
    d. 120 seconds

19. Which of the following must be included when one is obtaining informed consent for an invasive procedure?
    1. explanation of the examination techniques
    2. the possible risks and benefits of the examination
    3. alternatives to the procedure involved
    a. 1 only
    b. 1 and 2 only
    c. 1 and 3 only
    d. 1, 2, and 3

20. Which of the following may be considered a low-osmolar contrast medium?
    1. iothalamate meglumine
    2. diatrizoate sodium
    3. iohexol
    a. 1 only
    b. 3 only
    c. 1 and 2 only
    d. 1, 2, and 3

21. After the intrathecal injection of an iodinated contrast agent for a postmyelography CT study of the lumbar spine, the patient should be instructed to:
    a. take a cleansing enema
    b. resume normal activity
    c. rest for 8–24 hours with the head slightly elevated
    d. rest for 8–24 hours in the Trendelenburg position

22. Which of the following pharmaceuticals may be administered before a cardiac CT procedure in an effort to improve visualization of the coronary vessels?
    1. β-blocker
    2. nitroglycerin
    3. metformin
    a. 1 only
    b. 2 only
    c. 1 and 2 only
    d. 1, 2, and 3

SAFETY

23. During CT examinations of the chest and abdomen, the highly radiosensitive breast tissue can be protected with minimal image artifact with the use of specialized shielding composed of:
    a. barium
    b. aluminum
    c. lead
    d. bismuth

24. As part of a comprehensive approach to minimize CT radiation exposure to the pediatric patient, the technologist should:
    1. precisely limit the acquisition to the indicated anatomical area
    2. refuse to perform unnecessary CT examinations
    3. reduce the technical parameters (e.g., mA, kVp) based upon the body habitus
    a. 2 only
    b. 1 and 2 only
    c. 1 and 3 only
    d. 1, 2, and 3

25. An x-ray photon may lose some of its energy in an interaction with an outer-shell electron of a target atom within the patient in the interaction know as:
    a. Compton scatter
    b. Rayleigh scatter
    c. photoelectric absorption
    d. pair production

26. Which of the following may be used to calculate the dose length product of a CT acquisition?
    1. DLP = slice width (cm) × pitch
    2. DLP = MSAD × slice width (cm) × # of slices in scan volume
    3. DLP = $CTDI_{vol}$ × scan length (cm)
    a. 1 and 2 only
    b. 1 and 3 only
    c. 2 and 3 only
    d. 1, 2, and 3

27. If all other technical factors remain constant, which of the following would serve to decrease patient radiation dose during a helical single-slice CT (SSCT) examination?
    a. decreased scan field of view (SFOV)
    b. decreased filtration
    c. increased pitch
    d. increased matrix size

28. Electrocardiogram (ECG)-gated tube current modulation may effectively reduce patient radiation dose during which of the following procedures?
    a. CT colonography
    b. brain perfusion CT
    c. CT urogram
    d. cardiac CT

29. Which of the following radiation dose indices is a measure of the total radiation exposure for an entire series of CT images?
    a. $CTDI_{100}$
    b. dose length product (DLP)
    c. $CTDI_{vol}$
    d. multiple scan average dose (MSAD)

30. *Effective dose* is a relative radiation dose measurement term that accounts for the:
    a. beam pitch
    b. tissue radiosensitivity
    c. detector pitch
    d. collimation

31. The dose modulation capabilities of a CT scanner may include automatic control of:
    1. tube current (milliamperage)
    2. tube potential (applied kilovoltage)
    3. focus-to-isocenter distance (centimeters)
    a. 1 only
    b. 1 and 2 only
    c. 2 and 3 only
    d. 1, 2, and 3

32. Late effects of radiation, such as genetic mutations, may occur with even small doses of radiation and are termed:
    a. stochastic
    b. somatic
    c. nonstochastic
    d. chronic

33. Assuming no other technical changes are made, which of the following adjustments would result in *decreased* radiation dose to the patient for a given CT acquisition?
    1. Eliminate a clinically unnecessary contrast phase acquisition.
    2. Increase the tolerated noise level of the scan.
    3. Increase tube potential (kVp) from 100 to 140.
    4. Increase the pitch from 1.0 to 1.5.
    5. Decrease the scan length along the z-axis.
    a. 1, 3, and 5 only
    b. 2, 3, and 4 only
    c. 1, 2, 4, and 5 only
    d. All (1–5)

34. Which of the following statements is true regarding the relationship between multiple scan average dose (MSAD) and image spacing during axial (step-and-shoot) scanning?
    a. MSAD decreases with overlapping scans.
    b. MSAD increases with overlapping scans.
    c. MSAD increases with noncontiguous scans.
    d. MSAD equals the product of image spacing and pitch.

35. The dosimetry index used to approximate the radiation dose for CT sections acquired during a helical scan is called the:
    a. $CTDI_W$
    b. effective dose
    c. $CTDI_{vol}$
    d. equivalent dose

36. Which of the following techniques may be employed to reduce patient radiation dose during a cardiac CT examination?
    a. retrospective electrocardiogram (ECG) gating
    b. z-axis interpolation
    c. prospective ECG gating
    d. multisegment reconstruction

37. Which of the following reconstruction methods may be employed by a CT system for the purpose of reducing patient radiation dose?
    a. convolution reconstruction
    b. interpolation reconstruction
    c. back-projection reconstruction
    d. iterative reconstruction

38. The dose length product (DLP) is identical for a given CT scan acquired on two patients, each with a significantly different body habitus. Which of the following statements is correct?
    a. The absorbed dose is identical in each patient.
    b. The absorbed dose is greater in the patient with a larger body habitus.
    c. The absorbed dose is greater in the patient with a smaller body habitus.
    d. Dose length product is unrelated to absorbed dose in the patient.

39. Compared with single-slice CT (SSCT), patient radiation dose during a multidetector CT study may be higher because of:
    1. use of a cone beam of radiation
    2. acquisitions at thinner section widths
    3. higher-powered x-ray tubes
    a. 1 only
    b. 1 and 2 only
    c. 1 and 3 only
    d. 1, 2, and 3

40. Which of the following will *not* reduce patient exposure during CT?
    a. increase mA from 180 to 360
    b. increase pitch from 1.0 to 1.5
    c. increase tolerated noise level (index)
    d. increase table speed from 32 to 48 mm/sec

41. Model-based iterative reconstruction (MBIR) considers which of the following during CT image formation?
    a. the shape of the x-ray beam before (pre-) and after (post-) the patient
    b. a master image stored in the CT system's computer
    c. the detector configuration used for the acquisition
    d. the age, gender, and weight of the scanned patient

42. The reduction in intensity of an x-ray beam as it interacts with matter is called:
    a. scatter
    b. attenuation
    c. transmission
    d. luminescence

IMAGING PROCEDURES

43. A _____ is a benign, highly vascular mass commonly found in the liver.
    a. hematoid
    b. vasculoma
    c. hemogenic carcinoma
    d. hemangioma

44. Which of the following is the preferred contrast enhancement phase for CT acquisition of the spleen?
    a. precontrast phase
    b. equilibrium phase
    c. arterial phase
    d. portal venous phase

Use Fig. 8.1 to answer questions 45–48.

45. Number 2 on the figure corresponds to which of the following?
    a. capitate
    b. lunate
    c. hamate
    d. scaphoid

46. The anatomic plane of the image in the figure can be best described as the:
    a. coronal plane
    b. sagittal plane
    c. axial plane
    d. oblique axial plane

47. Number 1 on the figure corresponds to which of the following?
    a. capitate
    b. lunate
    c. hamate
    d. scaphoid

48. Number 5 on the figure corresponds to which of the following?
    a. capitate
    b. lunate
    c. hamate
    d. scaphoid

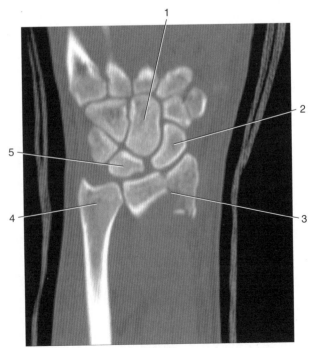

FIG. 8.1

49. Which of the following terms describes the appearance of an acute subdural hematoma on a CT image of the brain?
    a. radiolucent
    b. hyperdense
    c. hypodense
    d. isodense

50. The angiographic assessment known as a *CT runoff* evaluates the peripheral arterial tree from the renal arteries through the:
    a. aortic arch
    b. superior mesenteric artery
    c. aortic bifurcation
    d. distal lower extremity

51. During a PET-CT examination, the amount of fludeoxyglucose F 18 (FDG) uptake in an anatomic region is directly proportional to the area's:
    a. size
    b. central vs. peripheral location
    c. radiosensitivity
    d. metabolic activity

Use Fig. 8.2 to answer questions 52–54.

52. Number 2 on the figure corresponds to which of the following?
    a. left ovary
    b. bladder
    c. sigmoid colon
    d. uterus

53. Number 4 on the figure corresponds to which of the following?
    a. left ovary
    b. bladder
    c. sigmoid colon
    d. uterus

54. Number 5 on the figure corresponds to which of the following?
    a. left ovary
    b. bladder
    c. sigmoid colon
    d. uterus

55. Accurate demonstration of _____ would most likely require the intravenous injection of an iodinated contrast agent during a CT study of the chest.
    a. pneumonia
    b. asbestosis
    c. a dissecting aortic aneurysm
    d. a solitary pulmonary nodule

56. The benign mass of the eighth cranial nerve known as a *vestibular schwannoma* may also be termed a(n):
    a. acoustic neuroma
    b. hypoglossal adenoma
    c. olfactory neuroblastoma
    d. optic nerve glioma

Use Fig. 8.3 to answer questions 57–60.

57. Number 3 on the figure corresponds to which of the following?
    a. cricoid cartilage
    b. piriform sinus
    c. aryepiglottic fold
    d. vocal cord

58. Number 1 on the figure corresponds to which of the following?
    a. trachea
    b. piriform sinus
    c. aryepiglottic fold
    d. vocal cord

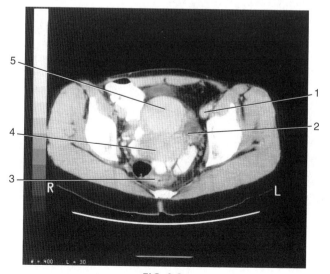

FIG. 8.2

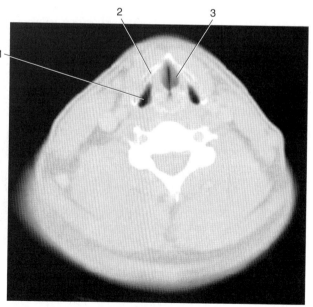

FIG. 8.3

59. Which of the following window settings was most likely used to display the image in the figure?
    a. WL −300, WW 1000
    b. WL −50, WW 50
    c. WL +50, WW 150
    d. WL +400, WW 3000
60. Number 2 on the figure corresponds to which of the following?
    a. hyoid bone
    b. cricoid cartilage
    c. thyroid cartilage
    d. mandible
61. The thick, layered portion of the peritoneum responsible for attaching portions of the intestines to the bowel wall is called the:
    a. Gerota fascia
    b. falciform ligament
    c. mesentery
    d. ligamentum teres
62. After initiation of rapid bolus administration of an iodinated contrast agent, the nephrographic phase of renal contrast enhancement occurs at approximately:
    a. 20–25 seconds
    b. 30–40 seconds
    c. 70–90 seconds
    d. 3–5 minutes

Use Fig. 8.4 to answer questions 63–66.

63. Number 9 on the figure corresponds to which of the following?
    a. ethmoid sinus
    b. nasal concha
    c. maxillary sinus
    d. sphenoid sinus
64. Number 5 on the figure corresponds to which of the following?
    a. optic nerve
    b. superior ophthalmic vein
    c. oculomotor nerve
    d. superior oblique muscle
65. Number 4 on the figure corresponds to which of the following?
    a. superior rectus muscle
    b. superior ophthalmic vein
    c. levator palpebrae superioris muscle
    d. superior oblique muscle
66. Number 6 on the figure corresponds to which of the following?
    a. optic nerve
    b. medial rectus muscle
    c. lateral rectus muscle
    d. oculomotor nerve
67. Which of the following is a common complication of CT-guided biopsy of the lung?
    a. pulmonary embolism
    b. aspiration
    c. pneumoconiosis
    d. pneumothorax

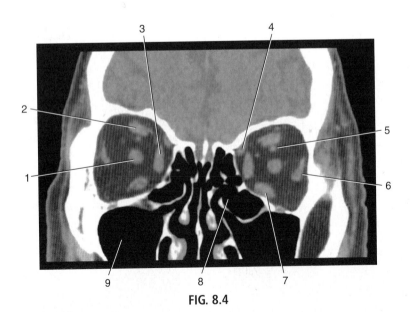

FIG. 8.4

Use Fig. 8.5 to answer questions 68–70.

68. Number 6 on the figure corresponds to which of the following?
    a. renal cortex
    b. renal pelvis
    c. renal calyx
    d. renal pyramid
69. Which of the following reformation techniques best describes the image in the figure?
    a. volume-rendered 3-D
    b. multiplanar reformation (MPR)
    c. minimum intensity projection (min-IP)
    d. maximum intensity projection (MIP)
70. Number 1 on the figure corresponds to which of the following?
    a. ureteropelvic junction
    b. ureterovesical junction
    c. ureterocalyceal junction
    d. ureteropyramidal junction
71. A common formula used to calculate the maximum dosage of intravenous iodinated contrast material used in any CT examination is:
    a. 5 mg per kg of body weight
    b. 5 mL per lb of body weight
    c. 2 mL per kg of body weight
    d. 1 mL per lb of body weight
72. Which of the following multidetector CT (MDCT) examinations may include endobrachial views?
    a. virtual colonoscopy
    b. high-resolution CT (HRCT) of the lungs
    c. virtual bronchoscopy
    d. computed tomography angiogram (CTA) of the aorta

73. During high-resolution CT (HRCT) of the lungs, edematous changes in the posterior lungs may be differentiated by positioning of the patient in the _____ position.
    a. supine
    b. right lateral decubitus
    c. left lateral decubitus
    d. prone
74. The firm, outer portion of each intervertebral disc is called the:
    a. nucleus pulposus
    b. nucleus prepositus
    c. anulus fibrosus
    d. anulus stapedius

Use Fig. 8.6 to answer questions 75–77.

75. Number 2 on the figure corresponds to which of the following?
    a. superior facet
    b. pedicle
    c. transverse process
    d. lamina
76. Number 1 on the figure corresponds to which of the following?
    a. spinal root
    b. superior articular recess
    c. anterior arch
    d. transverse foramen
77. Number 4 on the figure corresponds to which of the following?
    a. superior facet
    b. pedicle
    c. transverse process
    d. lamina
78. During which of the following IV contrast phases does the bladder wall enhance?
    a. early arterial
    b. corticomedullary
    c. nephrographic
    d. excretory

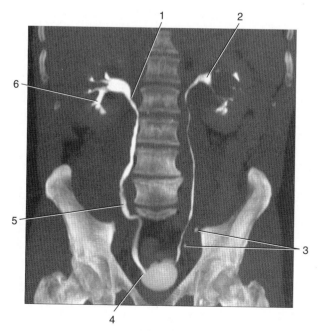

FIG. 8.5

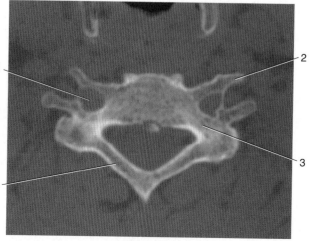

FIG. 8.6

79. Coronary artery calcium (CAC) quantitation by multidetector CT (MDCT) examination is used primarily to assess:
    a. aortic aneurysm
    b. atherosclerotic disease
    c. coronary artery stenosis
    d. ejection fraction

Use Fig. 8.7 to answer questions 80–83.

80. Number 4 on the figure corresponds to which of the following?
    a. left common iliac artery
    b. right common iliac artery
    c. left common iliac vein
    d. right common iliac artery

81. The best method for targeting the sacrum in the figure for detailed examination would be to:
    a. magnify the image 2×
    b. rescan the patient using a small scan field of view (SFOV)
    c. retrospectively reconstruct the image using a small display field of view (DFOV)
    d. decrease the matrix dimension

82. Number 5 on the figure corresponds to which of the following?
    a. right common iliac vein
    b. right ureter
    c. left common iliac vein
    d. inferior mesenteric vein

83. Number 1 on the figure corresponds to which of the following?
    a. psoas muscle
    b. gluteus medius muscle
    c. iliacus muscle
    d. rectus abdominis muscle

84. A specialized CT examination involving the administration of an enteral contrast agent directly into the small bowel via nasogastric tube is called:
    a. CT enteroclysis
    b. CT colonography
    c. CT enterography
    d. CT colonoscopy

85. The epithelial lining of the urinary tract is called the:
    a. omentum
    b. haustrum
    c. urothelium
    d. pyelocalyx

86. The primary drainage opening within the sinus cavities, which is a common area for inflammation, is referred to as the:
    a. mucosal fossa
    b. adenovestibular complex
    c. external olfactory canal
    d. ostiomeatal complex

Use Fig. 8.8 to answer questions 87–91.

87. Number 1 on the figure corresponds to which of the following?
    a. right brachiocephalic artery
    b. right pulmonary artery
    c. right pericardiacophrenic artery
    d. right subclavian artery

88. Which of the following best describes the type of image displayed in the figure?
    a. coronal maximum intensity projection (MIP)
    b. direct coronal acquisition
    c. coronal multiplanar reformation (MPR)
    d. coronal minimum intensity projection (min-IP)

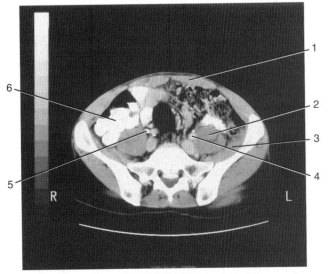

FIG. 8.7

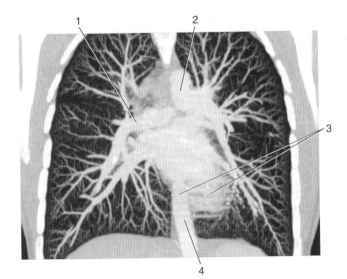

FIG. 8.8

89. Number 4 on the figure corresponds to which of the following?
    a. gastric artery
    b. inferior vena cava (IVC)
    c. superior mesenteric artery (SMA)
    d. descending aorta

90. The areas of image quality degradation indicated by number 3 on the figure are an example of:
    a. aliasing artifact
    b. windmill artifact
    c. pulsation artifact
    d. beam-hardening artifact

91. Number 2 on the figure corresponds to which of the following?
    a. aortic arch
    b. pulmonary trunk
    c. superior vena cava
    d. left anterior descending artery

92. During CT examination of the chest, the administration of a saline flush after the bolus injection of iodinated IV contrast media helps alleviate artifact from dense contrast in the:
    a. ascending aorta
    b. superior vena cava
    c. descending aorta
    d. inferior vena cava

93. Delayed postcontrast acquisition of the lower extremities after a CT angiogram (CTA) of the pulmonary arteries is termed:
    a. CT venography
    b. CT perfusion
    c. femoral CTA
    d. iliac CTA

Use Fig. 8.9 to answer questions 94–97.

94. Number 4 on the figure corresponds to which of the following?
    a. third ventricle
    b. quadrigeminal cistern
    c. fourth ventricle
    d. sagittal sinus

95. Number 2 on the figure corresponds to which of the following?
    a. left posterior cerebral artery
    b. left middle cerebral artery
    c. left anterior cerebral artery
    d. left posterior communicating artery

96. Number 5 on the figure corresponds to which of the following?
    a. posterior communicating artery
    b. anterior communicating artery
    c. internal carotid artery
    d. basilar artery

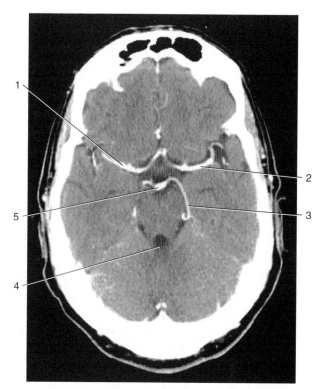

FIG. 8.9

97. Number 3 on the figure corresponds to which of the following?
    a. left posterior cerebral artery
    b. left middle cerebral artery
    c. left anterior cerebral artery
    d. left posterior communicating artery

98. The overall quality of multiplanar reformation (MPR) and volume-rendered 3-D images for a carotid artery CT angiogram (CTA) may be improved by:
    1. reducing the kVp for an increase in displayed vessel opacification and contrast
    2. retrospective reconstructions with a 50% overlap in section increment
    3. bolus-tracking software to maximize contrast enhancement
    a. 2 only
    b. 1 and 2 only
    c. 2 and 3 only
    d. 1, 2, and 3

99. Which of the following is the most common sign of gastrointestinal (GI) pathology on CT images?
    a. fluid collection
    b. wall thickening
    c. air distention
    d. dense fecal matter

Use Fig. 8.10 to answer questions 100–103.

100. Number 2 on the figure corresponds to which of the following?
   a. right brachiocephalic vein
   b. left subclavian artery
   c. left brachiocephalic vein
   d. brachiocephalic artery

101. Number 5 on the figure corresponds to which of the following?
   a. right brachiocephalic vein
   b. left subclavian artery
   c. left brachiocephalic vein
   d. brachiocephalic artery

102. Number 1 on the figure corresponds to which of the following?
   a. right brachiocephalic vein
   b. left subclavian artery
   c. left brachiocephalic vein
   d. brachiocephalic artery

103. Which number on the figure corresponds to the left common carotid artery?
   a. 1
   b. 6
   c. 4
   d. 3

104. Arterial phase CT imaging of the liver is used to optimally demonstrate which of the following?
   a. fatty infiltration
   b. hepatic cysts
   c. portal vein thrombosis
   d. hepatocellular carcinoma (HCC)

105. Noncontrast CT of the urinary tract is a valuable tool in the investigation of:
   a. transitional cell carcinoma (TCC)
   b. urinary tract lithiasis
   c. renal artery stenosis
   d. ureteral duplication

106. Which of the following techniques may be used to improve visualization of the vocal cords during a CT examination of the neck?
   1. oral administration of thick barium paste
   2. CT acquisition with the mouth open as widely as tolerable
   3. scanning while the patient phonates the letter "E"
   a. 2 only
   b. 3 only
   c. 1 and 3 only
   d. 1, 2, and 3

Use Fig. 8.11 to answer questions 107–109.

107. Which number on the figure corresponds to the superior mesenteric vein?
   a. 3
   b. 5
   c. 1
   d. 2

108. Number 4 on the figure corresponds to which of the following?
   a. descending colon
   b. spleen
   c. adrenal gland
   d. renal vein

109. Number 6 on the figure corresponds to which of the following?
   a. duodenum
   b. terminal ileum
   c. appendix
   d. pancreas

110. Percutaneous drainage under CT guidance may be used for the aspiration of which of the following pathologic processes?
   a. chronic subdural hematoma
   b. hydrocephalus
   c. abdominal abscess
   d. dissecting aortic aneurysm

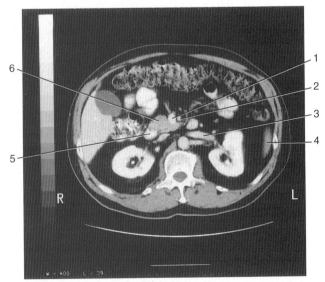

FIG. 8.10   **FIG. 8.11**

PHYSICS AND INSTRUMENTATION

111. The device constructed to house the x-ray tube and data acquisition system (DAS) for a CT scanner is called the:
    a. central processing unit (CPU)
    b. generator
    c. array processor
    d. gantry

112. Third-generation CT scanners use which of the following scan geometries?
    a. translate–rotate
    b. rotate–stationary
    c. transaxial
    d. rotate–rotate

113. A quality control procedure determines that the low-contrast resolution of a CT scanner is extremely poor. Likely causes are:
    1. tube arcing
    2. increased electronic noise
    3. decreased tube output
    a. 1 only
    b. 1 and 3 only
    c. 2 and 3 only
    d. 1, 2, and 3

114. When one is viewing a maximum intensity projection (MIP) image, each pixel represents:
    a. the maximum attenuation occurring within the voxel
    b. the average attenuation occurring within the voxel
    c. the minimum attenuation occurring within the voxel
    d. all attenuation occurring within the voxel above a set threshold value

115. A CT image is reconstructed using a 512^2 matrix and a display field of view of 40 cm. What is the linear dimension of each pixel?
    a. 0.0015 mm
    b. 0.08 mm
    c. 0.78 mm
    d. 1.28 mm

116. Which of the following statements about collimation of the CT x-ray beam is false?
    a. Collimation of the x-ray beam occurs both before and after the patient.
    b. Collimation of the beam occurs in the z-axis, thus affecting slice thickness.
    c. Increases in collimation increase the intensity of the primary beam.
    d. Collimation of the CT x-ray beam is used to limit the detection of scatter radiation.

117. Which of the following terms may be used to describe the quantity of radiation emitted from the CT x-ray tube toward the patient?
    a. effective mAs
    b. photon flux
    c. constant mAs
    d. photon fluence

118. Which of the following is the most common type of noise found in the CT image?
    a. quantum noise
    b. electronic noise
    c. artifactual noise
    d. filter noise

119. A picture archival and communications system (PACS) is connected with imaging modalities and other peripheral devices on a computerized communications system called a:
    a. network
    b. web
    c. radiology information system (RIS)
    d. hospital information system (HIS)

Use Fig. 8.12 to answer questions 120–122.

120. Which of the following artifacts is evident on the image in the figure?
    a. blooming
    b. aliasing
    c. edge gradient effect
    d. ring artifact

121. Which of the following would serve to reduce the image artifact present in the figure?
    1. increase in filtration
    2. increase in kVp
    3. increase in section width
    a. 1 only
    b. 1 and 2 only
    c. 1 and 3 only
    d. 1, 2, and 3

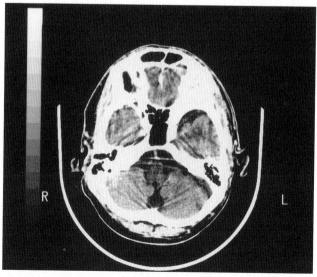

FIG. 8.12

122. The image in the figure was most likely displayed in a window with a level of:
    a. −150
    b. 0
    c. +50
    d. +400

123. The major disadvantage of the back-projection method of image reconstruction is the appearance of the:
    a. partial volume effect
    b. ring artifact
    c. Gibb phenomenon
    d. star artifact

124. The most effective method of reducing involuntary motion on a CT image is:
    a. immobilization
    b. thorough explanation of the examination to the patient
    c. reduced scan times
    d. physical restraint

125. The process of displaying CT images in a different orientation from the one used in the original reconstruction process is called:
    a. retrospective reconstruction
    b. prospective reconstruction
    c. multiplanar reformation
    d. multisegment reconstruction

126. The process of grayscale mapping of the CT image may be referred to as:
    a. analog-to-digital conversion
    b. retrospective reconstruction
    c. prospective reconstruction
    d. windowing

127. In the formula used to calculate the linear attenuation coefficient, $I = I_0 e^{-\mu x}$, the symbol I_0 identifies the:
    a. Euler constant
    b. incident intensity
    c. absorber thickness
    d. transmitted intensity

128. First-generation CT scanners possess which of the following characteristics?
    a. pencil-thin x-ray beam
    b. silver halide detectors
    c. rotate-rotate geometry
    d. nutating detector array

129. The intensity of the x-ray beam after it passes through an object to a detector is called the:
    a. incident intensity
    b. ray
    c. transmitted intensity
    d. primary beam

130. An accurate, modern CT scanner possesses a spatial resolution up to:
    a. 10 lp/mm
    b. 25 lp/mm
    c. 10 lp/cm
    d. 25 lp/cm

131. A high-resolution comb is utilized by a multidetector CT (MDCT) detector array in an effort to reduce:
    a. scatter radiation
    b. patient radiation dose
    c. low spatial frequency signal
    d. high spatial frequency signal

132. The distance between the centers of two adjacent reconstructed CT images is termed the:
    a. section width
    b. interpolation degree
    c. section interval
    d. sampling rate

133. The maximum number of simultaneous sections a multidetector CT (MDCT) system can acquire per gantry rotation is controlled by the number of:
    a. detector rows
    b. data channels
    c. focal spots
    d. x-ray tubes

134. *Matrix size* describes which of the following?
    a. aperture size used during data acquisition
    b. number of pixels used to display image
    c. relationship between the field of view and the algorithm
    d. the number of data channels available

Use Fig. 8.13 to answer questions 135–136.

135. The circle shown on the image in the figure is used to:
    a. magnify a portion of the image
    b. localize an area for percutaneous biopsy
    c. perform a region of interest (ROI) measurement
    d. produce a multiplanar reformation (MPR) image
136. The density measurement performed in the figure yielded an average CT number of zero. This area consists of:
    a. fat
    b. blood
    c. water
    d. air
137. The implementation of corrective actions to improve any identified performance inadequacies of the CT system is referred to as:
    a. quality control
    b. uniformity
    c. quality assurance
    d. linearity
138. The major disadvantage of the fan- or cone-shaped x-ray beams used in modern CT units in comparison with the "pencil-thin" beams of older units is:
    a. increased transmission measurements
    b. greater patient radiation dose
    c. decreased transmission measurements
    d. excess tube wear
139. When choosing a scan field of view (SFOV), the CT technologist is controlling the:
    1. diameter of data acquisition
    2. number of activated detectors within the array
    3. correction factors for the specific area of anatomic interest
    a. 2 only
    b. 1 and 2 only
    c. 1 and 3 only
    d. 1, 2, and 3
140. As the attenuation of a volume of tissue decreases, the transmitted intensity of a CT x-ray beam:
    a. increases
    b. remains unchanged
    c. decreases
    d. increases to a peak value and then rapidly decreases
141. Which of the following parameters or factors is improved by the selection of a smaller x-ray tube filament?
    a. scan time
    b. spatial resolution
    c. heat rating
    d. signal-to-noise ratio (SNR)
142. The geometric efficiency of a CT detector is influenced primarily by the:
    a. atomic number of the detector material
    b. size of the detector element
    c. size of the tube filament
    d. amount of interspace material between detectors
143. Which of the following factors may affect the attenuation of an object during CT data acquisition?
    a. beam pitch
    b. mA
    c. kVp
    d. algorithm
144. An image that is reconstructed a second time with some change in technical factor is said to be:
    a. reiterated
    b. postprocessed
    c. retrospective
    d. reformatted
145. The Feldkamp–Davis–Kress (FDK) algorithm may be applied to multidetector CT (MDCT) acquisition data to overcome image artifacts from:
    a. patient motion
    b. beam hardening
    c. partial volume averaging
    d. beam divergence

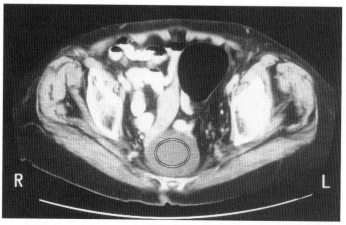

FIG. 8.13

146. Multidetector CT (MDCT) systems are typically capable of differentiating adjacent objects with attenuation differences as small as:
    a. 3 HU
    b. 10 HU
    c. 25 HU
    d. 60 HU

147. The ability of a multidetector CT (MDCT) system to freeze motion and provide an image free of blurring is called:
    a. in-plane spatial resolution
    b. longitudinal spatial resolution
    c. temporal resolution
    d. contrast resolution

148. Ring artifacts on the CT image are associated with which of the following tube-detector geometries?
    a. rotate–nutate
    b. rotate–stationary
    c. rotate–rotate
    d. translate–rotate

149. What is the maximum beam collimation for a multidetector CT (MDCT) system with 16 rows of 1.25-mm detectors?
    a. 2.5 mm
    b. 5.0 mm
    c. 20.0 mm
    d. 40.0 mm

150. The polyenergetic x-ray beam emitted from a CT x-ray tube is susceptible to artifacts resulting from the phenomenon known as:
    a. beam hardening
    b. density bloom
    c. kerma
    d. partial volume

151. In a multidetector CT (MDCT) system, which of the following technical parameters determines the reconstructed section width?
    a. detector collimation
    b. number of data channels
    c. beam collimation
    d. detector pitch

152. Daily air or water calibration of the CT system is performed to evaluate which of the following components of image quality?
    a. contrast resolution
    b. temporal resolution
    c. uniformity
    d. linearity

153. Pixels whose average attenuation coefficients are less than the coefficient of water have which of the following types of CT number values?
    a. extremely large
    b. high positive
    c. negative
    d. high contrast

154. Which of the following actions would serve to magnify the CT image on the display monitor?
    a. decrease matrix size
    b. increase scan field of view
    c. decrease display field of view
    d. increase display field of view

155. The bit depth of a digital imaging system defines the number of information bits contained within each:
    a. pixel
    b. matrix
    c. axial image
    d. multiplanar reformation (MPR)

156. The technical factor(s) necessary for the acquisition of an isotropic data set is/are:
    1. thin detector collimation
    2. high mA setting
    3. small DFOV
    a. 1 only
    b. 1 and 3 only
    c. 2 and 3 only
    d. 1, 2, and 3

Use Fig. 8.14 to answer questions 157–159.

157. The limiting resolution of the bone algorithm in the figure is:
    a. 6.1 lp/cm
    b. 9.5 lp/cm
    c. 14.6 lp/cm
    d. 15.5 lp/cm

158. At a modulation transfer function (MTF) of 20%, which reconstruction algorithm will demonstrate the greatest number of line pairs per centimeter (lp/cm)?
    a. bone
    b. standard
    c. smooth
    d. impossible to determine from the information provided

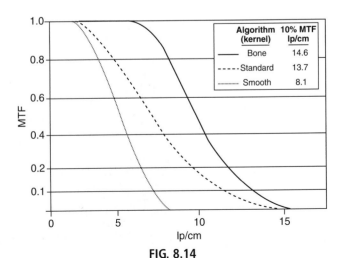

FIG. 8.14

159. When one is assessing a modulation transfer function (MTF) graph such as the figure, the limiting resolution is determined at a point where the signal frequency corresponding to a particular object has reached:
    a. 10%
    b. 20%
    c. 50%
    d. 100%

160. In multidetector CT (MDCT), the combined thicknesses of all of the sections simultaneously acquired with each gantry rotation are called the:
    a. detector configuration
    b. beam pitch
    c. detector pitch
    d. total collimation

161. Multidetector CT (MDCT) systems typically employ which of the following types of detectors?
    a. tungsten ring
    b. solid-state scintillation
    c. charged-coupled device (CCD)
    d. gas ionization

162. Which of the following technical adjustments may be employed to reduce step artifact in a multiplanar reformation CT image?
    1. acquisition of an isotropic data set
    2. overlapping section increment
    3. increase in effective mAs
    a. 1 only
    b. 1 and 2 only
    c. 2 and 3 only
    d. 1, 2, and 3

163. Which of the following is a manifestation of the partial volume artifact?
    a. cupping
    b. Hounsfield bar
    c. aliasing
    d. streaking

164. During volumetric CT acquisition, the slice sensitivity profile (SSP) graphically represents the:
    a. effective section width
    b. dose profile
    c. beam width
    d. detector collimation

165. An increase in the sampling rate during CT data acquisition corresponds to an increase in:
    a. views per rotation
    b. patient radiation dose
    c. image noise
    d. matrix size

Answer Key—Examination One

ANSWERS

1. C
The partial thromboplastin time (PTT) is a laboratory measure of blood coagulation. This value is used to screen patients for invasive procedures. Because of individual laboratory practices, the average range may fluctuate slightly.

2. B
A butterfly needle should be inserted at an angle of 15 degrees for the intravenous administration of contrast material. It is also important that the vein be properly stabilized and that the needle be inserted gently with the bevel facing upward.

3. D
The flow rate may be calculated by dividing the total contrast volume by the time of the injection. In this example, the total contrast volume is 125 mL and the time for the injection is 50 seconds. The flow rate programmed for this injection would be 125 ÷ 50, or 2.5 mL per second.

4. A
Hypoxemia refers to a condition whereby the patient suffers from a low concentration of oxygen in the blood. Hypoxia describes insufficient oxygenation of tissue at the cellular level. Hypotension refers to the condition of low blood pressure. Hyponatremia describes the condition of low sodium levels in the blood.

5. C
Prior reactions to contrast media and a history of asthma are factors that increase the incidence of adverse reaction to iodinated contrast media. It is therefore vital to question the patient regarding these factors before contrast agent administration. The presence of the human immunodeficiency virus (HIV) or hepatitis does not increase the incidence of adverse reaction to iodinated contrast media. Because universal precautions govern the protection of all patients and health care professionals, there is no need to question the patient regarding these factors.

6. D
Glomerular filtration rate (GFR) is calculated using the patient's measured serum creatinine level and takes into account the patient's age, sex, and race.

7. B
A bolus administration of contrast agent requires the entire volume of material to be injected over the shortest possible time. Accomplished by hand or with the use of an automatic injector, bolus administration provides the maximum plasma iodine concentration and subsequent tissue enhancement.

8. D
General signs and symptoms that a patient is going into shock include rapid breathing, tachycardia, hypotension, weak pulse, pallor, cyanosis, and cold, clammy skin.

9. D
SOLU-CORTEF is a brand name for hydrocortisone, which is a type of corticosteroid. This drug, or other types of corticosteroids, may be used during the treatment of anaphylactoid reactions to iodinated contrast materials.

10. C
Nonionic contrast media include iopamidol (Isovue), iohexol (Omnipaque), and iopromide (Ultravist).

11. B
The term *dyspnea* may be defined as the condition of difficult breathing.

12. D
Implied consent occurs when a patient is in need of immediate medical services but is unconscious or physically unable to consent to treatment. The assumption is made that the patient would consent if able.

13. D
Complete cardiac diastole is the period of atrial and ventricular relaxation after heart contraction. The T wave of an electrocardiogram (ECG) corresponds to cardiac diastole.

14. A

Iodinated water-soluble radiopaque contrast media (RCM) are injected directly into the joint space of interest during CT arthrography.

15. A

Iodixanol (Visipaque) is an example of a nonionic iso-osmolar contrast agent. Iohexol (Omnipaque), iopamidol (Isovue), and ioversol (Optiray) are all nonionic low-osmolar contrast media (LOCM).

16. D

Antecubital space refers to the anterior recess of the elbow. It contains the basilic vein medially and the cephalic vein laterally. Both veins are common sites for the IV administration of iodinated contrast media.

17. C

Contrast-induced nephrotoxicity (CIN) is a potentially serious delayed effect of contrast agent administration. It is a considerable decline in renal function that can occur after a patient receives an IV contrast agent. CIN is typically marked by an increase in serum creatinine concentration in comparison with a baseline measurement obtained before contrast agent administration.

18. D

The use of a saline flush also improves the overall contrast agent utilization efficiency of the CT examination.

19. A

If not contraindicated, sublingual nitroglycerine may be administered just before the cardiac multidetector CT (MDCT) study to cause dilation of the coronary vessels, improving their visualization. Please consult the referring physician and/or department protocol for further information regarding pharmaceutical administration for cardiac CT procedures.

20. B

The normal range for diastolic blood pressure in adults is 60–90 mm Hg. Diastolic pressure is the measurement of blood pressure at its lowest point, in between contractions of the heart.

21. B

Parenteral administration involves the injection of medication into the body. Common routes of parental medication administration include intramuscular, intravenous, intradermal, and subcutaneous.

22. C

Enteric precautions attempt to protect from the spread of infection through direct or indirect contact with fecal matter. Gowns and gloves are common protective devices used for enteric precautions. The use of a surgical mask is not warranted.

23. B

Ionic contrast media are salts consisting of sodium and/or meglumine.

24. B

In a lethargic state, the patient appears drowsy but can be aroused.

25. A

Several factors may be regarded as contraindications to administration of iodinated contrast material, including known allergy to iodine, prior severe reaction, and renal insufficiency. Multiple myeloma and diabetes, although not absolute contraindications to intravenous (IV) administration of iodinated contrast agents, do require attention to the patient's hydration level to limit renal complications.

26. C

The CT dose index (CTDI) is used to quantify the radiation dose received by the patient during a CT scan. It involves the use of an ionization chamber to accurately measure radiation exposure for a given set of technical factors.

27. A

Bismuth shields may be placed directly over radiosensitive tissues and organs during CT acquisition. Referred to as an "in-plane" type of shielding, the bismuth material may be placed within the acquisition area, resulting in minimal image artifact. The clinical use of bismuth shielding is controversial, with the American Association of Physicists in Medicine (AAPM) recommending against the use of bismuth shielding in favor of more comprehensive dose reduction techniques.

28. C

With no consideration of image quality, reductions in mA and/or scan time (seconds) are direct methods of decreasing patient dose during a CT examination.

29. C

An ionization chamber is a device used to accurately measure radiation exposure. Radiation causes ionization within the chamber, which is measured by an electrode. The amount of charged particles is proportional to the radiation exposure. The ionization chamber is an extremely accurate device that is used to quantify radiation exposure from a CT scan.

30. D

The National Electrical Manufacturers Association (NEMA) – Medical Imaging Technology Alliance (MITA) Standard XR-29, commonly referred to as the MITA Smart Dose standard requires a CT system to feature DICOM radiation dose structured reporting (RDSR), a dose check system that alerts the technologist that the scan parameters may result in a patient dose that is higher than acceptable, an automated tube current modulation

(ATCM) system that serves as an automatic exposure control (AEC), and reference protocols for both adult and pediatric patients.

31. B
Protocol optimization must include size-based dose adjustments by reducing the tube current (mAs). Optimal scans of pediatric patients can be achieved with substantially reduced mAs settings.

32. C
Effective dose may be used as a whole-body risk estimation, accounting for the type of tissue(s) exposed to ionizing radiation. Different tissues are assigned weighting factors on the basis of their individual radiosensitivities. Effective dose approximates the relative risk from exposure to low doses of ionizing radiation. The unit of measurement for effective dose is the sievert (Sv).

33. B
Iterative reconstruction techniques are used to increase the signal-to-noise ratio (SNR) of the reconstructed CT image. This reduction in image noise allows for reduced technical factors (tube milliamperage) and lower patient radiation dose. Iterative reconstruction techniques require increased reconstruction time, made acceptably short enough by today's powerful computer processors.

34. D
The selected mA should be adapted to each patient according to size and/or weight. The "child-sizing" of CT protocols is an important method of reducing radiation dose to the pediatric patient. Eliminating unnecessary CT scans at the discretion of the physician is an additional way to reduce pediatric dose.

35. A
Based on the design of a multidetector CT (MDCT) system, any reduction in the focus-to-detector distance would subsequently reduce the distance between the source (x-ray tube) and the patient positioned in the isocenter of the CT gantry. This reduced distance would cause an increase in the dose to the patient, according to the inverse square law.

36. A
$CTDI_w$ is calculated from measurements made with dosimeters positioned at the center and periphery of a phantom and accounts for the variance in dose distribution resulting from the effects of beam hardening.

37. C
The radiation dose structured report (RDSR) must include all pertinent information related to the x-ray tube's output during CT data acquisition. This includes the tube current and voltage, scan time, acquisition length, pitch, and collimation width.

38. C
Attenuation describes the reduction in x-ray intensity as the beam traverses the patient. The overall attenuation of the beam results from a combination of photon absorption and scatter.

39. D
Utilizing in-plane bismuth shielding with a CT system that employs real-time (angular and longitudinal) automatic tube current modulation can result in an increase in patient exposure as the system inappropriately measures patient density to include the shielding material. In-plane bismuth shielding should be avoided in this scenario. Increases in tube potential can result in an overall decrease in patient exposure if the tube current (mA) is decreased appropriately. To reduce patient dose, the reconstructed CT image should contain a tolerable amount of noise.

40. B
Dose length product (DLP) is used to estimate the radiation dose to the patient. During helical scanning, it can be calculated as the product of the $CTDI_{vol}$ and the acquisition (scan) length in centimeters. For an axial (nonhelical) acquisition, DLP is calculated as the product of the multiple scan average dose (MSAD), the section width (cm), and the total number of acquired sections.

41. C
The cone beam of a multidetector CT system extends beyond the width of the detector array along the z-axis, known as *overbeaming*. This penumbra can be minimized by a modern system's precise collimation of the beam.

42. D
The dose length product (DLP) is the total patient dose over a given scan acquisition length (z) and can be illustrated as the product of $CTDI_{vol}$ and scan length. The DLP is expressed in units of milligrays per centimeter (mGy-cm).

43. D
Found typically in the emergency setting, a comprehensive acute stroke CT imaging protocol begins with a precontrast sequence to evaluate for hemorrhage. After the IV administration of an iodinated contrast agent, a CTA acquisition is performed through the carotid vessels and brain. CTP is then performed to evaluate potential cerebral perfusion defects secondary to stroke.

44. A
Number 1 on the figure corresponds to the left pulmonary artery.

45. C
Number 4 on the figure corresponds to the superior vena cava.

46. D

Pleural effusions are commonly seen in the posterior portion of the lung field on images obtained with the patient in a supine position on the CT table. Differentiation between pleural effusion and pleural thickening is made when region of interest (ROI) measurements reveal fluid with density readings at or slightly above zero. Pleural effusion may be caused by multiple pathologic processes, including infection, neoplasm, and congestive heart failure.

47. B

Simple cysts contain primarily water and therefore exhibit CT numbers ranging from approximately 0 (or slightly below) to +20 Hounsfield units.

48. B

The arterial phase is the period of peak arterial enhancement typically occurring at 25 to 35 seconds after the initiation of contrast agent administration. During this phase, hypervascular tumors or tumors supplied by the hepatic artery undergo maximal enhancement.

49. C

Number 2 on the figure corresponds to the left internal carotid artery.

50. A

Number 5 on the figure corresponds to the right internal jugular vein.

51. D

Number 1 on the figure corresponds to the epiglottis.

52. D

The abdominal aorta descends to the level of the fourth lumbar vertebra (L4), where it bifurcates into the left and right common iliac arteries.

53. B

Small amounts of gas may appear in the areas of degenerated intervertebral discs. The accumulation of gases such as nitrogen occurs as a by-product of the physical breakdown of the disc material.

54. C

Because of their increase in CT number, subdural hematomas may be well visualized without the IV administration of an iodinated contrast agent.

55. D

Excretory phase acquisitions after a delay of 3 to 15 minutes demonstrate the urinary tract while it is opacified with a contrast agent. Transitional cell lesions of the urothelium appear as filling defects within the bladder, ureters, and/or renal pelvis.

56. B

Number 1 on the figure corresponds to the stomach.

57. D

The location of the liver on the inferior portion of the image indicates that this patient is in the right lateral decubitus position.

58. B

The right lateral decubitus position is often used to differentiate the pancreatic head and the duodenum.

59. A

Number 2 on the figure corresponds to the right ureter.

60. C

Penumbra is the ischemic, yet still viable, tissue immediately surrounding the infarct core. It can be described as the region of ischemic brain parenchyma where cerebral blood volume (CBV) is compromised but still higher than 2.5 mL per 100 g of tissue.

61. B

The wrist's scaphoid bone (navicular) is a common location for complex fracture.

62. D

Thin section (1–3 mm) images are required in both the axial and coronal planes to properly demonstrate the orbits. Isotropic multidetector CT (MDCT) axial-plane acquisition will yield multiplanar reformation images of sufficient quality to eliminate the need for an additional scan in a second (coronal) plane. Acquiring data in only a single plane will reduce patient dose.

63. C

High-resolution CT is a specialized technique using narrow section widths and a high-resolution algorithm for image reconstruction. It is used to maximize detail of high spatial frequency tissue, such as the lungs and bony structures.

64. B

The flow rate range 1.0 to 3.0 mL/sec should be sufficient to provide the enhancement necessary for proper evaluation of the abdomen. This is a general range that may be adjusted to meet the needs of the examination at the discretion of the physician and medical personnel involved for each patient.

65. B

Fatty liver disease, or hepatic steatosis, is a condition in which large quantities of fats (lipids) are retained within the liver. Whereas normal liver parenchyma exhibits attenuation values approximately 10 HU higher than those of the spleen, the liver with steatosis has attenuation values at least 10 HU below those of the spleen.

66. D
The renal pyramids are cone-shaped regions of the renal medulla. The wider bases of the renal pyramids border the renal cortex.

67. B
Beginning 30 to 40 seconds after the initiation of contrast agent administration, the corticomedullary phase demonstrates optimal enhancement of the renal cortex with maximum differentiation of the cortex from the renal medulla.

68. C
Number 2 on the figure corresponds to the right adrenal gland.

69. A
Number 6 on the figure corresponds to the psoas muscle.

70. A
Patient inspiration provides optimal chest expansion and allows for better demonstration of anatomic structures.

71. A
Routine CT scanning of the head should be performed with the gantry angled 15 degrees above the infraorbital-meatal line. This angle produces axial sections of the brain while limiting beam-hardening artifacts and direct orbital exposure.

72. D
The patient should be instructed to phonate the letter "E" during CT scanning of the larynx. As data are acquired during scanning, the patient's phonation requires vibration of the vocal cords, thus allowing for thorough evaluation of their mobility.

73. C
Number 2 on the figure corresponds to the cochlea.

74. D
Number 4 on the figure corresponds to the carotid canal.

75. A
Targeted reconstructions should be performed bilaterally utilizing a small display field of view (DFOV) or a higher zoom factor to maximize resolution of the small bony components of the inner ear.

76. A
Number 3 on the figure corresponds to the vestibule.

77. A
The *cul-de-sac* is the area posterior to the uterus and ovaries in the female patient. It is a common site for ascites in the patient with pelvic pathology.

78. A
Interstitial diseases of the lungs are usually diffuse pathologic processes involving the interstitium, or framework, of the lungs. Examples of interstitial diseases are bronchiectasis, emphysema, asbestosis, and sarcoidosis.

79. B
An enterovesical fistula is an abnormal communication between the bowel and the bladder. It typically results from inflammatory processes of the colon such as diverticulitis.

80. D
During a CT examination of the lumbar spine, a foam cushion should be placed under the patient's flexed knees. This maneuver reduces strain on the lower back, making the patient more comfortable and cooperative. It also reduces the lordotic curve of the lumbar spine, allowing for more accurate imaging of the intervertebral disc spaces.

81. C
The axial plane is parallel to the foot's plantar surface. The oblique axial plane is parallel to the metatarsals, approximately 20 to 30 degrees caudal from the direct axial plane.

82. B
Claudication refers to the condition of intermittent cramping pain in the legs resulting from poor circulation.

83. D
Ground-glass opacities are hazy areas of increased attenuation in the lungs and are often associated with the interstitial lung disease evaluated by high-resolution CT (HRCT).

84. C
Number 1 on the figure corresponds to the ascending aorta.

85. A
High-resolution CT (HRCT) acquisitions of the chest should be performed with thin sections, within the range of 1 to 2 mm.

86. B
Number 2 on the figure corresponds to the anterior segment of the left upper lobe bronchus.

87. B
The pituitary and other structures involving the sella turcica are usually imaged in the coronal plane with CT. The coronal plane provides the best visualization of the pituitary gland with regard to its position within the sella turcica and involves less partial volume averaging of the pituitary with surrounding structures than scans obtained in the axial plane.

88. C

The spleen is the most common site of organ injury resulting from blunt abdominal trauma. Hematoma, hemorrhage, and laceration are typical signs of traumatic splenic injury.

89. B

Number 7 on the figure corresponds to the pancreatic head.

90. A

Number 2 on the figure corresponds to the superior mesenteric vein.

91. D

Number 8 on the figure corresponds to the ascending colon.

92. B

The spinal cord extends to the lower margin of the first or upper margin of the second lumbar vertebra. At this level it tapers to a point known as the *conus medullaris*.

93. A

A *leiomyoma* is a benign mass of smooth muscle. It commonly occurs in the uterus and is readily identified on CT examination as a bulky, nonspecific uterine enlargement.

94. B

Number 4 on the figure corresponds to the ethmoid sinus.

95. A

The section thickness of a CT scan directly affects the detail and spatial resolution of the image. Narrow section widths result in greater detail for imaging of small anatomic parts such as the sinuses.

96. C

Number 2 on the figure corresponds to the zygomatic bone.

97. D

The peritoneal cavity is formed by the membranous sac called the *peritoneum*. It contains the stomach, liver, gallbladder, spleen, ovaries, transverse colon, and most of the small bowel.

98. C

Routine preparations for general studies of the abdomen and pelvis include the administration of an oral contrast agent for opacification of the gastrointestinal (GI) tract. Patients are typically instructed to refrain from eating or drinking anything else for up to 6 hours before the examination. Polyethylene glycol (PEG) is used for bowel cleansing before a colonoscopy and may have certain applications for CT preparation limited to CT colonography.

99. A

Complete CT scans of the pelvis should include from the iliac crests to the pubic symphysis. This scan range may be extended if clinically warranted. Scan parameters (i.e., slice thickness, incrementation) can be adjusted to correlate with the patient's clinical history.

100. B

Number 4 on the figure corresponds to the cuboid.

101. C

The figure is a multiplanar reformation (MPR) in the sagittal plane.

102. A

Number 6 on the figure corresponds to the navicular.

103. D

Number 1 on the figure corresponds to the talus.

104. C

In comparison with the surrounding soft tissues, the thyroid gland is hyperdense on CT because it naturally contains iodine. This density increases further with administration of an iodinated contrast agent.

105. D

In the minimum intensity projection technique, displayed pixels represent the minimum attenuation value encountered along each sampled ray. Also referred to as *min-IP*, this type of multiplanar volume reconstruction (MPVR) can be applied to a volume of the thorax to demonstrate air trapping within the trachea and bronchial tree.

106. B

Number 5 on the figure corresponds to the anterior horn of the lateral ventricle.

107. B

Number 3 on the figure corresponds to the thalamus.

108. C

Number 4 on the figure corresponds to the septum pellucidum.

109. D

The small bowel consists of the duodenum, the jejunum, and the ileum. The cecum is the proximal portion of the large bowel; it is connected to the small bowel at the ileocecal valve.

110. D

A CT cystogram involves the administration of an iodinated contrast agent directly into the bladder via a Foley catheter.

111. D

Multidetector CT (MDCT) utilizes a cone-shaped beam that is incident upon an expanded array of detectors. The detector array consists of multiple rows along the z-axis and requires a cone-shaped beam to measure incident radiation.

112. C

Collimation of the x-ray beam in CT is accomplished by both prepatient and predetector collimators, or detectors. The prepatient detectors restrict the field size, directly influencing the reconstructed section thickness. The predetector or postpatient detectors absorb scatter radiation before it contributes to the signal produced by the detector array.

113. A

The *CT number* is a relative value based on the attenuation that occurs within a voxel of tissue. The Hounsfield unit is used for this value.

114. C

Interpolation is the mathematical process whereby data from tube rotations just above and just below a given slice position are used for image reconstruction. Interpolation allows for the reconstruction of a thin, motion-free image from a volumetric data set acquired from a moving patient.

115. A

The spatial resolution of a CT scanner can be measured by studying the amount of blurring that occurs around a point within the CT image. Known as the *point spread function* (PSF), this image unsharpness may be graphically represented. The spatial resolution can then be quantified by measuring the graph at half its maximum value. This measurement, called the *full width at half-maximum (FWHM)*, is used to illustrate the spatial resolution of a CT scanner.

116. C

First-generation CT scanners were based on a translate–rotate principle. The x-ray tube and detectors would translate across the patient's head and then rotate 1 degree. This process would repeat in a semicircular fashion, for 180 degrees around the patient's head.

117. B

Picture archival and communications systems (PACSs) are computerized networks charged with the responsibility of storing, retrieving, distributing, and displaying CT and other digital medical images.

118. C

The operator may control the contrast and brightness of the CT image by adjusting the "window" setting. As a form of grayscale mapping, the window determines the pixels assigned shades of gray on the basis of their CT numbers.

119. B

Isotropic is used to describe voxels with equal dimensions along the x-, y- and z-axes. The ability to acquire an isotropic data set is a distinct advantage of multidetector CT (MDCT).

120. D

Although the CT technologist must be able to readily identify them, ring artifacts are caused by detector malfunction and are beyond his or her control. Patient motion, partial volume averaging, and edge gradient artifacts can all be limited by the CT technologist through adequate preparation and careful scan procedures.

121. B

A standard multiplanar reformation (MPR) image is 1 voxel thick, with the pixels facing the viewer, each representing the average attenuation occurring within the represented voxels.

122. D

Statistical noise is a term that may be used for quantum noise, or mottle. Caused by an insufficient number of photons being detected, this type of noise appears as graininess on the CT image.

123. C

The beam pitch for a given acquisition is equal to the table feed per rotation divided by the total collimation. The total collimation for this acquisition is equal to the total number of sections (detectors) multiplied by the detector dimension, or 64 × 0.625 mm. The table feed per rotation can be calculated as the product of the total collimation and the beam pitch, or 40 mm × 1.5, and equals 60 mm for the example provided.

124. B

The primary data-processing component of the CT system is the array processor. It is responsible for receiving scan data from the host computer, performing all of the major processing of the CT image, and returning the reconstructed image to the storage memory of the host computer.

125. B

Misregistration is an artifact that occurs when a patient suspends respiration at different depths during consecutive scans. It results in the loss of anatomic information.

126. B

The analog-to-digital converter is responsible for transforming the analog signal from the detectors into a digital form that may be used by the computer. Analog information is based on a scale, whereas digital information is in numerical form.

127. C

The back-projection method of image reconstruction involves the acquisition of attenuation values, which are then projected back onto a matrix for subsequent display.

128. B

The contrast of a CT image is controlled by the spatial frequencies of the tissue(s) within the section. Tissues of differing densities are represented electronically by different spatial frequencies. Adjacent tissues that greatly differ in density are represented by high spatial frequencies.

129. D

Noise is most commonly measured by scanning a water-filled phantom with a consistent set of technical factors. The image noise is equal to the standard deviation of pixel values within a region of interest (ROI) measurement of the image. Uniformity may also be evaluated by positioning several ROI measurements at different locations along the center and periphery of the image. The CT values should not differ by more than 2 HU from one location to another.

130. C

Beam hardening occurs as low-energy x-ray photons are absorbed while the beam passes through the patient. The average photon energy of the beam increases along the path and may result in a loss of system uniformity.

131. A

The image noise is equal to the standard deviation of pixel values within an ROI measurement of the image. ROI number 1 on the figure demonstrates the highest value for standard deviation (SD) (SD = 2.87).

132. B

An *algorithm* may be defined as a set of rules or steps used to solve a mathematical problem. The programs used by the CT computer to reconstruct the image are often referred to as *algorithms*.

133. C

The dimensions of a voxel are determined by multiplying the pixel dimensions by the slice thickness. The dimensions of a pixel are directly controlled by the matrix size and the field of view.

134. B

Increasing the display field of view (DFOV) for a reconstructed CT image decreases its displayed size. Electronically magnifying the image on the display system results in a larger displayed image but has no effect on pixel or voxel dimension.

135. B

The average photon energy of the primary beam used in CT is approximately 70 keV. The average photon energy of any radiographic primary beam is typically 30% to 40% of the applied kilovoltage. The average photon energy of the CT beam is increased through beam filtration.

136. C

All multidetector CT (MDCT) systems utilize third-generation geometry and solid-state scintillation detectors.

137. B

Cine CT acquisition involves multiple axial scans obtained at a single anatomic level over a predetermined period. Clinical applications of cine CT acquisition include contrast bolus tracking; dynamic imaging of physiologic processes such as respiration, swallowing, and the cardiac cycle; and for CT perfusion studies.

138. B

The rate at which a quantity of radiation (photon fluence) passes through a unit area over unit time is termed the *photon flux*. It may also be referred to as the *fluence rate*.

139. C

An average CT number value for bone is approximately +1000 HU. This may vary widely with the density of the particular bone in question and with the beam quality of the CT scanner.

140. A

Each CT image reconstructed on a 512^2 matrix is approximately 0.5 megabytes (MB) in digital size.

141. A

Linearity describes the relationship between the CT number and actual linear attenuation coefficients of an object. It is used to measure the accuracy of a CT scanner.

142. A

It is important that the calibration of a CT scanner be checked daily by the operator. CT units should be calibrated with their reference CT number for water at approximately zero. The CT number for air should be at approximately −1000.

143. D

Volume rendering adjusts the opacity of voxels included in the 3-D model according to their tissue characteristics. Unlike the thresholding concept used for shaded-surface display (SSD), or surface rendering, volume rendering does not exclude voxels, but instead alters their appearance so that the 3-D model contains the entire volume data set.

144. A

The high-frequency generator used to produce the three-phase power used in modern CT scanners is located inside the gantry. It may be positioned in a corner of the gantry or fixed to the rotating tube assembly.

145. A

The *bit* is the smallest unit of information within the binary system. Its name is derived from the term "*binary* digi*t*" and can appear as either a number 1 or 0. A sequence of eight bits constitutes a byte.

146. C

Eliminating the need for cables, slip-ring technology allows for continuous gantry rotation by utilizing a system of contact brushes that supply electricity to power the system, enabling the passage of transmission data to the computer system.

147. A

The process known as *convolution* is applied to reduce image unsharpness. An algorithm, or convolution kernel, acts as a mathematical filter, modifying the ray sum data and removing the unwanted blurring effect of the back-projection.

148. C

Contiguous images are those acquired with equal section thickness and interval. For example, 3.75-mm sections reconstructed every 3.75 mm completely cover a given volume of tissue with no unmeasured tissue.

149. B

When calculated by a formula comparing the attenuation coefficient of tissue with that of water, materials whose coefficients are greater than that of water are assigned positive CT numbers.

150. D

The Digital Imaging and Communications in Medicine (DICOM) standard confirms the process of recording, storing, printing, and transmitting medical image data.

151. A

The contrast resolution of a CT scanner depends on several factors, including section width, algorithm selection, detector sensitivity, and noise. The focal spot size is a geometric factor that influences the spatial resolution of a CT scanner.

152. B

The artifact present in the figure most likely represents an out-of-field artifact. This relatively large patient was incorrectly positioned, and a portion of the anatomy lies outside the scanned field of view. This improperly centered anatomy interferes with the reference detectors, thus causing a streak artifact near the unscanned area.

153. D

The out-of-field artifact present in this image could be easily reduced by properly centering the patient within the scan field of view.

154. B

Increases in filtration cause a greater amount of low-energy x-ray photons to be absorbed, thereby increasing the average photon energy of the beam. Higher mAs values increase the intensity of the beam but do not affect average photon energy.

155. C

Scintillation crystals are used in cooperation with photodiodes in a scintillation-type CT detector. The *photodiode* is a solid-state device that absorbs the light flashes given off by the crystal. The photodiode then emits an electrical signal in response to this light.

156. A

Automatic tube current modulation (ATCM) programs adjust the mA throughout an acquisition to reduce patient radiation dose to a minimum. ATCM automatically alters the applied mA on the basis of a predetermined noise index that is acceptable for appropriate image quality.

157. A

A uniform matrix array consists of multiple detectors in the longitudinal direction, each with the same dimensions.

158. B

The width of a window determines the range of pixel values that will be assigned shades of gray around a given level. In this example, all pixels within the range of −250 to +250 HU will be assigned shades of gray. Pixels below −250 HU will appear black, and pixels above +250 HU will appear white.

159. B

Orthogonal planes are at right angles to each other. Orthogonal reformations are perpendicular to the original plane of data acquisition.

160. A

The controlling factors of the temporal resolution of a CT system are the gantry rotation speed and reconstruction method. Temporal resolution can be improved by segmenting the data acquisition process into separate components of smaller rotation angles. Single-segment or half-scan acquisitions reconstruct data obtained from half of the rotation time. For example, this type of segmentation would yield a 250-msec temporal resolution from a 0.5-sec gantry rotation time.

161. D

Cone beam artifacts are unique to the cone beam geometry of multidetector CT (MDCT) systems and typically manifest much like partial volume artifacts.

162. C

The analytic methods of CT image reconstruction include the filtered back-projection and the Fourier transform method. These techniques are called *analytic* because they utilize precise formulas for image reconstruction.

163. B

The number of data channels controls the number of sections the scanner can simultaneously acquire with each gantry rotation. A 16-slice system possesses 16 data channels and is capable of acquiring 16 images per gantry rotation. The configuration of the detector array with regard to the size of individual detector elements controls the possible section widths for each reconstructed CT image.

164. D

The measurement of transmitted radiation made by an individual detector is called a *ray sum*. It equals the total attenuation occurring along a straight-line path from tube to detector.

165. C

The threshold setting is used to include and exclude information during the 3-D reconstruction of a CT scan. For example, a high threshold (+150 HU) may be set to produce a 3-D model of a bony structure. This threshold eliminates any density value below +150 HU from the data set. The reconstructed 3-D model would include only bone tissue or any other substance with a Hounsfield value above +150.

Answer Key—Examination Two

ANSWERS

1. A

Diastole refers to the relaxation of heart muscle. It is the period of the cardiac cycle that occurs between successive contractions of the heart muscle, which are known as *systole*.

2. C

High-osmolar contrast media (HOCM) are ionic agents that dissociate into charged particles (ions) in solution. Ionic contrast media are salts consisting of sodium and/or meglumine. Iothalamate meglumine and diatrizoate sodium are commonly known by the brand names Conray and Hypaque, respectively. Another HOCM, Gastrografin is a solution of diatrizoate meglumine and diatrizoate sodium.

3. C

Epinephrine (Adrenalin) is an adrenergic drug used as a bronchodilator. Diphenhydramine (Benadryl) may be used to block the physiologic effects of the body's release of histamine, thus reducing the allergic effect of the contrast material. Atropine should be used only to combat bradycardia during a vagal reaction to contrast material.

4. D

The escape of contrast material from a needle or blood vessel into the subcutaneous tissues is called *extravasation*. It is also sometimes referred to as *infiltration*.

5. D

Good communication between the technologist and patient is an extremely important factor in the production of high-quality CT examinations. Patients can be made to feel more comfortable, and when they are given detailed instructions, their greater cooperation can improve the CT results.

6. B

Risk factors for contrast-induced nephrotoxicity (CIN) include preexisting renal function compromise, dehydration, diabetes, myeloma, advanced age, and cardiovascular disease.

7. D

Normal range of O_2 saturation as measured by a pulse oximeter is between 95% and 100%. Saturation levels below 95% may indicate respiratory insufficiency.

8. C

The laboratory measurements blood urea nitrogen (BUN) and serum creatinine (a component of urine) can be used to indicate the status of a patient's renal function.

9. D

Angiocatheters and higher-gauge needles are preferred for administration of a contrast agent with the use of a power injector. The stability of an angiocatheter maintains proper placement within the vein while withstanding the high pressure applied by the power injector.

10. D

The technologist and/or radiologist should always ask the patient about allergic history as well as current renal function status and history of cardiac illness (high blood pressure, congestive heart failure, and so on) before administration of any contrast material.

11. B

Nosocomial infections may be commonly referred to as *health care–associated infections*. They occur within the first 48 hours of a patient's stay in a health care facility.

12. B

The normal range for a creatinine level is 0.5 to 1.5 mg/dL. The normal range for blood urea nitrogen (BUN) levels is 7 to 25 mg/dL. Creatinine and BUN are laboratory measurements that may be used to evaluate the renal function of a patient scheduled to undergo a CT examination that involves intravenous administration of an iodinated contrast agent.

13. A

Larger-lumen (lower-gauge) needles allow for more rapid intravenous administration of contrast media. The lumen is considerably larger in a 19-gauge needle than in a 25-gauge needle. The viscosity of contrast material necessitates the use of a relatively large-bore needle.

14. C

Patients may be assigned to a higher-risk group for an adverse reaction to iodinated contrast material on the basis of several factors, including previous allergic history and physical condition. Patients considered to be at high risk for adverse reactions should be administered nonionic contrast material. Iso-osmolar contrast material is an alternative choice that may also reduce the risk of adverse reactions.

15. D
Examples of mild adverse reactions to iodinated contrast material are nausea, vomiting, mild urticaria, and a warm, flushed sensation. Dyspnea is a moderate reaction, whereas pulmonary edema and shock are severe reactions to contrast media.

16. D
The patient is required to provide informed consent before the start of any invasive procedure. The administration of intravascular contrast material is invasive in nature and requires the informed consent of the patient.

17. A
Because of the inherent differences in manufactured batches of tissue factor, the international normalized ratio (INR) is calculated to standardize prothrombin time (PT) results. The INR compares a patient's PT with a control sample for a more accurate result.

18. B
Insertion of any intravenous line requires the use of sterile technique to prevent microorganisms from entering the bloodstream.

19. D
Common sites for intravenous contrast injection are the antecubital, basilic, cephalic, and accessory cephalic veins.

20. A
Intrathecal injections of iodinated contrast material are used in the CT evaluation of the lumbar spine. This type of injection introduces contrast material directly into the subarachnoid space, which is located between the arachnoid and pia mater. The subarachnoid space contains the cerebrospinal fluid.

21. A
The serum iodine concentration is a measure of the amount of iodine within the bloodstream. The specific dose depends on the patient's age, weight, and renal function, as well as on the clinical indication for the CT procedure. The specific criteria of intravenous contrast administration must always be directed by a physician.

22. A
Additional components of the aseptic technique include cleaning the site of venipuncture in a circular motion with alcohol swab before injection, and applying pressure with an alcohol swab to the site after removal of the needle or catheter. It is *sterile* technique that involves establishing a sterile field around the area of an invasive procedure.

23. B
Automatic tube current modulation (ATCM) programs adjust the mA throughout an acquisition to reduce patient radiation dose to a minimum. ATCM automatically alters the applied mA on the basis of a predetermined noise index that is acceptable for appropriate image quality.

24. B
Kerma may be used to describe absorbed dose. *Air kerma* is the amount of radiation absorbed in a quantity of air. The term is an acronym for "kinetic energy released per unit mass."

25. C
Many CT scanners allow the technologist to reduce the total rotation of the x-ray tube, thus reducing the scan time and subsequent patient radiation dose. This type of partial scan, commonly referred to as a *"half-scan" or segmenting,* is most often used to improve the temporal resolution of the acquisition.

26. C
For all patients, regardless of age or sex indication, the CT protocol should be optimized according to size or weight.

27. A
Multiple scan average dose (MSAD) accounts for the effects of image spacing, or bed index, on patient radiation dose during axial scanning. MSAD increases when slice thickness is greater than image spacing and decreases when slice thickness is less than the bed index.

28. A
Because of the rotational nature of the x-ray tube, a patient receives exposure from all sides during a CT examination. Therefore lead shielding should be placed above and below the patient.

29. A
As the beam traverses the patient, beam hardening alters the penetrability of the beam and affects the absorption across the field of view. The $CTDI_w$ is calculated by summing two-thirds of the exposure recorded at the periphery of the field with one-third of the centrally recorded radiation dose. This weighting yields a more accurate dose approximation.

30. A
The fetus is most susceptible to the harmful effects of ionizing radiation during the first trimester of the gestation period.

31. B
All detectors of the multidetector CT (MDCT) array must be exposed to x-rays of equal intensity. The beam must be expanded even further to avoid exposing the detectors to undesirable "penumbra." This process is referred to as *overbeaming.*

32. C

Automatic tube current modulation (ATCM) is a form of automatic exposure control for a CT system. It manages patient radiation dose on the basis of the size, density, and overall attenuation of the part being examined.

33. A

An automated dose alert (CT dose check) function is a common feature of a modern CT system. This function automatically alerts the CT operator if the selected scan parameters may result in a patient dose that exceeds the predefined dose index value. Dose alert, or dose check, is a required system function to meet current industry standards (NEMA XR 29-2013) for patient radiation dose reduction during CT.

34. B

The *focus-to-isocenter distance* describes the distance from the x-ray source (CT tube) to the center of the gantry opening, where the patient should be positioned. A structural decrease in this distance would result in a decrease in patient dose, based upon the inverse square law.

35. D

Photoelectric (effect) absorption occurs when the energy of an incoming (incident) x-ray photon is completely absorbed through the ionization of an inner-shell electron of the target atom.

36. B

The CT x-ray beam is heavily filtered to remove low energy x-ray photons, hardening the beam to reduce patient dose and to improve image quality. The inherent structure of the CT x-ray tube (housing, cooling oil, etc.) typically amounts to 3.0 mm of Al-equivalent filtration.

37. C

Adaptive collimation technology may also be employed in a modern CT system to reduce z-axis overscanning or overranging that may occur at the start and end of a helical acquisition.

38. A

Pitch values greater than 1 allow for the acquisition of a given scan volume in a shorter time, resulting in a reduction in patient radiation dose. All other factors remaining consistent, the higher the pitch, the greater the dose savings at a cost of x-axis resolution. A multidetector CT (MDCT) system may automatically increase the tube current (mA) when the pitch is increased to maintain a predetermined image noise level. To maintain dose savings when pitch is increased, the operator will need to manually reduce the mA setting or increase the amount of noise tolerated in the reconstructed image.

39. D

A comprehensive CT dose reduction program includes the minimization of acquisition volumes, tailoring the dose to the size of the patient, and restricting public and nonessential personnel access to the CT scan room.

40. A

A thin foam spacer may be placed between the patient surface and the bismuth shield to reduce the scatter artifact that may occur when using in-plane bismuth shielding.

41. B

$CTDI_{vol}$ is used to approximate the radiation dose for each section obtained during a helical scan.

It corresponds to the axially acquired $CTDI_w$ divided by the helical pitch.

42. D

Low values for kVp and mA and short CT fluoroscopy time all reduce occupational radiation exposure. Greater distance from the source, as with the use of a needle holder to keep the operator's hands out of the CT fluoroscopy field, also greatly diminish exposure. Additional methods of exposure reduction are lead shielding, leaded patient drapes, and the utilization of a last-image-hold function to cut down on continuous CT fluoroscopy.

43. D

Number 4 in the figure corresponds to the large colon (splenic flexure).

44. C

Number 2 in the figure corresponds to the portal vein.

45. A

Morison pouch is the common name for the hepatorenal recess, which is indicated by number 7 in the figure. This space between the liver and right kidney is a common location for the abnormal collection of fluid known as *ascites*.

46. B

Number 6 in the figure corresponds to the superior mesenteric artery.

47. D

Number 3 in the figure corresponds to the pancreas.

48. A

Thin sections are required to properly assess abnormalities of the minute structures of the inner ear. The thinnest sections possible provide maximum detail.

49. A

The *Lisfranc joint* is the articulation between the tarsals and metatarsals; it can be the site of complex fractures and dislocations of the foot.

50. C

The Agatston scoring system quantifies the volume and density of calcium within the coronary arteries.

51. B

Adnexa is used to describe an appendage of an organ. The ovaries and fallopian tubes constitute the uterine adnexal region.

52. D

Opacification of the stomach and bowel loops is imperative during general CT examinations of the abdomen and pelvis. Effervescent agents may be used to ensure proper gastric distention. Intravenous contrast agents are used to opacify blood vessels and are helpful in anatomic differentiation and evaluation of mass vascularity.

53. C

The liver has a dual blood supply, receiving 75% of its supply from the portal vein and the remaining 25% from the hepatic artery.

54. A

Number 3 on the figure corresponds to the superior rectus muscle.

55. B

Number 2 on the figure corresponds to the optic nerve.

56. D

The image is a multiplanar reformation (MPR) image through the orbit in the oblique sagittal plane.

57. C

Number 1 on the figure corresponds to the inferior oblique muscle.

58. B

Number 6 on the figure corresponds to the azygos vein.

59. B

Number 4 on the figure corresponds to the pectoralis minor muscle.

60. C

With the lung fields black, the bony structures white, and the mediastinum and muscles gray, the image in the figure is displayed in a soft tissue window.

61. A

Number 1 on the figure corresponds to the superior vena cava.

62. C

It is widely recommended that volumetrically acquired CT sections be reconstructed with the use of at least a 50% overlap to improve the quality of 3-D and multiplanar reformation (MPR) images.

63. B

Positron emission tomography (PET) provides a map of normal and abnormal tissue function. It offers excellent sensitivity for malignancy, but suffers from an inability to accurately localize tumor activity. Fusion of PET with CT provides such precise anatomic localization. CT data is also used to correct the differences in attenuation that occur as fluorodeoxyglucose (FDG) decay occurs throughout the patient. For example, decay photons emerging from the center of the patient will be attenuated more than those from the periphery of the patient. CT data during a PET-CT is used to correct this potential artifact.

64. A

Spondylolisthesis refers to the forward "slipping" of an upper vertebral body over the lower as a result of degenerative changes of the facet joints.

65. B

Number 2 on the figure corresponds to the sigmoid colon.

66. C

Number 3 on the figure corresponds to the seminal vesicles.

67. A

Number 1 on the figure corresponds to the rectus abdominis muscle.

68. C

Number 4 on the figure corresponds to the ureterovesical junction (UVJ).

69. C

Contrast enhancement greatly improves demonstration of lymphadenopathy within the chest in comparison with other mediastinal structures.

70. C

Thin-section (0.5–2.0 mm) helical acquisition specific to the larynx should extend from just above the hyoid bone inferiorly through the cricoid cartilage.

71. C

Number 3 on the figure corresponds to the glenoid process.

72. A

The image is a multiplanar reformation (MPR) of the right shoulder in the coronal plane. This perspective demonstrates the relationship between the humeral head and the glenoid fossa (4).

73. B

Number 2 on the figure corresponds to the acromion.

74. B

The administration of an oral contrast agent is subject to specific departmental protocol considerations. Generally, 400 to 600 mL of oral contrast administered 45 to 90 minutes before the examination should opacify the small bowel. An additional dose of contrast agent (250 mL) immediately before the examination should ensure gastric opacification. Administration of contrast agents via enema is indicated for evaluation of the distal large bowel.

75. B
Cerebral blood flow (CBF) describes the quantity of blood (in mL) that moves through 100 g of brain tissue each minute. Normal CBF range in gray matter is 50 to 60 mL/100 g/min.

76. B
Number 3 in the figure corresponds to the trapezius muscle.

77. C
A total contrast agent volume between 100 and 150 mL is sufficient for imaging the neck. The precise volume and administration technique vary from one institution to another.

78. A
Number 1 on the figure corresponds to the common carotid artery.

79. D
Number 4 on the figure corresponds to the levator scapulae muscle.

80. B
Differentiation between a metastatic lesion and a benign adenoma of the adrenal masses can be accomplished by calculating the percentage of enhancement washout after a 10- to 15-minute delay. Precontrast, portal venous phase, and delayed acquisitions are obtained. On delayed postcontrast imaging, metastatic lesions of the adrenal gland remain enhanced longer than adrenal adenomas.

81. C
Ileus is used to describe an area of intestine that has lost normal contractile motion, resulting in obstruction.

82. B
Number 5 on the figure corresponds to the descending colon.

83. C
Number 3 on the figure corresponds to the abdominal aorta.

84. A
Demonstrating the same density and contrast as a conventional helically acquired axial image, the coronal display in the figure is a standard MPR image. Multiplanar reformation (MPR) describes the process of displaying CT images in a different orientation from the one used in the original reconstruction process. The reformatted image is 1 voxel thick, with the pixels facing the viewer, each representing the average attenuation occurring within the represented voxels.

85. C
Number 6 on the figure corresponds to the bladder.

86. C
The third and fourth ventricles communicate through the cerebral aqueduct, which is commonly referred to as the aqueduct of Sylvius.

87. C
Complete CT examination of the chest for bronchogenic carcinoma consists of an acquisition from the apices through the liver. The adrenal gland and liver are common sites for metastatic disease in patients with primary lung neoplasm. Scanning may be done in a caudocranial direction to ensure maximum contrast enhancement of the liver and adrenals when indicated.

88. C
The mediastinum is a potential space located between the two lungs. It contains the heart, great blood vessels, thymus, and portions of the trachea and esophagus.

89. D
The scan field of view (SFOV) chosen must be larger than the width of the patient in order to eliminate out-of-field artifacts. Some CT scanners may have limited choices for SFOV values. Other common terminology includes full-field or half-field, and body-cal and head-cal.

90. D
The kidneys are located in a portion of the retroperitoneum known as the perirenal space. They are held in place by fibrous connective tissue commonly referred to as Gerota's fascia.

91. C
The portal (or hepatic) venous phase is the period of peak hepatic parenchymal enhancement, when contrast material redistributes from the blood into the extravascular spaces. It occurs at approximately 60 to 70 seconds after the initiation of rapid bolus contrast agent administration.

92. D
Number 1 on the figure corresponds to the genu of the corpus callosum.

93. B
Number 6 on the figure corresponds to the falx cerebri.

94. B
Number 2 on the figure corresponds to the internal capsule.

95. A
Number 3 on the figure corresponds to the pineal gland.

96. C

The prone position during a postmyelogram CT study of the lumbar spine reduces pooling or layering of the intrathecal contrast material.

97. D

Bolus duration, or the time required to inject a specific volume of contrast agent, may be calculated as the product of injection flow rate and total contrast volume.

98. B

Number 4 on the figure corresponds to the lamina.

99. A

Number 1 on the figure corresponds to the pedicle.

100. B

Intrathecal administration of an iodinated contrast agent allows for greater visualization of the spinal cord and nerve roots after its introduction into the subarachnoid space.

101. D

Number 3 on the figure corresponds to the spinous process.

102. B

The pancreatic phase of contrast enhancement is a delayed arterial phase occurring approximately 35 to 45 seconds after the start of contrast agent administration, assuming an adequate volume injected at a rate of 3 mL/sec or greater.

103. A

Upon IV contrast enhancement, a tumor may be described as *hypovascular* if it is lower in density than the surrounding organ parenchyma or *hypervascular* if it is higher in density.

104. B

The "*triple rule-out*" *MDCT procedure* is a comprehensive evaluation of the chest for cardiac and noncardiac pain. The single acquisition consists of a coronary computed tomography angiogram (CTA) for coronary artery disease, a CTA of the aorta for aneurysm, and a CTA of the pulmonary arteries for embolism.

105. B

There is often significant artifact within the mediastinum from high concentrations of iodine in the superior vena cava. This artifact may be alleviated by administering a bolus of a contrast agent with reduced iodine concentration, which is achieved by diluting a full-strength contrast agent with saline.

106. D

Number 3 on the figure corresponds to the left primary bronchus.

107. B

Dense contrast opacification of the aorta and pulmonary arteries indicates that this image was obtained during the arterial phase, most likely within the first 20 to 30 seconds after bolus injection of contrast material.

108. A

Number 2 on the figure corresponds to the left pulmonary artery.

109. C

Number 6 on the figure corresponds to the ascending aorta.

110. B

The density of the mass in question indicates that it consists of fatty tissue. A *lipoma* is a benign mass consisting of fat cells. An *angiomyolipoma,* a common benign mass found in the kidney, consists of muscle cells, blood vessels, and fat. The average CT value range for fat is −50 to −100 Hounsfield units.

111. D

The *array processor* is a specialized component of the CT computer system. It is capable of performing the massive calculations required for CT image reconstruction.

112. A

Modern CT system x-ray tubes utilize dual-filament systems with focal spot sizes ranging between 0.5 and 1.2 mm in diameter.

113. B

The spatial resolution of a CT examination can be improved with the use of small focal spots, narrow sections, and large matrices.

114. C

The back-projection method of image reconstruction involves the acquisition of attenuation values, which are then projected back onto a matrix for subsequent display.

115. D

Multiple–detector row CT systems utilize the process called *z-filtering* during image reconstruction. Z-filtering allows for thin sections to be reconstructed at any point along the acquired z-axis volume. This interpolation technique utilizes multiple complementary rays beyond those immediately above and below the particular slice plane.

116. C

Fourth-generation CT scanners operate with a rotating x-ray tube and a stationary ring of detectors. Some fourth-generation scanners also use a rotating x-ray tube with a nutating detector ring.

117. D

Aliasing is a type of streak artifact caused when an insufficient number of views (data samples) is obtained during data acquisition. It is typically because of a technical failure of the CT system.

118. C

Quality assurance refers to the measurement of the scanner's performance through quality testing procedures and evaluation of the test results. *Quality control* refers to the implementation of corrective actions to improve any identified performance inadequacies of the CT system found through quality assurance procedures.

119. D

The mA setting in coordination with the scan time (seconds) gives the constant mAs for a CT acquisition.

120. B

The filtered back-projection, or convolution, method of image reconstruction had previously been the most common type of CT reconstruction. Today, improved processing speeds have allowed iterative reconstruction to become a primary method of CT image reconstruction. Many CT systems now employ iterative techniques, which offer reduced image noise, allowing for decrease technical parameters (mA, kVp) and reduced patient dose.

121. D

The matrix size used to reconstruct an image can be calculated by dividing the display field of view (DFOV) by the pixel dimension. A pixel whose area is 0.25 mm^2 has a linear dimension of 0.5 mm. Dividing the DFOV of 250 mm by the pixel dimension 0.5 mm gives a matrix size of approximately 512 × 512 pixels.

122. C

Minimum intensity projection (min-IP) images display the minimum pixel value along each ray to the viewer. As the viewer faces a min-IP image, each pixel represents the minimum attenuation that occurs in the associated voxel. Min-IP reformations are used primarily during the evaluation of the biliary tree, colon, lungs, and trachea.

123. D

The purposes of predetector or postpatient collimation are to remove scatter radiation and to shape the portion of the beam that is incident on each detector.

124. D

The Lambert–Beer law or equation is properly written as $I = I_0 e^{-\mu x}$. This important exponential equation illustrates the mathematical relationship between the primary beam, the object thickness (density), and the radiation measured by each detector in the calculation of the linear attenuation coefficient (μ).

125. B

The longitudinal spatial resolution is usually qualified by the extent of broadening that occurs to the slice sensitivity profile (SSP) during volumetric acquisition. The section width (slice) for a volumetric acquisition may be graphically represented as an SSP.

126. C

The section width (slice) for a volumetric acquisition may be graphically displayed as a slice sensitivity profile (SSP). The effective section width is defined as the full width at half maximum (FWHM) of the SSP. The FWHM is labeled in the figure as C. At this point of the graph, the section width of B is wider than that of A.

127. A

Thorough communication between the technologist and the patient is vital in ensuring superior examination quality. If the patient has been informed of the examination process, his or her anxiety may be reduced and cooperation improved. During all CT procedures, the patient must be instructed to hold still in an effort to reduce motion artifact on the CT images.

128. D

The power output of modern multidetector CT (MDCT) systems is vendor specific, within a typical range of 60 to 100 kilowatts (kW).

129. D

The terms *algorithm*, *kernel*, and *mathematical filter function* may all be used interchangeably in describing the mathematical process used for the complex calculations required during CT image reconstruction.

130. C

The scan field of view (SFOV) size is determined by the number of detectors activated along the in-plane (x-, y-) axes during data acquisition.

131. C

An average range of CT numbers for blood is +42 to +58. The CT number of any material is based on many factors, including the beam quality of a particular scanner.

132. A

Binning refers to the electronic combination of signal from adjacent detectors to form a reconstructed slice that is thicker than the individual detector width. For example, transmission data from four adjacent 1.25-mm detectors is combined to produce a CT section 5.0 mm thick.

133. D

Technical adjustments to improve the temporal resolution of the CT system may help reduce involuntary motion artifacts. Reductions in scan time (gantry rotation), image segmentation, and physiologic gating can be used to reduce the effects of involuntary motion.

134. D

The dense bony areas of the posterior fossa of the skull are especially prone to beam-hardening artifacts. *Hounsfield bar* is commonly used to describe this particular artifact.

135. A

The relative accuracy between calculated CT numbers and their respective linear attenuation coefficients is termed *linearity*. Calibration and routine vendor maintenance procedures work to establish and maintain CT system linearity.

136. D

Digital encryption is used to encode data that is transferred across a network into a form decipherable only by software at the destination location.

137. C

Perspective volume rendering provides one a viewpoint of being within the lumen of the object, similar to an endoscopic view. Also referred to as *immersive rendering*, this type of 3-D reconstruction is commonly used during CT colonography and CT bronchography.

138. D

Thin-section reconstruction using the smallest display field of view (DFOV) possible results in the smallest pixel and voxel dimensions. Voxels with equal dimensions along the x-, y- and z-axes are described as *isotropic*.

139. B

CT does not employ silver halide crystal as a detector material.

140. B

Interpolation is a mathematical technique used in the reconstruction process of the spiral CT image. It involves the estimation of an unknown value from information above and below it.

141. D

Misregistration is the loss of anatomic information that occurs when a patient suspends respiration at different depths during consecutive scans. It occurs only during CT examinations in which suspended respiration of the patient is necessary. The ability of multidetector CT (MDCT) systems to volumetrically acquire entire anatomic areas in a single, short breath-hold has greatly reduced the occurrence of misregistration artifact.

142. C

Single-slice helical geometry allows for volumetric data acquisition. The reconstruction of CT sections at any point along the scanned volume is possible. The section width must be the same, however, and is controlled by the collimation (slice thickness) chosen before data acquisition. The advancement of multislice CT (MDCT) allows for retrospective reconstruction of sections at varying thicknesses.

143. C

Bow-tie filters, which are thicker at the ends than in the middle, help shape the beam to reduce patient radiation exposure. Because most body parts are circular or cylindrical, less radiation is necessary at the periphery than in the center. Bow-tie filters reduce beam intensity toward the outer margins, resulting in a reduction in patient radiation dose.

144. D

The thickness of the reconstructed section is controlled primarily by the detector configuration in a multidetector CT (MDCT) system. Beam collimation also exerts an indirect effect on section width by controlling the portion of the detector array exposed to transmitted radiation.

145. B

Noise appears on the CT image as an inaccuracy in CT number. The noise of a CT scanner may be measured by scanning a homogeneous object such as a water phantom. Fluctuations in CT number from pixel to pixel indicate the presence of noise.

146. D

The region of interest (ROI) measurement provides a quantitative analysis of the Hounsfield values of a specific anatomic area. System software calculates the average CT number in HUs within the defined ROI. The average ROI measurement provides information regarding tissue characteristics that may be helpful for clinical diagnosis.

147. A

The linear dimension of the pixel must first be calculated by dividing the display field of view (DFOV), in mm, by the matrix (380 mm ÷ 512 = 0.74 mm). This linear pixel dimension is squared to yield the pixel area in mm^2 (0.74 × 0.74 = 0.55 mm^2). The volume of the voxel may be calculated by multiplying the pixel area by the section width 0.55 mm^2 × 1.25 mm = 0.69 mm^3).

148. B

The presence of metal within the patient causes a streak artifact on the image. The artifact occurs when the dense metal absorbs a large amount of the radiation, interfering with the signal produced.

149. A

Metallic dental fillings often cause a streak artifact during CT examinations of the head.

150. C

An isotropic axial acquisition of the paranasal sinuses from the hard palate superiorly through the frontal sinus avoids artifact from dental fillings while providing excellent multiplanar reformations (MPRs) in any plane. Direct coronal acquisition may not be required because the detail provided by the reformatted images is usually sufficient. This technique also aids in reducing patient radiation dose.

151. C

The first-generation CT scanner acquired data through a process based on the principle of tube translation and rotation around the patient's head.

152. D

At a maximum, the multidetector CT (MDCT) cone beam may be collimated to a dimension equal to the entire multirow detector array. In the example, the total dimension of the detector array along the z-axis is 40.00 mm, or 64 × 0.625 mm.

153. A

Computed tomography has better low-contrast resolution over conventional radiography. The CT system is extremely sensitive to small changes in tissue density and removes the problem of superimposition, both leading to greater contrast resolution.

154. C

Write-once, read-many (WORM) describes certain CD and DVD media capable of storing data only once. The stored images can be read multiple times, but once recorded on, the media may not be reused.

155. A

The CT number of a pixel may be calculated by subtracting the linear attenuation coefficient of water from the linear attenuation coefficient of the tissue within the voxel (0.008 − 0.181 = −0.173). This number is divided by the linear attenuation coefficient of water (−0.173 ÷ 1.81 = −0.956). The quotient is multiplied by a contrast factor of 1000 to yield the value of the pixel in Hounsfield units.

156. B

Because of its solid nature, the scintillation detector interacts with a higher percentage of incident x-ray photons, giving it a better capture efficiency.

157. D

The data acquisition system (DAS) of a CT scanner consists of the detector array, the analog-to-digital convertor, and a transmission device used to send the converted digital information to the computer for image reconstruction.

158. A

During CT image reconstruction using the back-projection method, the data are manipulated with a convolution kernel or algorithm to remove image unsharpness (blurring). This method is called the *filtered back-projection.*

159. D

The oversampling technology known as *flying focal spot* involves the electromagnetic steering of the electron beam emitted from the cathode. The beam of electrons is directed toward two separate locations on the rotating anode, resulting in two sources of x-radiation. As the tube rotates around the patient, the number of data samples is essentially doubled because of the electronic switching between the two focal spots, improving the system's temporal and spatial resolution.

160. D

Water has a CT number at or near zero. This area in the region of interest (ROI) in the figure most likely represents a hepatic cyst.

161. C

At the range of photon energies employed during most CT examinations, water exhibits an approximate attenuation coefficient value of 0.206.

162. B

The width of a window used to display a CT image of the abdomen should be within the range of 350 to 600 HU. This range allows for excellent visualization of the soft tissue structures.

163. D

The contrast of a CT image is controlled by the spatial frequencies of the tissue(s) within the section. Tissues of differing densities are represented electronically by different spatial frequencies. Adjacent tissues with similar densities or areas of tissue with minimal differences in density are represented by low spatial frequencies.

164. C

The width of a window determines the range of pixel values that will be assigned a shade of gray around a given level. In this example, all pixels within the range of −300 to +700 HU will be assigned shades of gray. Pixels below 300 HU will appear black, and pixels above +700 HU will appear white. This calculation is performed by dividing the width in half (1000/2 = 500) and subtracting and adding this value to the level (+200 HU + 500 = +700 HU, +200 HU − 500 = −300 HU).

165. C

A *byte* is a series of eight bits. Bits and bytes are part of the binary language used by computers to process information.

Answer Key—Examination Three

ANSWERS

1. D
The use of water as a negative contrast agent is becoming increasingly common for many CT applications for the abdomen and pelvis.

2. A
The top number of a blood pressure measurement is the systolic pressure. This is a measure of the pressure exerted on the arterial walls during a contraction of the heart.

3. B
Nonionic contrast materials do not dissociate into charged particles (ions) when placed in solution. Ionic contrast materials are salts that form independent particles in aqueous solutions.

4. C
CT manufacturers routinely supply comfortable, nonadhesive straps and cushions to help maintain motion-free patient positioning. Adhesive tape should not be routinely used because of the abrasive effects of tape removal. Good patient communication is a key immobilization technique. Proper instructions for remaining still, suspending respiration, not swallowing, and so on help ensure patient cooperation and yield higher-quality CT examinations.

5. C
Normal range of glomerular filtration rate (GFR) is 70 ± 14 mL/min/m^2 for men and 60 ± 10 mL/min/m^2 for women.

6. C
Risk factors for contrast-induced nephrotoxicity (CIN) include preexisting compromise of renal function, dehydration, diabetes, myeloma, advanced age, and cardiovascular disease.

7. A
Medical asepsis is the reduction in number of infectious agents without the complete elimination of the organisms. It is accomplished through the use of soap, water, and many other types of disinfectant materials.

8. A
Patients with slower heart rates exhibit longer diastolic phases, which yield higher-quality cardiac CT examinations. The preferred heart rate for optimal imaging on most multidetector CT (MDCT) systems is 65 beats per minute (bpm). Newer systems at the 64-slice level and beyond are capable of acquiring adequate cardiac CT images at higher heart rates.

9. C
Urticaria is a common adverse reaction to iodinated intravenous contrast material. Characterized by the presence of wheals or localized skin eruptions, it is commonly referred to as *hives*.

10. B
Barium sulfate is not water soluble and is not easily absorbed by the body. If it leaks out of the digestive tract because of perforation, this agent may cause peritonitis.

11. C
The use of automatic injectors does not decrease the risk of contrast-induced nephrotoxicity (CIN) in comparison with the manual bolus technique. Automatic injectors do offer shorter injection times, more consistent administration, and greater enhancement.

12. A
Severe reactions to iodinated contrast material include anaphylaxis, shock, cardiac arrest, and death. Urticaria and vomiting may be considered mild or moderate reactions, depending on their severity.

13. B
Serum creatinine levels are the most accurate and dependable laboratory measures of renal function. The blood urea nitrogen (BUN) level may be affected by many variables and is not a suitable test of renal function by itself. BUN levels are usually evaluated in conjunction with creatinine levels for a more accurate measurement of renal function.

14. C
Twenty-two-gauge angiocatheters are sufficient for flow rates up to 3 mL/sec. Twenty-gauge or larger angiocatheters should be utilized whenever flow rates exceed 3 mL/sec.

15. A

Atrial systole refers to the contraction of the left and right atria. The onset of the P wave on an electrocardiogram (ECG) corresponds to atrial systole.

16. B

A bolus injection is one in which the entire volume of medication or contrast agent is administered at once over a short period.

17. B

Osmolality, or osmotic concentration, is the number of ions or particles formed when a substance (solute) dissociates in a given solution. It is described as the number of particles in solution per kg of water.

18. C

The total injection time may be calculated by dividing the contrast agent volume by the flow rate. In this example, the flow rate is 1.5 mL/sec, for a total of 150 mL. The time required for this injection would be 100 seconds.

19. D

Informed consent must be obtained from the patient before any invasive procedure. The components of informed consent are thorough explanations of the procedure, any possible risks in addition to the proposed benefits, and alternatives to the procedure.

20. B

Low-osmolar contrast media (LOCM) are nonionic agents that do not dissociate into charged particles (ions) in solution. Examples of LOCM are iohexol (Omnipaque), iopamidol (Isovue), and ioversol (Optiray).

21. C

In an effort to reduce the possibility of headaches after a CT examination involving an intrathecal injection of contrast material, the patient should rest for 8 to 24 hours with the head slightly elevated (35–45 degrees).

22. C

β-Adrenergic receptor blocking agents (β-blockers) may be used to reduce a patient's heart rate, and sublingual nitroglycerin may be administered to cause dilation of the coronary vessels. The use of these pharmaceuticals may improve the overall visualization of the coronary vessels during a cardiac CT examination. Please consult the physician and/or department protocol for further information regarding pharmaceutical administration for cardiac CT procedures.

23. D

In-plane bismuth shielding of particularly radiosensitive areas such as the orbits, thyroid, and breast tissue can substantially reduce effective radiation dose.

24. C

"Child-sizing" protocols, minimizing the anatomic scan area, and eliminating unnecessary enhancement phase acquisitions are all valuable components of a comprehensive dose reduction approach for pediatric patients. Rather than refuse to perform an ordered CT examination, technologists are encouraged to discuss the justification for a pediatric CT procedure with a supervising physician or other independent licensed practitioner and to make every effort to minimize dose when the clinical indication for the procedure is confirmed.

25. A

Compton scatter occurs when an incident x-ray photon interacts with an outer-shell electron of a target atom. The photon loses some energy in this ionization interaction and undergoes a resultant change in direction.

26. C

Dose length product (DLP) is a measure of the weighted radiation dose ($CTDI_{vol}$) over a given scan length (CM) and is typically given in units of a subunit of gray (cGy or mGy) per centimeter (i.e., cGy-cm). Current CT systems will typically report the DLP as part of the radiation dose structured report (RDSR), as a means of providing an estimation of patient dose for a given CT acquisition. DLP is estimated from either the $CTDI_{vol}$ or the multiple scan average dose (MSAD) over a specific number of slices, taken from comparable dose measurements using an anthropomorphic phantom.

27. C

With a single-slice CT (SSCT) system, pitch equals the ratio of the table speed with the section thickness. As the detector pitch is increased, the patient translates through the gantry at a greater rate relative to each rotation of the x-ray tube, resulting in the acquisition of a given volume of anatomy with fewer tube-detector rotations and shorter scan times. Increases in pitch therefore allow for reduced patient radiation dose while covering the necessary anatomic area.

28. D

During multidetector CT (MDCT) cardiac studies, prospective gating can be used to reduce the patient radiation dose. Electrocardiogram (ECG)-triggered tube current modulation allows for pulses of x-ray energy rather than continuous exposure to be used. Tube current is reduced during the cardiac phase not utilized for image reconstruction.

29. B

The $CTDI_{vol}$ is a measure of dose to each slice along a helically acquired volume. The dose length product (DLP) is calculated by multiplying the $CTDI_{vol}$ by the total scan length.

30. B

Effective dose accounts for the type of tissue that the radiation is deposited in. Different tissues are assigned weighting factors on the basis of their individual radiosensitivities.

31. B

Modern CT systems employ automated systems controlling both tube milliamperage (mA) and applied potential (kVp) for the purpose of patient dose reduction. These systems act as a means of automatic exposure control (AEC) for CT. The focus-to-isocenter distance of a given CT system is predetermined in the system design and cannot be adjusted. A manufactured decrease in focus-to-isocenter distance will result in an increase in patient dose, according to the inverse square law.

32. A

A stochastic, or random, effect of radiation exposure is one having no threshold dose. Common examples of stochastic radiation effects are genetic mutations and cancer.

33. C

An increase in kVp, with no other compensating adjustment in technical parameters, will result in greater tube output and a higher subsequent patient dose. Decreases in kVp will significantly lower patient dose (according to radiography's 15% rule) if the mAs is not increased to compensate.

34. B

During axial scanning, overlapping scans increase the patient radiation dose, whereas gaps between slices decrease the dose.

35. C

$CTDI_{vol}$ is used to approximate the dose from a helical scan. It corresponds to the axially acquired $CTDI_w$ divided by the helical pitch. Whereas $CTDI_w$ approximates the dose along the x- and y-axes of the acquired CT image, $CTDI_{vol}$ also includes the dose along the z-axis of the scan acquisition. As pitch increases, the dose per section, or $CTDI_{vol}$, decreases.

36. C

During multidetector CT (MDCT) cardiac studies, prospective gating can be used to reduce patient radiation dose. In this technique, electrocardiogram (ECG)-triggered tube current modulation allows for pulses of x-ray energy to be used rather than continuous exposure. Both retrospective ECG gating and multisegment reconstruction require constant radiation exposure throughout multiple heartbeats.

37. D

Iterative reconstruction uses multiple image reconstruction passes (iterations) to arrive at a final image with reduced noise and artifacts, leading to improved overall quality. This reduction in noise allows technical factors to be significantly reduced, resulting in decreased patient radiation dose.

38. C

It is important to remember that $CTDI_{vol}$ and dose length product (DLP) do not account for patient size and so overestimate the radiation dose to the larger patient and underestimate the dose to the smaller patient. For a given DLP, absorbed dose will be less in the larger patient, as the radiation is distributed over a larger mass than in the smaller patient. This concept forms the basis of why customized, size-based protocols are an important component of dose-reduction efforts.

39. B

Dose can be considerably higher with multidetector CT (MDCT) due to a decrease in the focal spot–detector distance, the use of a cone beam instead of a more z-axis–collimated fan beam, an increase in number of imaging phases enabled by shorter scan times, and the acquisition of thinner sections for improvement of 3-D and multiplanar reformation (MPR) images.

40. A

Increased pitch, noise level (index), and table speed will all result in a measurable radiation dose savings. Increasing the tube current (milliamperage, mA) will result in a direct and proportionate increase in tube output and subsequent patient radiation dose.

41. A

Model-based iterative reconstruction (MBIR) considers the shape of the CT x-ray beam both prepatient and postpatient and uses complex statistical analyses in both a forward and backward series of reconstructions to arrive at an improved image with reduced noise.

42. B

Attenuation is the reduction in intensity of an x-ray beam as it interacts with matter. Several interactions are responsible for the attenuation of primary radiation, including Compton scatter and photoelectric effect. Each of these interactions reduces the energy and/or number of the x-ray photons in a primary beam.

43. D

A hemangioma is a congenital, benign mass containing blood-filled spaces. It is commonly found in the liver and spleen.

44. D

The preferred timing for CT acquisition of the spleen is the portal venous phase (60–70 sec), when a more homogeneous pattern of enhancement is demonstrated.

45. D
Number 2 on the figure corresponds to the scaphoid.

46. A
The image in the figure is a multiplanar reformation (MPR) of the wrist in the coronal plane. MPR images are particularly helpful for trauma indications, such as fracture of the distal radius, labeled number 3 on the figure.

47. A
Number 1 on the figure corresponds to the capitate.

48. B
Number 5 on the figure corresponds to the lunate.

49. B
Subdural hematomas are collections of blood that occur throughout the subdural space after traumatic injury to the head. An acute subdural hematoma is one that has manifested clinically during the first 24 hours after the injury. During this stage, the hematoma appears hyperdense compared with normal brain tissue because of the initial clotting that has occurred and the concentration of hemoglobin in fresh blood.

50. D
The angiographic assessment of the peripheral arterial tree from the renal arteries through the feet is commonly referred to as a *CT runoff.*

51. D
Malignant cells demonstrate an increase in metabolic activity and glucose utilization. Once administered, fludeoxyglucose F 18 (FDG) mimics glucose and is taken up by normal and abnormal tissue. The amount of FDG uptake is directly proportional to the area's metabolic activity. Malignant cells will take up a disproportionately larger amount of FDG than metabolically normal tissue.

52. A
Number 2 on the figure corresponds to the left ovary.

53. D
Number 4 on the figure corresponds to the uterus.

54. B
Number 5 on the figure corresponds to the bladder.

55. C
Intravenous administration of an iodinated contrast agent is vital to making an accurate diagnosis of a dissecting aortic aneurysm. The contrast agent helps outline the wall of the aorta and improves visualization of any division within it. Because of differences in blood flow, CT numbers within the actual lumen of the aorta are different from those in the dissected portion.

56. A
The eighth cranial nerve is the vestibulocochlear nerve responsible for both hearing and balance. Vestibular schwannoma may also be referred to as *acoustic neuroma.* This type of mass most often involves the vestibular portion of the nerve bundle, with deleterious effects on balance and equilibrium.

57. D
Number 3 on the figure corresponds to the vocal cord.

58. B
Number 1 on the figure corresponds to the piriform sinus.

59. A
A wide window setting (WL −300, WW 1000) may be used to properly demonstrate the small soft tissue vocal structures from the surrounding air-filled endolarynx.

60. C
Number 2 on the figure corresponds to the thyroid cartilage.

61. C
The mesentery is a double fold of the peritoneum that attaches the jejunum and ileum of the small bowel to the abdominal wall.

62. C
The nephrographic phase occurs between 70 and 90 seconds after the start of injection. Enhancement of the renal cortex and medulla reaches equilibrium, providing optimal sensitivity for parenchymal lesions.

63. C
Number 9 on the figure corresponds to the maxillary sinus.

64. B
Number 5 on the figure corresponds to the superior ophthalmic vein.

65. D
Number 4 on the figure corresponds to the superior oblique muscle.

66. C
Number 6 on the figure corresponds to the lateral rectus muscle.

67. D
Pneumothorax is one of the most common complications of CT-guided needle biopsy of the lung. The term describes a collection of air in the pleural space. A pneumothorax causes a portion of the lung to collapse, often resulting in the placement of a chest tube to reinflate the lung.

68. C
Number 6 on the figure corresponds to the renal calyx.

69. D
Maximum intensity projection (MIP) images display only the maximum pixel value along a ray traced through the object to the viewer's assumed perspective in front of the viewing monitor. Tissues with lower attenuation values are not displayed, leaving high-attenuation structures such as bone and contrast-enhanced soft tissue structures free of superimposition.

70. A
Number 1 on the figure corresponds to the ureteropelvic junction (UPJ).

71. C
Dosage calculations for intravenous contrast agent administration should adhere to the general guiding principle of injecting the smallest quantity of contrast agent possible to meet the technical requirements of the examination. The maximum dose for any procedure should not exceed 2 mL per kg of body weight.

72. C
CT bronchography is a three-dimensional examination of the tracheobronchial tree. It may include detailed endobrachial views, on which the viewer has the perspective of flying through the trachea and bronchi, as in conventional bronchoscopy. These specialized 3-D reconstructions are commonly referred to as *virtual bronchoscopy*.

73. D
High-resolution CT (HRCT) images with the patient in the prone position can be acquired to differentiate the dependent edematous changes often seen in the lung bases.

74. C
The outer portion of an intervertebral disc is the anulus fibrosus.

75. C
Number 2 on the figure corresponds to the transverse process.

76. D
Number 1 on the figure corresponds to the transverse foramen.

77. D
Number 4 on the figure corresponds to the lamina.

78. C
Nephrographic (70–90 sec) imaging provides enhancement of the bladder wall, which is used to evaluate the extent of tumor infiltration.

79. B
The primary clinical indication for multidetector CT (MDCT) coronary artery calcium (CAC) quantitation is the assessment of atherosclerotic disease. The presence of CAC is a specific indicator of atherosclerotic disease.

80. C
Number 4 on the figure corresponds to the left common iliac vein.

81. C
Portions of the CT image may be enlarged on the display screen by either of two methods. The image may be magnified to offer the viewer a closer, enlarged look at a specific area. A CT image may also be "targeted" through a decrease in the display field of view (DFOV) size. A targeted image places the area of interest over the entire display matrix, providing greater resolution and more detail than a magnified image.

82. B
Number 5 on the figure corresponds to the right ureter.

83. D
Number 1 on the figure corresponds to the rectus abdominis muscle.

84. A
CT enteroclysis is a specialized evaluation of the small bowel whereby a nasogastric catheter is placed into the duodenum under fluoroscopic guidance. Then 1.5 to 2.0 L of enteral contrast agent is administered directly into the small intestine for maximal opacification. Non–IV contrast, thin-section (0.6–1.25 mm) CT images are acquired through the abdomen and pelvis.

85. C
The urothelium lines most of the urinary tract, including the renal pelvis, ureters, and bladder. The transitional portion of the urothelium can be the site of transitional cell carcinoma (TCC), a common malignancy of the bladder, ureters, and kidneys.

86. D
The ostiomeatal complex is an important sinus opening that allows for drainage of the frontal, ethmoid, and maxillary sinuses. It is a common area for sinusitis, or inflammation of the sinuses.

87. B
Number 1 on the figure corresponds to the right pulmonary artery.

88. A
Maximum intensity projection (MIP) images are a routine component of CT angiogram (CTA) examinations of the chest. This CTA of the pulmonary arteries (CTPA)

demonstrates the well-opacified pulmonary vasculature in coronal thick-slab format. From the perspective of the viewer, each pixel displays the maximum attenuation value contained within the thickness of the slab.

89. D
Number 4 on the figure corresponds to the descending aorta.

90. C
Pulsation artifacts are unique to cardiac imaging and CT angiogram (CTA) procedures of the mediastinum. They appear as a type of stair-step artifact and result from the diastolic heart motion occurring during relatively long exposure times. Improving the temporal resolution of the scan and electrocardiogram (ECG) gating are methods employed to reduce pulsation artifact.

91. B
Number 2 on the figure corresponds to the pulmonary trunk.

92. B
The use of a saline flush reduces artifact from dense contrast in the superior vena cava. The streaking artifact can hamper visualization of the upper mediastinum and surrounding lung tissue.

93. A
Shortly after a CT angiogram (CTA) of the pulmonary arteries (CTPA) study, CT venography (CTV) of the lower extremities for the identification of deep vein thrombosis (DVT) may also be performed. After the CTPA acquisition, a delay of 2 to 3 minutes is employed, and an acquisition is made from the iliac crest to the ankles. This may be commonly referred to as a CT runoff.

94. C
Number 4 on the figure corresponds to the fourth ventricle.

95. B
Number 2 on the figure corresponds to the left middle cerebral artery.

96. D
Number 5 on the figure corresponds to the basilar artery.

97. A
Number 4 on the figure corresponds to the left posterior cerebral artery.

98. D
Reductions in kVp, overlapping axial sections, and precise bolus timing are all important factors in the production of high-quality CT angiogram (CTA) examinations.

99. B
The most important identifying sign of gastrointestinal (GI) pathology on CT examination is wall thickening. The ability to evaluate the gastric and bowel walls is a crucial component of the successful CT evaluation of the GI system. Distention and opacification with oral media, coupled with contrast enhancement through intravenous (IV) administration, offer the best demonstration of the GI wall.

100. B
Number 2 on the figure corresponds to the left subclavian artery.

101. A
Number 5 on the figure corresponds to the right brachiocephalic vein.

102. C
Number 1 on the figure corresponds to the left brachiocephalic vein.

103. C
Number 4 on the figure corresponds to the left common carotid artery.

104. D
Hepatocellular carcinomas (HCCs) are hypervascular lesions that appear hyperdense in comparison with surrounding normal hepatic parenchyma during the arterial phase of contrast enhancement.

105. B
Lithiasis refers to the presence of stones. Unenhanced helical CT of the urinary tract has become the standard for the investigation of urinary tract lithiasis.

106. B
Phonation during acquisition may be used to demonstrate abnormal mobility of the vocal cord(s). A thin-section (0.5–2 mm) sequence is obtained during which the patient is instructed to phonate a low, steady "E" sound during the entire scan duration.

107. C
Number 1 on the figure corresponds to the superior mesenteric vein.

108. B
Number 4 on the figure corresponds to the spleen.

109. D
Number 6 on the figure corresponds to the pancreas.

110. C
Computed tomography is commonly used during percutaneous aspiration and drainage procedures. CT images enable the radiologist to view the precise location of abnormal fluid collections and allow for accurate planning of a safe access route for the aspiration procedure. When performed properly, CT-guided aspiration of an abdominal

abscess can be a valuable nonsurgical therapeutic technique. This type of procedure can also be used to reduce other types of abnormal fluid collections, including cysts, bilomas, urinomas, and lymphoceles.

111. D

The x-ray tube and data acquisition system (DAS) are housed within the gantry of a CT scanner. The gantry aperture is the circular opening through which the patient moves during scanning.

112. D

Both the x-ray tube and detector array rotate around the patient during scanning with a third-generation CT unit.

113. C

The scanner's reduced low-contrast resolution is most likely the cause of increased noise. When the noise level of a CT image increases, the low-contrast resolution decreases. Decreased patient radiation dose implies that the signal-to-noise ratio has decreased, thus raising the noise level of the image. The same situation would apply for an increase in electronic noise.

114. A

Maximum intensity projection (MIP) images display only the maximum pixel value along a ray traced through the object to the viewer's assumed perspective in front of the viewing monitor. As the viewer faces an MIP image, each pixel represents the maximum attenuation that occurs in the associated voxel.

115. C

The dimension of a pixel may be calculated by dividing the field of view by the matrix size. The display field of view (DFOV) of 40 cm must first be converted into 400 mm. This is then divided by 512 mm, for a pixel dimension of 0.78 mm. Keep in mind that the pixel is a square, two-dimensional item and that the measurement of 0.78 mm corresponds to only one side.

116. C

Collimation occurs as lead shutters close down upon the beam, limiting its projected area. Constructed of lead, the collimator shutters absorb portions of the primary beam, thereby reducing its intensity.

117. D

Photon fluence may be described as the quantity of x-radiation passing through a unit area.

118. A

The most common cause of CT image noise is the fluctuation in the number of x-ray photons measured by the detectors. When a CT scanner attempts to reconstruct an image from an insufficient amount of transmitted radiation measurements, quantum noise occurs.

119. A

A computer network is a communication system designed to facilitate the transfer of data between computers. A picture archival and communications system (PACS) works on a network, which connects each of the involved imaging modalities, viewing stations, printers, and so on.

120. C

The edge gradient effect occurs when the CT x-ray beam passes through areas of abrupt changes in density that are represented by high spatial frequencies. This type of streak artifact commonly occurs at the interface of dense bone and soft tissue in anatomic areas such as the brain.

121. B

Streaking edge gradient artifacts may be reduced with increases in the beam's average photon energy. Increases in kVp and filtration would accomplish this. This type of artifact may also be reduced with a decrease in reconstructed section width, which helps minimize the edge gradient effect. A decrease in partial volume averaging may lessen the streaking that is apparent from edge gradient inconsistencies.

122. C

The level chosen for a given window setting should correspond to the average density value of the tissue(s) of interest. Areas of soft tissue, such as the brain, are often displayed at window levels of approximately +50 HU.

123. D

The star artifact was an unwanted by-product of the back-projection method of image reconstruction used in older CT scanners. It is now removed by the process of convolution used in the modern reconstruction method known as *filtered back-projection*.

124. C

Involuntary motion is beyond control of the patient and includes peristalsis, cardiac contraction, and tremors. The most effective method of reducing involuntary motion on a CT scan is reduction of scan times. Many scanners offer segmenting, or "half-scan," options whereby images may be reconstructed after a partial revolution of the tube-detector system. In the case of digestive involuntary motion, glucagon administration is an additional option.

125. C

Multiplanar reformation (MPR) describes the process of displaying CT images in a different orientation from the one used in the original reconstruction process. Unlike retrospective reconstruction, reformation does not change the makeup of the image voxels. Reformation merely alters the viewing perspective of the images to a different anatomic plane.

126. D
Windowing is used to describe the process of grayscale mapping the CT image, during which the display system assigns a shade of gray to an individual pixel on the basis of its CT number (HU).

127. B
The Lambert–Beer law, $I = I_0 e^{-\mu x}$, is used to calculate the attenuation coefficient of a volume of material. The symbol "I_0" represents the intensity of the radiation incident upon the tissue being imaged. It is compared with the intensity of the radiation passing through the tissue (I) during the calculation of the linear attenuation coefficient.

128. A
The x-ray beam of a first-generation CT scanner was highly collimated to the size of a single detector. It was often referred to as a *pencil beam*.

129. C
The transmitted intensity is the amount of energy that passes through the patient onto a detector.

130. D
The limiting resolution of a modern CT scanner is approximately 25 lp/cm. This resolution varies greatly with scan factors and is considerably less than that of projection radiography.

131. A
Postpatient collimation occurs through a high-resolution comb placed over the detector array. Functioning like a grid, it removes unwanted scatter radiation and off-axis photons that result from the more divergent nature of the multidetector CT (MDCT) beam.

132. C
Section interval describes the spacing between two adjacent CT images. It is measured as the distance between the center of one section and the center of the adjacent section.

133. B
The number of data channels controls the number of sections the scanner can simultaneously acquire with each gantry rotation. For example, a four-slice multidetector CT (MDCT) system has sixteen 1.25-mm detectors in its array. However, with only four data channels, the maximum number of sections that may be reconstructed from each gantry rotation is four. The system combines transmission information from the individual detectors through its four data channels, resulting in the acquisition of four sections per gantry rotation.

134. B
Consisting of an arrangement of pixels in rows and columns, the matrix is used to organize the attenuation information from the anatomic section into a digital image. The size of the matrix is given as the number of pixels across multiplied by the number of pixels down.

135. C
Region of interest (ROI) measurements may be made by superimposing a cursor over an area and instructing the computer to average the CT numbers included within the region.

136. C
The CT number for water has an average value of zero.

137. A
Quality control refers to the implementation of corrective actions to improve any identified performance inadequacies of the CT system found through quality assurance procedures.

138. B
The use of a fan- or cone-shaped x-ray beam during CT increases the total volume of tissue irradiated, thereby increasing the amount of scatter radiation produced. This change results in a significantly higher patient radiation dose than the "pencil beam" radiation used in older CT scanners.

139. D
Each CT scanner has several choices for scan field of view (SFOV). The choice made by the technologist activates a certain percentage of the detector array so that information is acquired from a circular portion of the anatomic section. Built into the SFOV selection are additional correction factors used to process different types of tissue. For example, a CT scanner may have a specific selection for scans of the head, which attempts to limit the artifact occurring at the delineation of bone from brain tissue.

140. A
The transmitted intensity of a CT x-ray beam and the attenuation of the tissue imaged are inversely related. As the tissue begins to attenuate less radiation, the transmitted intensity of the beam increases. Areas of less dense tissue allow more radiation to pass onto the detectors, and vice versa.

141. B
Smaller focal spots improve the geometric efficiency of the x-ray beam, leading to greater spatial resolution.

142. D
The geometric efficiency of a CT detector is influenced primarily by the amount of interspace material necessary between adjacent detectors. Although valuable in limiting interference (crosstalk) between adjacent detectors, the interspace material reduces geometric efficiency by absorbing transmitted x-ray energy.

143. C

The degree of attenuation depends on multiple factors, including the x-ray energy and the atomic structure and density of the exposed tissue.

144. C

Retrospective reconstruction occurs when an image is reconstructed a second time with an adjustment in a technical factor. The scan data, or "raw" data, are used to reconstruct the image with a different display matrix, display field of view, algorithm, and so on.

145. D

The beam divergence inherent to the cone beam geometry of multidetector CT (MDCT) can cause difficulty during the image reconstruction process. Specific cone beam algorithms such as the Feldkamp–Davis–Kress (FDK) and advanced single-slice rebinning (ASSR) algorithms attempt to overcome the issues resulting from the divergent path of the x-ray beam from the tube to the widened detector array.

146. A

Each 1.0% difference in contrast between adjacent objects amounts to a difference in pixel value of approximately 10 HU. Multidetector CT (MDCT) systems are typically capable of differentiating adjacent objects with attenuation differences as small as 3 HU.

147. C

The stop-motion capability of a CT system is referred to as *temporal resolution*. Temporal resolution quantifies the CT system's ability to freeze motion and provide an image free of blurring.

148. C

Ring artifacts are associated with the use of third-generation CT scanners. Both the x-ray tube and the detector array rotate around the patient with third-generation scanners. A malfunctioning detector or series of detectors in a third-generation CT scanner causes a ring artifact to appear on the image as a result of the rotational nature of the detector array.

149. C

At a maximum, the multidetector CT (MDCT) cone beam may be collimated to a dimension equal to the entire multirow detector array. In the example, the total dimension of the detector array along the z-axis is 16×1.25 mm, or 20.0 mm.

150. A

The polyenergetic CT x-ray beam consists of photons of varying energy. As the beam traverses the patient, low-energy photons are absorbed first, increasing the average intensity of the beam as it travels along its path. This change, referred to as *beam hardening,* can have an artifactual result on the CT image.

151. A

With multidetector CT (MDCT), detector collimation determines the width of the reconstructed section. By electronically adjusting the detector dimension, the operator can control the width of the x-ray beam contributing to a reconstructed section. Beam collimation no longer directly controls section width.

152. D

The accuracy between calculated CT numbers and their respective linear attenuation coefficients is termed *linearity.* Daily system calibration and routine vendor maintenance procedures work to establish and maintain CT system linearity.

153. C

When a formula comparing the attenuation coefficient of tissue with that of water is used, materials whose coefficients are less than that of water are assigned negative CT numbers.

154. C

Referred to as *targeting,* decreasing the display field of view (DFOV) causes an increase in the image size on the monitor. The DFOV controls the amount of scanned information to be displayed on the matrix. If a small portion of information is to be displayed on the entire matrix, it will appear larger to the viewer.

155. A

The bit depth of a digital imaging system defines the number of information bits contained within each pixel. This parameter ultimately controls the total range of CT values that may be assigned to a given pixel. For example, a bit depth of 12 results in 4096 possible CT values ($2^{12} = 4096$).

156. B

Isotropic voxels have equal dimensions along the x-, y-, and z-axes. Use of a thin reconstructed section width and small display field of view (DFOV) minimizes each voxel dimension.

157. C

The limiting resolution of a particular CT scan is determined at a point on the graph where the signal frequency corresponding to a particular object has reached 10% (modulation transfer function [MTF] = 0.1).

158. A

According to the modulation transfer function (MTF) diagram, the bone algorithm has a resolution of approximately 12 lp/cm. The standard algorithm and smooth algorithm are approximately 10 and 7 lp/cm, respectively.

159. A

The limiting resolution of a particular CT scan is determined at a point on the graph where the signal frequency corresponding to a particular object has reached 10%. When the modulation transfer function (MTF) is lower than 10% (0.1), the object is no longer resolved.

160. D
Total collimation equals the combined thicknesses of all the sections that are simultaneously acquired with each gantry rotation. For example, a given multidetector CT (MDCT) system has an array of 64 detectors, each 0.625 mm wide. If the beam is collimated to expose the entire array, the total collimation for the acquisition is equal to 0.625 mm × 64, or 40 mm.

161. B
All modern multidetector CT (MDCT) systems utilize solid-state detectors consisting primarily of a scintillating crystal material. Solid-state detectors are preferred for MDCT because of their ability to accurately record incident x-ray energy from any angle. This flexibility is important when one considers the widened cone beam geometry inherent to MDCT systems.

162. B
In modern multidetector CT (MDCT) systems, the highest-quality 3-D and multiplanar reformation (MPR) images are obtained with the acquisition of an isotropic or near-isotropic data set. The other equally important piece is an overlapping data set, for which the reconstruction interval is less than the section width.

163. A
The cupping artifact that occurs at the superior portion of the skull is another form of partial volume artifact. The dense skull table averages with the low-attenuating brain tissue, causing an artifact by which the brain parenchyma may appear abnormally dense.

164. A
The effective section width corresponds to the slice sensitivity profile (SSP) of the reconstructed section in consideration of the widening that occurs during helical data acquisition.

165. A
The sampling rate may be quantified as views per rotation (VPR). As the sampling rate rises, the number of VPR increases.

180-degree linear interpolation (180LI) Type of algorithm used for multislice computed tomography (MSCT) image reconstruction in which data acquired from a shorter distance (180 degrees) away from the reconstructed slice location are interpolated.

360-degree linear interpolation (360LI) Type of algorithm used for MSCT image reconstruction in which two sets of projection data acquired 360 degrees apart are used to form an image at a precise z-axis location.

absorbed dose The amount of x-ray energy absorbed in a unit of mass. It is measured in grays (Gy).

absorption efficiency The ability of an individual CT detector to absorb and measure the transmitted x-ray intensity incident upon it. Primarily controlled by the characteristics and physical makeup of the detector material.

adaptive array The type of MSCT detector array configured with the thinnest detectors at the center, surrounded by detectors of incrementally increasing widths along the z-axis.

advanced single-slice rebinning (ASSR) algorithm Cone beam correction algorithm utilized to overcome potential attenuation calculation errors from the divergent beam of MSCT systems.

afterglow The tendency of a scintillation-type CT detector to continue to glow in response to x-radiation after the exposure source has been terminated.

Agatston score Quantification of the volume and density of calcium within the coronary arteries. As calculated during a CT coronary artery calcification (CAC) examination, the Agatston score is used to indicate a patient's risk of suffering a cardiac event.

ALARA Acronym for *as low as reasonably achievable*, the cardinal principle of radiation dose reduction for all radiologic procedures, including CT.

algorithm Mathematical filter applied to raw data during CT image reconstruction to remove blurring artifact inherent to back-projection. May also be referred to as a *kernel*.

aliasing A form of streak artifact caused by an insufficient number of views (data samples) obtained during data acquisition.

analog-to-digital converter (ADC) Component of the data acquisition system (DAS) responsible for converting the electronic signal emitted by the CT detectors into digital form.

archival The storage of CT data in either hard (film) or soft (digital) form.

array processor (AP) Component of the CT computer system responsible for receiving raw scan data, performing all of the major processing of the CT image, and returning the reconstructed image to the storage memory of the host computer.

arterial phase Period of peak arterial enhancement after the bolus IV administration of iodinated contrast material. For example, the hepatic arterial phase occurs approximately 25 to 35 seconds after the initiation of contrast agent administration.

artifact A form of noise on the CT image resulting from errors during the measurement of transmitted radiation by the detectors.

ataxia A neurologic sign characterized by a loss of muscular coordination.

attenuation The reduction in intensity of a radiation beam as it passes through a substance.

attenuation coefficient The value assigned to an object quantifying its ability to attenuate an x-ray beam.

automatic tube current modulation (ATCM) CT system software used to adjust the milliamperage (mA) throughout an acquisition to reduce patient radiation dose to a minimum.

automatic tube voltage selection (ATVS) CT system software used to adjust the tube voltage (kVp) based upon the changing patient attenuation along the scan acquisition range to reduce patient radiation dose to a minimum.

back-projection The mathematical process of CT image reconstruction whereby ray sum data are projected back onto a matrix.

beam hardening The phenomenon whereby low-energy photons are absorbed as the x-ray beam passes through an object, resulting in an increase in the average photon energy of the beam.

beam pitch The ratio of table feed per gantry rotation to the total collimation used during acquisition with an MSCT system.

beam width The dimension of the primary beam in the longitudinal or z-axis as controlled by the prepatient collimator.

binning The process of electronically combining signal from adjacent detector elements to produce a reconstructed CT image that is thicker than the individual detector width.

bit depth The number of information bits contained within each pixel.

blood urea nitrogen (BUN) A measurement of renal function, determined as the amount of nitrogen in the blood in the form of the waste product urea. The normal range of BUN in adults is 7 to 25 mg/dL.

bow-tie filter A type of filter added to the CT x-ray tube to compensate for the cylindrical shape of most body parts. The filter is thicker at the ends and helps shape the beam to reduce patient radiation exposure.

cardiac cycle The series of blood flow–related events that occur from the beginning of one heartbeat to that of the next.

cerebral blood flow (CBF) A common measurement during CT perfusion studies of the brain. CBF is the quantity of blood (mL) that moves through 100 g of brain tissue each minute. Normal range in gray matter is 50 to 60 mL/100 g/min.

cerebral blood volume (CBV) A common measurement during CT perfusion studies of the brain. CBV is the quantity of blood (mL) contained within a 100-g volume of brain tissue. Normal range is 4 to 5 mL/100 g.

cerebral perfusion The level of blood flow throughout brain tissue.

coma A state of unconsciousness where the individual is completely unresponsive to stimuli.

constant mAs The product of milliamperage (mA) and scan time (seconds) utilized for a CT acquisition.

contiguous images   CT images acquired with equal section thicknesses and reconstruction intervals.

contrast resolution   The ability of a CT system to detect an object with a small difference in linear attenuation coefficient from the surrounding tissue. May also be referred to as *low-contrast detectability* or *sensitivity*.

contrast-induced nephrotoxicity (CIN)   A substantial decline in renal function that can occur after a patient receives IV contrast material. It is usually signified by a marked increase in serum creatinine over a baseline measurement obtained before contrast agent administration.

convolution   Mathematical filtration used by the CT system to remove blurring artifact during the back-projection method of image reconstruction.

corticomedullary phase   A late arterial phase of renal enhancement beginning 30 to 40 seconds after the initiation of contrast agent administration. Optimal enhancement of the renal cortex and renal veins occurs during this period.

creatinine   A waste product of metabolism found in the bloodstream and measured as an indicator of renal function. Normal range of creatinine is 0.5 to 1.5 mg/dL.

CT arthrography   CT evaluation of a joint after the intra-articular injection of iodinated contrast material.

CT bronchography   Specialized MSCT examination of the tracheobronchial tree consisting of multiplanar reformation (MPR) and volume-rendered three-dimensional (3D) images reconstructed from thin, overlapping MDCT axial images through the airways.

CT colonography   Specialized CT evaluation of the large intestine used primarily for colon cancer screening. The large intestine is extended and scanned with thin-section CT. Two-dimensional (2D) and 3D models are constructed, including virtual endoscopic fly-through views.

CT cystography   Specialized CT examination of the bladder whereby iodinated contrast material is administered directly under gravity into the bladder via Foley catheter.

CT dose index (CTDI)   An approximate measure of the radiation dose received in a single CT section or slice.

CT enteroclysis   Specialized CT evaluation of the small bowel whereby enteral contrast material is administered directly into the duodenum through a nasogastric catheter placed under fluoroscopic guidance.

CT enterography   Specialized CT evaluation of the small bowel after the oral administration of low-density (0.1%) barium.

CT fluoroscopy   Continuous, real-time CT imaging used predominantly for CT-guided interventional procedures.

CT myelography   CT evaluation of the spinal cord and nerve roots after the intrathecal administration of iodinated contrast material.

CT number   Relative value assigned to each pixel to quantify the attenuation occurring in each voxel in comparison with the attenuation of water. The calculated CT number for a given pixel is given in Hounsfield units (HU). May also be referred to as *pixel value*.

CT runoff   The CT angiographic assessment of the peripheral arterial tree from the renal arteries through the lower extremities.

CT simulation   The process of obtaining anatomic information with CT imaging that is used to calculate the beam arrangement for radiotherapy.

CT urogram   A comprehensive, multiphasic CT evaluation of the urinary tract. Consists primarily of precontrast, postcontrast, and delayed CT acquisitions through the kidneys, ureters, and bladder. It may also be commonly referred to as a *CT-IVP*.

cupping artifact   An error occurring in the superior portion of the skull, where dense bone averages with the low-attenuating brain tissue. This partial volume artifact may result in abnormally dense-appearing brain parenchyma.

data acquisition system (DAS)   The electronic components of a CT system responsible for measuring the transmitted x-radiation absorbed by the detectors.

data channel   Pathway of data transmission from the detectors to the computerized components of the system's data acquisition system. The number of data channels of a CT system determines the maximum number of sections that may be acquired with each gantry rotation.

data transfer rate   The speed at which a computerized storage drive is able to transfer data.

deconvolution   Mathematical image processing technique used to generate blood perfusion maps during CT perfusion studies of the brain.

detector   Device responsible for measuring transmitted radiation and converting it into a proportionate electronic signal to be used for image reconstruction.

detector array   The CT image receptor, consisting of a series of detectors arranged in varying configurations.

detector collimation   The process of determining section width in the MSCT system as determined by the defined beam width and the number and thickness of detectors utilized for image reconstruction.

detector configuration   The number, length, and organization of the individual detector elements in an MSCT system.

detector pitch   The ratio of table feed per gantry rotation to the acquired section width. This definition of pitch is used for helical single-slice CT (SSCT).

diastole   Portion of the cardiac cycle when the heart muscle is relaxed. Diastolic blood pressure reflects the force exhibited on the arterial walls during relaxation of the heart muscle. It is the bottom or second number provided during the assessment of blood pressure.

DICOM   Acronym for the Digital Imaging and Communications in Medicine standard for the process of recording, storing, printing, and transmitting medical image data.

display field of view (DFOV)   The diameter of the acquired attenuation data displayed across the image matrix. May also be referred to as the *zoom factor* or *target view*.

dose length product (DLP)   The measurement of dose for an entire series of CT images. DLP is equal to the calculated dose per section multiplied by the length of a CT acquisition along the z-axis.

dose profile   The section of the patient exposed to radiation at the gantry isocenter.

dual-energy CT   Simultaneous acquisition, by an MSCT system, of attenuation data for a single anatomic section with two x-ray beams, each having a different energy spectrum. Dual-energy CT systems rapidly switch between or alternate kVp settings during data acquisition, allowing for improved contrast between substances of differing densities.

dual-source CT   CT system that consists of two separate x-ray tubes and detector arrays mounted 90 degrees from each other within the gantry, allowing for dual-energy CT acquisition.

edge gradient   Streak artifact that occurs at the interface between a high-density object and the lower-attenuation material surrounding it.

effective dose   Approximation of the relative risk from exposure to ionizing radiation; it is calculated by assigning weighting factors to different tissues on the basis of their individual radiosensitivities. It is measured in sieverts (Sv).

effective mAs   The calculated mAs per acquired slice with a MSCT system.

effective section width   The slice sensitivity profile (SSP) of the reconstructed CT section. It is measured at the full width at half maximum (FWHM) of the SSP for a given CT acquisition.

electrocardiogram (ECG)   A graphical representation of the electrical activity of the heart recorded over time through electrodes placed on the patient's skin.

electron beam CT (EBCT)   Specialized CT design devoid of moving parts. Utilizes a beam of electrons bombarding a tungsten target to produce x-radiation. EBCT systems are capable of extremely short exposure times and have their greatest application in cardiac imaging.

equilibrium phase   Contrast phase of the liver when hepatic parenchymal enhancement dissipates and there is minimal attenuation difference between the intravascular and extravascular spaces. Usually occurs at 2 to 3 minutes after the initiation of contrast agent administration.

excretory phase   A delayed imaging renal enhancement phase that begins approximately 3 minutes after the initiation of contrast agent administration. Contrast material has been excreted into the renal calyces, opacifying the renal pelvis and the remainder of the urinary collecting system (i.e., ureters, bladder).

exposure   The ability of x-rays to ionize a volume of air. It is measured in roentgens (R).

extravasation   The escape of contrast material outside the blood vessel into the surrounding soft tissue.

fan angle   Angle of coverage by the x-ray beam as it emerges from the tube housing and exposes the detector array within the scan plane (x-y axis).

Feldkamp–Davis–Kress (FDK) algorithm   Cone beam correction algorithm utilized to overcome potential attenuation calculation errors from the divergent beam of MSCT systems.

filtered back-projection   The mathematical process of CT image reconstruction that involves convolution of the raw data before their projection back onto a matrix.

filtration   Removal of the low-energy x-ray photons emitted from the x-ray tube to improve beam quality and reduce patient radiation dose.

flat-panel detector   Large-area detector consisting of a film of scintillating crystals bonded to a matrix of silicon photosensors. May be used in place of the segmented detector rows found in MDCT systems.

flying focal spot   Electronic switching technique whereby the electron beam is electromagnetically steered toward two separate locations on the rotating anode. Results in the emission of two sources of x-radiation from the CT

x-ray tube and a doubling of the data samples acquired from each gantry rotation.

focus-to-detector distance   Characteristic of the CT gantry described as the distance between the x-ray source (CT tube) and the detector array.

focus-to-isocenter distance   Characteristic of the CT gantry described as the distance from the x-ray source (CT tube) to the center of the gantry opening, where the patient should be positioned.

full width at half maximum (FWHM)   The midpoint of an SSP, where the effective section width for a CT acquisition is determined.

gantry   The assembly that houses the x-ray tube, detectors, and additional data acquisition components of a CT system. The patient is positioned within the gantry during CT data acquisition.

geometric efficiency   The ability of a detector array to absorb and measure the transmitted x-ray intensity incident upon it. Primarily controlled by the physical arrangement of detectors within the array and the amount of interspace material required between adjacent detectors.

glomerular filtration rate (GFR)   An approximation of creatinine clearance or the rate by which creatinine is filtered from the bloodstream. GFR is utilized as a measure of renal function with normal ranges of 70 ± 14 mL/min/m^2 for men and 60 ± 10 mL/min/m^2 for women.

Half-value layer (HVL)   The thickness of material that is capable of reducing the intensity of the x-ray beam to one-half of its original value.

helical   The type of CT acquisition whereby the x-ray tube and patient continuously move during scanning, yielding a data set in the form of a helix. May also be commonly referred to as *spiral*.

Hounsfield bar   Specific type of streaking beam-hardening artifact that occurs in the posterior fossa of the brain.

Hounsfield unit (HU)   The unit of the CT number scale assigned to each pixel to quantify relative attenuation.

hybrid array   The type of MSCT detector array with narrower detectors positioned midline, flanked by the wider detectors.

hyperdense   Possessing CT attenuation values greater than the values of the surrounding tissue.

hypodense   Possessing CT attenuation values less than the values of the surrounding tissue.

hypoxemia   Condition of low concentration of oxygen in the blood.

hypoxia   Condition of insufficient oxygenation of tissue at the cellular level.

image compression   Complex computer technique that reduces the size of digital CT image data.

image data   The reconstructed data that have been projected back onto a matrix after convolution by an algorithm and displayed on a monitor as a grayscale CT image.

immersive rendering   *See* perspective volume rendering.

insufflation   The introduction of air into an organ or cavity for distention and improved visualization.

interpolation   The mathematical process used for helical CT image reconstruction whereby data from tube rotations just above and just below a given slice position are used for image reconstruction.

isocenter   The center point of gantry rotation.

isodense   Possessing CT attenuation values equal to the values of the surrounding tissue.

isotropic   Having equal dimensions along the x-, y-, and z-axes; in CT, describes voxels with this property.

iterative reconstruction   A mathematical CT reconstruction method that uses multiple passes (iterations) to arrive at a final image with reduced noise and artifacts, leading to improved overall quality at reduced patient dose.

kerma   Quantity of energy deposited in a unit of mass. *Kerma* is used to describe the absorbed dose of x-radiation.

kernel   Mathematical filter applied to raw data during CT image reconstruction to remove the blurring artifact inherent to back-projection. May also be referred to as an *algorithm*.

lethargy   A level of consciousness characterized by feelings of fatigue, drowsiness or apathy.

linear attenuation coefficient (μ)   The value assigned to an object to quantify the extent to which it attenuates x-ray.

linearity   The relative accuracy between calculated CT numbers and their respective linear attenuation coefficients.

lossless compression   The reversible process whereby the CT image is digitally compressed in size without loss of data and is identical to the original.

lossy compression   The irreversible process whereby data are lost during the compression process and the CT image does not exactly match the original.

matrix   Two-dimensional grid of numbers arranged in rows and columns.

maximum intensity projection (MIP)   Multiplanar reformation technique that displays only the maximum pixel value along a ray traced through the object to the viewer's assumed perspective in front of the viewing monitor.

mean transit time (MTT)   A common measurement during CT perfusion studies of the brain. MTT refers to the average transit time, in seconds, needed for blood to pass through a given region of brain tissue.

minimum intensity projection (min-IP)   Multiplanar reformation technique that displays the minimum pixel value along each ray to the viewer.

misregistration   Artifact that occurs when patient motion between consecutive acquisitions causes misalignment of data and the potential loss of anatomic information.

modulation transfer function (MTF)   A graphical representation of a CT system's response to a spatial frequency that serves as a measurement of the system's in-plane spatial resolution.

monoenergetic   Consisting of a uniform photon energy; used in CT to describe a beam of x-radiation.

multiphase   CT data acquisition during multiple timed phases of contrast enhancement.

multiplanar reformation (MPR)   The process of displaying CT images in a different orientation from the one used in the original reconstruction.

multiple scan average dose (MSAD)   A calculation of the average cumulative radiation dose to each anatomic slice within the center of a CT scan consisting of multiple slices.

multisegment reconstruction   A method of improving the temporal resolution of a CT system whereby the data acquisition process is subdivided into separate components of smaller rotation angles.

multislice CT (MSCT)   A CT system with a detector array capable of acquiring more than one section for each gantry rotation. May also be referred to as *multidetector CT (MDCT)*.

nephrographic phase   Renal enhancement phase occurring between 70 and 90 seconds after the start of injection of a contrast agent. Enhancement between renal cortex and medulla reaches equilibrium, providing optimal sensitivity for parenchymal lesions.

noise   Grainy appearance on the CT image due primarily to an insufficient x-ray photon flux per voxel. May also be described as any portion of the signal that contains no useful information, as evident in certain CT image artifacts.

Nyquist theorem   A sampling law dictating that the data sampling frequency must be at least twice the object's spatial frequency in order for the object to be resolved by the CT system.

O-arm   Portable CT-fluoroscopy unit with a telescoping gantry used to acquire 3D CT images and standard fluoroscopy during invasive or surgical procedures.

obtundation   A depressed level of consciousness characterized by dulled feelings, with slowed response to stimuli.

opacification   The increase in CT density of a structure due to filling with positive contrast material.

operating system (OS)   The main software of the CT computer, controlling the utilization of the hardware resources including the available memory, central processing unit time, disk space, and so on.

orthogonal   Imaging planes that are perpendicular to each other.

orthographic volume rendering   Technique yielding a 3D model with the perspective of externally viewing the reconstructed object.

osmolality   The propensity of an iodinated contrast medium to cause fluid from outside the blood vessel to move into the bloodstream.

out-of-field artifact   Hyperdense streaking that occurs when a portion of the patient has been positioned outside the scan field of view (SFOV).

overbeaming   Expansion of the primary beam in an MSCT system to ensure that all detectors of the array are exposed to x-rays of equal intensity.

overlapping images   CT images produced with a reconstruction interval that is less than the section width.

overranging   The process of applying radiation dose before and after the acquisition volume to ensure sufficient data collection for the interpolation algorithms of helical CT reconstruction.

PACS   Acronym for a picture archival and communications system. Responsible for storing, retrieving, distributing, and displaying CT and other digital medical images.

pancreatic phase   A delayed arterial enhancement phase occurring approximately 35 to 45 seconds after the start of contrast agent administration, if an adequate volume has been injected at a rate of 3 mL/sec or greater.

parallel processing   The ability of a computer to perform multiple functions simultaneously.

partial volume artifact   An error that occurs when a structure is only partly positioned within a voxel and the attenuation for the object is not accurately represented by a pixel value.

partial volume averaging   Inaccuracy in pixel values that occurs when the associated voxels contain attenuation coefficients for multiple tissue types. The values are averaged together to yield a single pixel value that attempts to represent an assortment of different materials.

perspective volume rendering Technique yielding a 3D model with the perspective of being within the lumen of the object, similar to an endoscopic view. May also be referred to as *immersive rendering*.

phantom A quality control device typically composed of a radiolucent plastic material containing specialized inserts that is used to measure specific image quality criteria.

photodiode Device used by a solid-state CT detector to convert the light emitted by a scintillation crystal into a proportional electronic signal.

photon fluence Quantity of x-ray photons passing through a specified area.

photon flux The rate at which a quantity of x-ray photons (fluence) passes through a unit area over a unit time.

pipelining A form of parallel processing used by a computer to improve computation speed.

pitch The relationship between collimation and table movement per gantry rotation.

pixel Abbreviation of *picture element*. Refers to the individual boxes arranged in the matrix used to display the CT image.

pixel value *See* CT number.

point spread function (PSF) A measure of a CT system's in-plane spatial resolution that evaluates the amount of spread inherent in an orthogonal image of a thin wire.

polyenergetic Consisting of a spectrum of differing energies; used in CT to describe the beam of x-radiation.

portal venous phase Period of peak hepatic parenchymal enhancement when contrast material redistributes from the blood into the extravascular spaces. Typically occurs 60 to 70 seconds after the initiation of contrast agent administration.

prospective ECG gating Method of improving the temporal resolution of an MSCT system during examinations of the heart and mediastinum. Data are acquired in an axial "step-and-shoot" mode and only during the diastolic portion of the R-R interval.

prospective reconstruction The initial construction of the acquired raw data into CT image data with selected display field of view, algorithm, image center, and so on.

pseudoenhancement Minimal increase in attenuation demonstrated by a structure that typically does not enhance after intravenous contrast administration. Most common during MSCT evaluation of cysts.

pulmonary embolism The condition where a thrombus (blood clot) breaks free from elsewhere in the venous system (usually the lower extremities) and migrates into a pulmonary artery. The pulmonary artery becomes blocked, causing reduced blood flow to the lung tissue.

pulmonary hypertension A condition of increased blood pressure in the pulmonary vasculature (i.e., the pulmonary artery, pulmonary vein, and/or pulmonary capillaries).

pulse oximeter An electronic device placed on a patient's finger, toe, or earlobe to measure pulse and blood oxygen levels.

quality assurance The measurement of the scanner's performance through quality testing procedures and evaluation of the test results.

quality control The implementation of corrective actions to improve any identified performance inadequacies of the CT system.

raw data The transmission measurements obtained by the detectors used to mathematically reconstruct the CT image.

ray The portion of the x-ray beam transmitted through the patient and incident upon a single detector.

ray sum The measurement of transmitted radiation made by an individual detector used to determine the attenuation occurring along a ray.

region of interest (ROI) A user-defined graphic outline that calculates the average CT number of a given anatomic area.

rendering Use of 3D algorithms to provide a specific perspective to the construction of a 3D model.

response time The ability of a CT detector to quickly measure x-ray and then recover before the next measurement.

retrospective ECG gating Method of improving the temporal resolution of an MSCT system during CT examinations of the heart and mediastinum. Only data acquired during diastole are used for image reconstruction, allowing for a reduction of motion artifact in the CT image.

retrospective reconstruction Reconstruction performed after the initial prospective reconstruction. Multiple retrospective reconstructions of raw data are possible, with changes to display field of view, algorithm, image center, and so on.

ring artifact An incorrect ring of density on the reconstructed CT image resulting from detector malfunction.

saddle pulmonary embolism A condition where a large clot (thrombus) straddles the main trunk of the pulmonary artery as it bifurcates into the left and right pulmonary arteries.

saline flush Injection of a volume of normal saline solution immediately after the bolus administration of an iodinated contrast agent. The saline flushes any remaining contrast agent through the automated injector tubing, improving the efficiency of contrast agent utilization.

scan delay The time between the initiation of contrast agent administration and CT data acquisition. The chosen scan delay determines the phase of contrast enhancement for a given CT acquisition.

scan field of view (SFOV) A parameter that controls the diameter of the circular data acquisition field within the CT gantry as determined by the number of activated detectors along the x-y axis. May also be referred to as the *calibration field*.

scintillation The production of light energy by a CT detector material in response to absorbed x-ray energy.

scout image Digital survey radiograph acquired by the CT system for the purpose of prescribing the cross-sectional acquisition. Similar to a conventional radiograph, the scout view is produced by translating the patient through the gantry without tube and detector rotation. May also be referred to as a *topogram, scanogram,* or *survey radiograph*.

section interval The distance between the center of one CT section and the center of the next adjacent section.

section width The dimension of a reconstructed CT slice along the longitudinal direction of acquisition (z-axis). Commonly referred to as *slice thickness*.

shaded surface display (SSD) *See* surface rendering.

signal Electronic current emitted by the CT detector in response to the absorption and measurement of transmitted radiation.

signal-to-noise ratio (SNR)   Quantification of the amount of noise in a displayed CT image. SNR is calculated as the standard deviation in the ROI measurement of a water phantom image.

single-slice CT (SSCT)   A CT system with a single row of detectors capable of acquiring only one image section for each gantry rotation.

slice sensitivity profile (SSP)   Graph demonstrating the broadening of the section width that is inherent to volumetric (helical) CT acquisition.

slice thickness   *See* section width.

slip-ring   The rotating assembly used to enable the passage of electrical signal during continuous rotation of the helical CT system.

spatial frequency   The waveform of signal that represents the varied objects imaged by a CT system.

spatial resolution   The ability of a CT imaging system to display fine details separately. Given in units of line pairs per centimeter (lp/cm).

spiral   *See* helical.

step artifact   The unwanted appearance of individual sections on a multiplanar or 3D reformation image resulting in a loss of sharpness and detail.

stranding   Hazy increase in density of the fat surrounding an organ on CT examination that usually indicates an inflammatory process.

stupor   A semicomatose state of consciousness where the individual is nearly unresponsive to stimuli.

surface rendering   Construction of a 3D model of a specific tissue type by limiting the displayed volumetric data on the basis of an attenuation threshold. May also be referred to as *shaded surface display (SSD)*.

systole   Portion of the cardiac cycle when the heart muscle is in contraction. Systolic blood pressure reflects the force exhibited on the arterial walls during ventricular contraction. It is the top or first number provided during the assessment of blood pressure.

teleradiology   The transmission of image data across networks from the imaging facility to an off-site location for review and interpretation.

temporal resolution   The ability of a CT system to freeze motion and provide an image free of blurring.

total collimation   The combined thickness of all of the sections that are simultaneously acquired with each gantry rotation during MSCT acquisition.

triple rule-out   Comprehensive MSCT examination of the chest for cardiac and noncardiac pain. The single acquisition evaluates for coronary artery disease, aortic aneurysm, and pulmonary embolism.

tube arcing   Short circuiting within the x-ray tube during data acquisition that results in severe streak artifacts in the CT image.

uniform matrix array   The type of MSCT detector array that utilizes multiple detectors in the longitudinal direction, each of the same length.

uniformity   Maintenance of relatively consistent CT values across the entire image of an object of equal density.

urticaria   Itchy, red rash commonly referred to as *hives*.

Valsalva effect   Temporary rise in blood pressure that may occur during forceful exhalation.

view   Each data sample made by the DAS during CT data acquisition.

views per rotation (VPR)   The sampling rate of transmission measurements acquired during each gantry rotation.

virtual bronchography   Three-dimensional fly-through endobrachial views included in a CT bronchography examination.

volume rendering   A 3D modeling technique that utilizes the entire acquired data set but adjusts the opacity of voxels included in the 3D image according to their tissue characteristics.

voxel   Abbreviation of *volume element*. Refers to the volume of tissue represented by a pixel in the matrix used to display the CT image.

window   The user-defined range of pixel values that will be assigned a particular shade of gray.

window level (WL)   The pixel value, given in HU, at the center of the window width. Window level controls the brightness (density) of the CT image.

window width (WW)   The range of pixel values assigned a shade of gray in the displayed CT image. Window width controls the contrast of the CT image.

windowing   The process of grayscale mapping of the CT image on the basis of the CT number (Hounsfield value) assigned to each pixel.

x-y axis   The plane perpendicular (orthogonal) to the axis of data acquisition (z-axis). The x-y axis is parallel to the plane of the CT gantry.

z-axis   Longitudinal direction of the coordinate system used to spatially describe the location of acquired CT sections. The z-axis corresponds to the axis of data acquisition.

z-filtering   Mathematical process utilized by MSCT systems to reconstruct thin sections at any point along the acquired z-axis volume.

Abbara S, Soni AV, Cury RC: Evaluation of cardiac function and valves by multidetector row computed tomography, *Semin Roentgenol* 43:145–153, 2008.

Achenbach S, Kondo T, Narula J: Computed Tomography Imaging in 2012, *Cardiol Clin* 30(1):1–160, 2012.

American College of Radiology: *Manual on contrast media, version 10.2*, Reston, VA, 2016, American College of Radiology.

Adler AM, Carlton RR: *Introduction to radiologic sciences and patient care*, ed 5, Philadelphia, 2012, Elsevier.

Agarwal PP, Chughtai A, Matzinger FRK, Kazerooni EA: Multidetector CT of thoracic aortic aneurysms, *Radiographics* 29:537–552, 2009.

Aird EGA, Conway J: CT simulation for radiotherapy treatment planning, *Br J Radiol* 75:937–949, 2002.

Akbar SA, Mortele KJ, Baeyens K, et al: Multidetector CT urography: techniques, clinical applications, and pitfalls, *Semin Ultrasound CT MRI* 25:41–54, 2004.

American Association of Physicists in Medicine. *AAPM position statement on the use of bismuth shielding for the purpose of dose reduction in CT scanning*. http://www.aapm.org/publicgeneral/BismuthShielding.pdf. Published February 7, 2012. Accessed December August 1, 2016.

American College of Radiology: *ACR practice guideline for the performance of high-resolution computed tomography (HRCT) of the lungs in adults*, Reston, VA, 2005, American College of Radiology.

Bae KT, Heiken JP, Siegel GL, Bennett HF: Renal cysts: is attenuation artifactually increased on contrast-enhanced CT images?, *Radiology* 216:792–796, 2000.

Barrett CP, Anderson LD, Holder L, Poliakoff S: *Primer of sectional anatomy with MRI and CT correlation*, ed 2, Baltimore, 1994, Williams & Wilkins.

Barrett JF, Keat N: Artifacts in CT: recognition and avoidance, *Radiographics* 24:1679–1691, 2004.

Bauhs JA, Vrieze TJ, Primak AN, et al: CT dosimetry: comparison of measurement techniques and devices, *Radiographics* 28:245–253, 2008.

Becker CR, Wintersperger B, Jakobs TF: Multi-detector-row CT angiography of peripheral arteries, *Semin Ultrasound CT MR* 24:268–279, 2003.

Belden CJ, Zinreich SJ: Orbital imaging techniques, *Semin Ultrasound CT MR* 18:413–422, 1997.

Belfiore G, Tedeschi E, Ronza FM, et al: CT-guided radiofrequency ablation in the treatment of recurrent rectal cancer, *AJR Am J Roentgenol* 192:137–141, 2009.

Berland LL: *Practical CT: technology and techniques*, New York, 1987, Raven Press.

Bettmann MA: Frequently asked questions: iodinated contrast agents, *Radiographics* 4:S3S10, 2004.

Bhalla S, West OC: CT of nontraumatic thoracic aortic emergencies, *Semin Ultrasound CT MR* 26:281–304, 2005.

Blake MA, Kalra MK, Sweeney AT, et al: Distinguishing benign from malignant adrenal masses: multi-detector row CT protocol with 10-minute delay, *Radiology* 238:578–585, 2006.

Blebea JS, Meilstrup JW, Wise SW: Appendiceal imaging: which test is best?, *Semin Ultrasound CT MR* 24:91–95, 2003.

Blodgett T: Best practices in PET/CT: consensus on performance of positron emission tomography-computed tomography, *Semin Ultrasound CT MR* 29:236–241, 2008.

Blodgett TM, Meltzer CC, Townsend DW: PET/CT: form and function, *Radiology* 242:360–385, 2007.

Bluemke DA, Urban B, Fishman EK: Spiral CT of the liver: current applications, *Semin Ultrasound CT MR* 15:107–121, 1994.

Bo WJ, Wolfman NT, Krueger WA, Meschan I: *Basic atlas of sectional anatomy with correlated imaging*, ed 2, Philadelphia, 1990, Saunders.

Boone JM: Multidetector CT: opportunities, challenges, and concerns associated with scanners with 64 or more detector rows, *Radiology* 241:334–337, 2006.

Boonn WW, Litt HI, Charagundla SR: Optimizing contrast injection for coronary CT angiography and functional cardiac CT: applications in cardiac imaging, *Appl Radiol (Suppl)* 2007.

Brink M, deLange F, Oostveen LJ, et al: Arm raising at exposure-controlled multidetector trauma CT of thoracoabdominal region: higher image quality, lower radiation dose, *Radiology* 249:661–670, 2008.

Broder J: *Diagnostic imaging for the emergency physician*, 2011, Elsevier Health Sciences.

Brown MA: Imaging acute appendicitis, *Semin Ultrasound CT MR* 29:293–307, 2008.

Budoff MJ, Gul K: Computed tomographic cardiovascular imaging, *Semin Ultrasound CT MR* 27:32–41, 2006.

Bushberg JT, Seibert JA, Leidholdt EM, Boone JM: *The essential physics of medical imaging*, Baltimore, 2001, Williams & Wilkins.

Bushong SC: *Computed tomography*, New York, 2000, McGraw-Hill.

Bushong SC: *Radiologic science for technologists*, ed 10, St. Louis, 2013, Elsevier.

Buzug TM: *Computed tomography: from photon statistics to modern cone-beam CT*, Berlin, 2008, Springer-Verlag.

Cademartini F, Luccichenti G, van Der Lugt A, et al: Sixteen-row multislice computed tomography: basic concepts, protocols, and enhanced clinical applications, *Semin Ultrasound CT MR* 25:2–16, 2004.

Carr DH: *Contrast media*, London, 1988, Churchill Livingstone.

Chen JS: Noninvasive coronary plaque evaluation by cardiac CT: applications in cardiac imaging, *Appl Radiol (Suppl)* 2007.

Chen MY: Coronary artery disease assessment with cardiac CT: applications in cardiac imaging, *Appl Radiol (Suppl)* 2007.

Chiu LC, Lipcamon JD, Yiu-Chiu VS: *Clinical computed tomography for the technologist*, New York, 1995, Raven Press.

Christian PE, Waterstram-Rich KM: *Nuclear medicine and PET/CT*, ed 6, St. Louis, 2007, Mosby.

Chung JJ, Cho ES, Kang SM, et al: Usefulness of a lead shielding device for reducing the radiation dose to tissues outside the primary beams during CT, *Radiol Med (Torino)* 119(12):951–957, 2014.

Coakley FV, Gould R, Yeh BM, Arenson RL: CT radiation dose: What can you do right now in your practice?, *AJR Am J Roentgenol* 196(3):619–625, 2011.

Cody DD: AAPM/RSNA physics tutorial for residents: topics in CT: image processing in CT, *Radiographics* 22:1255–1268, 2002.

Cody DD, Mahadevappa M: Technologic advances in multi-detector CT with a focus on cardiac imaging, *Radiographics* 27:1829–1837, 2007.

Colletti PM, Micheli OA, Lee KH: To shield or not to shield: application of bismuth breast shields, *AJR Am J Roentgenol* 200(3):503–507, 2013.

Copstead LEC, Banasik JL: *Pathophysiology*, ed 5, St. Louis, 2013, Elsevier.

Costello JE, Cecava ND, Tucker JE, Bau JL: CT radiation dose: current controversies and dose reduction strategies, *AJR Am J Roentgenol* 201(6):1283–1290, 2013.

Costello P: Spiral CT of the thorax, *Semin Ultrasound CT MR* 15:90–106, 1994.

Creager MA, Beckman JA, Loscalzo J: *Vascular medicine: a companion to Braunwald's heart disease*, 2012, Elsevier Health Sciences.

Crim JR, Moore K, Brodke D: Clearance of the cervical spine in multitrauma patients: the role of advanced imaging, *Semin Ultrasound CT MR* 22:283–305, 2001.

Crim JR, Tripp D: Multidetector CT of the spine, *Semin Ultrasound CT MR* 25:55–66, 2004.

Curry TS, Dowdey JE, Murry RE: *Christensen's physics of diagnostic radiology*, ed 4, Philadelphia, 1990, Lea & Febiger.

Dalrymple NC, Prasad SR, El-Merhi FM, Chintapalli KN: Price of isotropy in multidetector CT, *Radiographics* 27:49–62, 2007.

Dalrymple NC, Srinivasa RP, Prasad SR, Freckleton MW, Kedar NC: Informatics in radiology (infoRAD): introduction to the language of three-dimensional imaging with multidetector CT, *Radiographics* 25:1409–1428, 2005.

DeMaio D: *Registry review in computed tomography*, Philadelphia, 1996, Saunders.

DeMaio DN, Turk J, Palmer E: Shielding in Computed Tomography: An Update, *Radiol Technol* 85(5):563–570, 2014.

Desser TS, Gross M: Multidetector row computed tomography of small bowel obstruction, *Semin Ultrasound CT MR* 29:308–321, 2008.

De Wever W, Bogaert J, Verschakelen JA: Virtual bronchoscopy: accuracy and usefulness—an overview, *Semin Ultrasound CT MR* 26:364–373, 2005.

Ehrlich RA, McCloskey ED, Daly JA: *Patient care in radiography*, ed 9, St. Louis, 2017, Mosby.

Einstein AJ, Elliston CD, Groves DW, et al: Effect of bismuth breast shielding on radiation dose and image quality in coronary CT angiography, *J Nucl Cardiol* 19(1):100–108, 2012.

Einstein AJ, Moser KW, Thompson RC, et al: Radiation dose to patients from cardiac diagnostic imaging, *Circulation* 116:1290–1305, 2007.

El-Khoury GY, Montgomery WJ, Bergman RA: *Sectional anatomy by MRI and CT*, ed 3, Philadelphia, 2007, Churchill Livingstone.

Fefferman NR, Roche KJ, Pinkney LP, et al: Suspected appendicitis in children: focused CT technique for evaluation, *Radiology* 220:691–695, 2001.

Filipek MS, Gosselin MV: Multidetector pulmonary CT angiography: advances in the evaluation of pulmonary arterial diseases, *Semin Ultrasound CT MR* 25:83–98, 2004.

Firooznia H, Golimbu CN, Rafii M, et al: *MRI and CT of the musculoskeletal system*, St. Louis, 1992, Mosby-Year Book.

Fishman EK, Jeffrey RB: *Spiral CT: principles, techniques and clinical applications*, New York, 1995, Raven Press.

Fiss DM: Normal coronary anatomy and anatomic variations: applications in cardiac imaging, *Appl Radiol (Suppl)* 2007.

Fleischmann D: A practical approach to contrast delivery for peripheral CTA, *Appl Radiol (Suppl)* 2004.

Fletcher JG, Kofler JM, Coburn JA, et al: Perspective on radiation risk in CT imaging, *Abdom Imaging* 38(1):22–31, 2013.

Flohr TG, Schaller S, Stierstorfer K, et al: Multi-detector row CT systems and image-reconstruction techniques, *Radiology* 235:756–773, 2005.

Flukinger T, White CS: Multidetector computed tomography in the evaluation of chest pain in the emergency department, *Semin Roentgenol* 43:136–144, 2008.

Foley WD, Kerimoglu U: Abdominal MDCT: liver, pancreas, and biliary tract, *Semin Ultrasound CT MR* 25:122–144, 2004.

Frank ED, Long BW, Smith BJ: *Merrill's atlas of radiographic positioning and procedures*, ed 13, St. Louis, 2015, Mosby.

Frush DP: Review of radiation issues for computed tomography, *Semin Ultrasound CT MR* 25:17–24, 2004.

Frush DP, Soden B, Frush KS, Lowry C: Improved pediatric multidetector body CT using a size-based color-coded format, *AJR Am J Roentgenol* 178:721–726, 2002.

Furlow B: *Computed tomography and magnetic resonance angiography*, 1999, American Society of Radiologic Technologists (ASRT).

Gao SY, Tang L, Cui Y, et al: Tumor angiogenesis-related parameters in multi-phase enhanced CT correlated with outcomes of hepatocellular carcinoma patients after radical hepatectomy, *Eur J Surg Oncol* 42(4):538–544, 2016.

Gedgaudas-McClees RK, Torres WE: *Essentials of body computed tomography*, Philadelphia, 1990, Saunders.

Gerber TC, Breen JF, Kuzo RS, et al: Computed tomographic angiography of the coronary arteries: techniques and applications, *Semin Ultrasound CT MR* 27:42–55, 2006.

Geyer LL, et al: State of the art: iterative CT reconstruction techniques, *Radiology* 276(2):339–357, 2015.

Goldman LW: Principles of CT and CT technology, *J Nucl Med Technol* 35:115–128, 2007.

Goldman LW: Principles of CT: radiation dose and image quality, *J Nucl Med Technol* 35:213–225, 2007.

Goldman LW: Principles of CT: multislice CT, *J Nucl Med Technol* 36:57–68, 2008.

Gonzalez-Beicos A, Nunez DB Jr: Role of multidetector computed tomography in the assessment of cervical spine trauma, *Semin Ultrasound CT MR* 30:159–167, 2009.

Green D, Parker D: CTA and MRA: visualization without catheterization, *Semin Ultrasound CT MR* 24:185–191, 2003.

Grenier PA, Beigelman-Aubry C, Fetita C, Martin-Bouyer Y: Multidetector-row CT of the airways, *Semin Roentgenol* 38:146–157, 2003.

Gruden JF, Tigges S, Baron MG, Pearlman H: MDCT pulmonary angiography: image processing tools, *Semin Roentgenol* 40:48–63, 2005.

Gupta R, Cheung AC, Bartling SH, et al: Flat-panel volume CT, fundamental principles, technology, and applications, *Radiographics* 28:2009–2022, 2008.

Guyton AC, Hall JE: *Textbook of medical physiology*, ed 11, Philadelphia, 2006, Saunders.

Haaga JR, Lanzieri CF, Gilkeson RC: *CT and MR imaging of the whole body*, ed 4, St. Louis, 2003, Mosby.

Haage P, Schmitz-Rode T, Hübner D, et al: Reduction of contrast material dose and artifacts by a saline flush using a double power injector in helical CT of the thorax, *AJR Am J Roentgenol* 174:1049–1053, 2000.

Herts BR, O'Malley CM, Wirth SL, et al: Power injection of contrast media using central venous catheters: feasibility, safety, and efficacy, *AJR Am J Roentgenol* 176:447–453, 2001.

Hoeffner EG, Case I, Jain R, et al: Cerebral perfusion CT: technique and clinical applications, *Radiology* 231:632–644, 2004.

Hofer M: *CT teaching manual*, ed 3, New York, 2007, Thieme.

Hofmann LK, Becker CR, Flohr T, Schoepf UJ: Multidetector-row CT of the heart, *Semin Roentgenol* 38:135–145, 2003.

Hollingsworth C, Frush DP, Cross M, Lucaya J: Helical CT of the body: a survey of techniques used for pediatric patients, *AJR Am J Roentgenol* 180:401–406, 2003.

Hopper KD: CT bronchoscopy, *Semin Ultrasound CT MR* 20:10–15, 1999.

Hopper KD: Orbital, thyroid, and breast superficial radiation shielding for patients undergoing diagnostic CT, *Semin Ultrasound CT MR* 23:423–427, 2002.

Horn AE, Ufberg JW: Appendicitis, diverticulitis, and colitis, *Emerg Med Clin North Am* 29(2):347–368, 2011.

Huda W, Ogden KM, Khorasani MR: Converting dose-length product to effective dose at CT, *Radiology* 248:995–1003, 2008.

Huda W, Ravenel JG, Scalzetti EM: How do radiographic techniques affect image quality and patient doses in CT?, *Semin Ultrasound CT MR* 23:411–422, 2002.

Hunsaker AR: Multidetector-row CT and interstitial lung disease, *Semin Roentgenol* 38:176–185, 2003.

Hurwitz LM, Yoshizumi TT, Goodman PC, et al: Radiation dose savings for adult pulmonary embolus 64-MDCT using bismuth breast shields, lower peak kilovoltage, and automatic tube current modulation, *AJR Am J Roentgenol* 192:244–253, 2009.

Hutchison SJ, Merchant N: *Principles of cardiac and vascular computed tomography: expert consult*, 2014, Elsevier Health Sciences.

Iball GR, Brettle DS: Organ and effective dose reduction in adult chest CT using abdominal lead shielding, *Br J Radiol* 2014.

Israel GM, Bosniak MA: How I do it: evaluating renal masses, *Radiology* 236:441–450, 2005.

Jacobs JE, Birnbaum BA: CT imaging in acute appendicitis: techniques and controversies, *Semin Ultrasound CT MR* 24:96–100, 2003.

Jakobs TF, Wintersperger BJ, Becker CR: MDCT-imaging of peripheral arterial disease, *Semin Ultrasound CT MR* 25:145–155, 2004.

Jeffrey RB Jr: CT angiography of the abdominal and thoracic aorta, *Semin Ultrasound CT MR* 19:405–412, 1998.

Jensen SC, Peppers MP: *Pharmacology and drug administration for imaging technologists*, ed 2, St. Louis, 2006, Elsevier.

Judy PF: Multidetector-Row CT image quality and radiation dose: imaging the lung, *Semin Roentgenol* 38:186–192, 2003.

Kalender WA: Technical foundations of spiral CT, *Semin Ultrasound CT MR* 15:81–89, 1994.

Kalender WA: Thin-section three-dimensional spiral CT: is isotropic imaging possible?, *Radiology* 197:578–580, 1995.

Kalender WA: *Computed tomography*, ed 3, Erlangen, 2011, Germany, Publicis Corporate Publishing.

Kalender WA: Dose in x-ray computed tomography, *Phys Med Biol* 59(3):R129, 2014.

Kalra MK, Maher MM, Toth TL, et al: Strategies for CT radiation dose optimization, *Radiology* 230:619–628, 2004.

Kalra MK, Maher MM, Toth TL, et al: Techniques and applications of automatic tube current modulation for CT, *Radiology* 233:649–657, 2004.

Kanada D, Catanzano TM: The role of cardiac CT for function: evaluation of perfusion, volumetric analysis, and regional wall motion assessment: applications in cardiac imaging, *Appl Radiol (Suppl)* 2007.

Kapoor V, McCook BM, Torok FS: An introduction to PET-CT imaging, *Radiographics* 24:523–543, 2004.

Katz DS, Loud PA, Hurewitz AN, et al: CT venography in suspected pulmonary thromboembolism, *Semin Ultrasound CT MR* 25:67–80, 2004.

Katzberg RW: *The contrast media manual*, Baltimore, 1992, Williams & Wilkins.

Kawamoto S, Johnson PT, Fishman EK: Three-dimensional CT angiography of the thorax: clinical applications, *Semin Ultrasound CT MR* 19:425–438, 1998.

Kawashima A, Vrtiska TJ, LeRoy AJ, et al: CT urography, *Radiographics* 24:S35S58, 2004.

Kelley LL, Petersen CM: *Sectional anatomy for imaging professionals*, ed 3, St. Louis, 2013, Mosby.

Knollman F, Coakley FV: *Multislice CT: principles and protocols*, Philadelphia, 2006, Elsevier.

Kok M, et al: Automated Tube Voltage Selection for Radiation Dose Reduction in CT Angiography Using Different Contrast Media Concentrations and a Constant Iodine Delivery Rate, *AJR Am J Roentgenol* 205(6):1332–1338, 2015.

Kuszyk BS, Beauchamp NJ, Fishman EK: Neurovascular applications of CT angiography, *Semin Ultrasound CT MR* 19:394–404, 1998.

Kuszyk BS, Fishman EK: Technical aspects of CT angiography, *Semin Ultrasound CT MR* 19:383–393, 1998.

Lake DR, Kavanagh JJ, Ravenel JG, et al: Computed tomography and pulmonary embolus: a review, *Semin Ultrasound CT MR* 26:270–280, 2005.

Lane A, Sharfaei H: *Modern sectional anatomy*, Philadelphia, 1992, Saunders.

Lane JI, Lindell EP, Witte RJ, et al: Middle and inner ear: improved depiction with multiplanar reconstruction of volumetric CT data, *Radiographics* 26:115–124, 2006.

Laudicina P, Wean D: *Applied angiography for radiographers*, Philadelphia, 1994, Saunders.

Lawler LP, Pannu HK, Fishman EK: MDCT evaluation of the coronary arteries, 2004: how we do it—data acquisition, postprocessing, display, and interpretation, *AJR Am J Roentgenol* 184:1402–1412, 2005.

Lee CH, Goo JM, Ye HJ, et al: Radiation dose modulation techniques in the multidetector CT era: from basics to practice, *Radiographics* 28:1451–1459, 2008.

Lee JKT, Sagel SS, Stanley RJ, Heiken JP: *Computed body tomography with MRI correlation*, ed 4, Philadelphia, 2006, Lippincott Williams & Wilkins.

Lee MJ, Kim S, Lee SA, et al: Overcoming artifacts from metallic orthopedic implants at high-field-strength MR imaging and multidetector CT, *Radiographics* 27:791–803, 2007.

Lell MM, Anders K, Uder M, et al: New techniques in CT angiography, *Radiographics* 26:S45S62, 2006.

Lewis MA: Patient dose reduction in CT, *Br J Radiol* 78:880–883, 2005.

Lira D, Padole A, Kalra MK, Singh S: Tube potential and CT radiation dose optimization, *AJR Am J Roentgenol* 204(1):W4–W10, 2015.

Loud PA, Katz DS, Belfi L, Grossman ZD: Imaging of deep venous thrombosis in suspected pulmonary embolism, *Semin Roentgenol* 40:33–40, 2005.

Luetmer PH, Mokri B: Dynamic CT myelography: a technique for localizing-high-flow spinal cerebrospinal fluid leaks, *AJNR Am J Neuroradiol* 24:1711–1714, 2003.

MacDonald SLS, Mayo JR: Computed tomography of acute pulmonary embolism, *Semin Ultrasound CT MR* 24:217–231, 2003.

Madden ME: *Introduction to sectional anatomy*, 3rd ed, 2013, Lippincott Williams & Wilkins.

Maglinte DD, Sandrasegaran K, Lappas JC, Chiorean M: CT enteroclysis, *Radiology* 245:661–671, 2007.

Mahesh M: The AAPM/RSNA physics tutorial for residents: search for isotropic resolution in CT from conventional through multiple-row detector, *Radiographics* 22:949–962, 2002.

Mahesh M, Scatarige JC, Cooper J, Fishman EK: Dose and pitch relationship for a particular multislice CT scanner, *AJR Am J Roentgenol* 177:1273–1275, 2001.

Mangold S, et al: Automated tube voltage selection for radiation dose and contrast medium reduction at coronary CT angiography using 3rd generation dual-source CT, *Eur Radiol* 26(10):3608–3616, 2016.

Mason RJ, Broaddus VC, Martin TR, et al: *Murray and Nadel's textbook of respiratory medicine: 2-volume set*, 6th ed, 2015, Elsevier Health Sciences.

Mayo JR, Leipsic JA: Radiation dose in cardiac CT, *AJR Am J Roentgenol* 192:646–653, 2009.

Mayo-Smith WW, Hara AK, Mahesh M, et al: How I do it: managing radiation dose in CT, *Radiology* 273(3):657–672, 2014.

McCollough CH: Standardization in CT terminology: a physicist's perspective, *Radiology* 241:661–662, 2006.

McCollough CH, Bruesewitz MR, Kofler JM: CT dose reduction and dose management tools: overview of available options, *Radiographics* 26:503–512, 2006.

McCollough CH, Wang J, Gould RG, Orton CG: The use of bismuth breast shields for CT should be discouraged, *Med Phys* 39(5):2321–2324, 2012.

McNitt-Gray MF: AAPM/RSNA physics tutorial for residents: topics in CT: radiation dose in CT, *Radiographics* 22:1541–1553, 2002.

Medical Imaging and Technology Alliance. [Internet] 2015 (Accessed 21 Apr 2017). http://www.medicalimaging.org/policy-and-positions/mita-smart-dose/.

Menke J: Comparison of different body size parameters for individual dose adaptation in body CT of adults, *Radiology* 236:565–571, 2005.

Mikla VI, Mikla VV: *Medical imaging technology*, 2013, Elsevier.

Mochizuki T, Hosoi S, Higashino H, et al: Assessment of coronary artery and cardiac function using multidetector CT, *Semin Ultrasound CT MR* 25:99–112, 2004.

Moloo J, Shapiro MD, Abbara S: Cardiac computed tomography: technique and optimization of protocols, *Semin Roentgenol* 43:90–99, 2008.

Mosby's Dictionary of Medicine: *Nursing & health professions*, ed 10, St. Louis, 2017, Mosby.

Moser JB, et al: Radiation dose-reduction strategies in thoracic CT, *Clin Radiol* 2017.

Moser T, Dosch JC, Moussaoui A, et al: Multidetector CT arthrography of the wrist joint: how to do it, *Radiographics* 28:787–800, 2008.

Moss AA, Gamsu GG, Genant HK: *Computed tomography of the body with magnetic resonance imaging*, ed 2, Philadelphia, 1992, Saunders.

Mullins ME, Kircher MF, Ryan DP, et al: Evaluation of suspected appendicitis in children using limited helical CT and colonic contrast material, *AJR Am J Roentgenol* 176:37–41, 2001.

Murray JG, Gean AD, Evans SJ: Imaging of acute head injury, *Semin Ultrasound CT MR* 17:185–205, 1996.

Naidich DP, Webb WR, Müller NL, et al: *Computed tomography and magnetic resonance of the thorax*, ed 4, Philadelphia, 2007, Lippincott Williams & Wilkins.

Newbold K, Partridge M, Cook G, et al: Advanced imaging applied to radiotherapy planning in head and neck cancer: a clinical review, *Br J Radiol* 79:554–561, 2006.

Newman J, Hladik WB: Pharmacology for the radiologic technologist. Part 2: intravascular radiopaque contrast media, *ASRT Homestudy Series* 2(2):1997.

Nghiem HV, Jeffrey RB Jr: CT Angiography of the visceral vasculature, *Semin Ultrasound CT MR* 19:439–446, 1998.

Nguyen BT, Mulins ME: Computed tomography follow-up imaging of stroke, *Semin Ultrasound CT MR* 27:168–176, 2006.

Nguyen L, Cook SC: Coarctation of the aorta: strategies for improving outcomes, *Cardiol Clin* 33(4):521–530, 2015.

Nickoloff EL, Lu ZF, Dutta AK, So JC: Radiation dose descriptors: bERT, COD, DAP, and other strange creatures, *Radiographics* 28:1439–1450, 2008.

Niederhuber JE: *Abeloff's Clinical Oncology*, Philadelphia, 2014, Churchill Livingstone Elsevier, p 2014.

Nørgaard BL, Leipsic J, Gaur S, et al: Diagnostic performance of noninvasive fractional flow reserve derived from coronary computed tomography angiography in suspected coronary artery disease: the NXT trial (Analysis of Coronary Blood Flow Using CT Angiography: Next Steps), *J Am Coll Cardiol* 63(12):1145–1155, 2014.

Padole A, et al: CT radiation dose and iterative reconstruction techniques, *AJR Am J Roentgenol* 204(4):W384–W392, 2015.

Parry RA, Glaze SA, Archer BR: The AAPM/RSNA physics tutorial for residents: typical patient radiation doses in diagnostic radiology, *Radiographics* 19:1289–1302, 1999.

Patel S: Normal and anomalous anatomy of the coronary arteries. In *Seminars in roentgenology*, vol 43, No. 2, 2008, WB Saunders, pp 100–112.

Patel S, Lieberman S: Computed tomography of coronary artery disease, *Semin Roentgenol* 43:122–135, 2008.

Paulsen SR, Huprich JE, Fletcher JG, et al: CT enterography as a diagnostic tool in evaluating small bowel disorders: review of clinical experience with over 700 cases, *Radiographics* 26:641–662, 2006.

Pickhardt PJ: Screening CT colonography: how I do it, *AJR Am J Roentgenol* 189:290–298, 2007.

Pomerantz SR, Harris GJ, et al: Computed tomography angiography and computed tomography perfusion in ischemic stroke: a step-by-step approach to image acquisition and three-dimensional postprocessing, *Semin Ultrasound CT MR* 27:243–270, 2006.

Prat-Gonzalez S, Sanz J, Garcia MJ: Cardiac CT: indications and limitations, *J Nucl Med Technol* 36:18–24, 2008.

Primak AN, McCollough CH, Bruesewitz MR, et al: Relationship between noise, dose, and pitch in cardiac multi-detector row CT, *Radiographics* 26:1785–1794, 2006.

Putman CE, Ravin CE: *Textbook of diagnostic imaging*, ed 2, Philadelphia, 1994, Saunders.

Raman SP, Mahesh M, Blasko RV, Fishman EK: CT scan parameters and radiation dose: practical advice for radiologists, *J Am Coll Radiol* 10(11):840–846, 2013.

Ramirez-Giraldo JC, Fuld M, Grant K, et al: New approaches to reduce radiation while maintaining image quality in multi-detector-computed tomography, *Curr Radiol Rep* 3(2):1–15, 2015.

Ravenel JG, Kipfmueller F, Schoepf UJ: CT angiography with multidetector-row CT for detection of acute pulmonary embolus, *Semin Roentgenol* 40:11–19, 2005.

Renne J, et al: CT angiography for pulmonary embolism detection: the effect of breathing on pulmonary artery enhancement using a 64-row detector system, *Acta Radiology* 55(8):932–937, 2014.

Rivitz SM, Drucker EA: Power injection of peripherally inserted central catheters, *J Vasc Interv Radiol* 8:857–863, 1997.

Rubin GD: CT angiography of the thoracic aorta, *Semin Roentgenol* 38:115–134, 2003.

Rubin GD, Rofsky NM: *CT and MR angiography: comprehensive vascular assessment*, Philadelphia, 2008, Lippincott Williams & Wilkins.

Rumberger JA: Coronary artery calcium scanning using computed tomography: clinical recommendations for cardiac risk assessment and treatment, *Semin Ultrasound CT MR* 29:223–229, 2008.

Samei E: Pros and cons of organ shielding for CT imaging, *Pediatr Radiol* 44(3):495–500, 2014.

Saini S: Multi-detector row CT: principles and practice for abdominal applications, *Radiology* 233:323–327, 2004.

Saini S, Rubin GD, Kalra MK: *MDCT: a practical approach*, Milan, 2006, Springer-Verlag.

Schnapauff D, Zimmermann E, Dewey M: Technical and clinical aspects of coronary computed tomography angiography, *Semin Ultrasound CT MR* 29:167–175, 2008.

Schoepf UJ, Costello P: Multidetector-row CT imaging of pulmonary embolism, *Semin Roentgenol* 38:106–114, 2003.

Schoepf UJ, Costello P: CT angiography for diagnosis of pulmonary embolism: state of the art, *Radiology* 230:329–337, 2004.

Schwartz RB: Neuroradiological applications of spiral CT, *Semin Ultrasound CT MR* 15:139–147, 1994.

Sechopoulos I, Trianni A, Peck D: The DICOM radiation dose structured report: what it is and what it is not, *J Am Coll Radiol* 12(7):712–713, 2015.

Seeram E: *Computed tomography: a study guide and review*, Philadelphia, 1997, Saunders.

Seeram E: *Computed tomography*, ed 4, St. Louis, 2016, Saunders.

Semba CP, Rubin GD, Dake MD: Three-dimensional spiral CT angiography of the abdomen, *Semin Ultrasound CT MR* 15:133–138, 1994.

Servaes S, Zhu X: The effects of bismuth breast shields in conjunction with automatic tube current modulation in CT imaging, *Pediatr Radiol* 43(10):1287–1294, 2013.

Shaked O, Siegelman ES, Olthoff K, Reddy KR: Biologic and clinical features of benign solid and cystic lesions of the liver, *Clin Gastroenterol Hepatol* 9(7):547–562, 2011.

Shanmuganathan K: Multi-detector row CT imaging of blunt abdominal trauma, *Semin Ultrasound CT MR* 25:180–204, 2004.

Sheth S, Fishman EK: Multi-detector row CT of the kidneys and urinary tract: techniques and applications in the diagnosis of benign disease, *Radiographics* 24:e20, 2004.

Shetty SK, Lev MH: CT perfusion in acute stroke, *Semin Ultrasound CT MR* 26:404–421, 2005.

Shreve P, January 29–30, 2005 *PET/CT: changing the practice of medical imaging—PET-CT protocols and techniques. Program and abstracts of the society of nuclear medicine mid-winter educational symposium Tampa, FL.*

Silverman PM: *Multislice computed tomography,* Philadelphia, 2002, Lippincott Williams & Wilkins.

Silverman SG, Leyendecker JR, Amis ES Jr: What is the current role of CT urography and MR urography in the evaluation of the urinary tract?, *Radiology* 250:309–323, 2009.

Singh J, Daftary A: Iodinated contrast media and their adverse reactions, *J Nucl Med Technol* 36:69–74, 2008.

Sistrom CL, Gay SB, Peffley L: Extravasation of iopamidol and iohexol during contrast-enhanced CT: report of 28 cases, *Radiology* 180:707–710, 1991.

Smith AB, Dillon WP, Lau BC, et al: Radiation dose reduction strategy for CT protocols: successful implementation in neuroradiology section, *Radiology* 247:499–506, 2008.

Smith PA, Fishman EK: Three-dimensional CT angiography: renal applications, *Semin Ultrasound CT MR* 19:413–424, 1998.

Snopek AM: *Fundamentals of special radiographic procedures,* ed 5, St. Louis, 2006, Elsevier.

Spearman JV, Schoepf UJ, Rottenkolber M, et al: Effect of automated attenuation-based tube voltage selection on radiation dose at CT: an observational study on a global scale, *Radiology* 279(1):167–174, 2015.

Srinivasan A, Goyal M, Al Azri F, Lum C: State-of-the-art imaging of acute stroke, *Radiographics* 26:S75S95, 2006.

Staffey KS, van Beek EJR, Jagasia D: Clinical performance and considerations in coronary CTA: applications in cardiac imaging, *Appl Radiol (Suppl)* 2007.

Standring S: *Gray's anatomy,* ed 40, St. Louis, 2008, Elsevier.

Strauss KJ, Goske MJ, Frush DP, et al: Image gently vendor summit: working together for better estimates of pediatric radiation dose from CT, *AJR Am J Roentgenol* 192:1169–1175, 2009.

Taber's Cyclopedic: *Taber's cyclopedic medical dictionary,* ed 23, Philadelphia, 2013, FA Davis.

Tack D, Gevenois PA: Efforts for lowering radiation dose delivered with CT: raising arms, or is there more?, *Radiology* 249:413–415, 2008.

Takakuwa KM, Halpern EJ: Evaluation of a "triple rule-out" coronary CT angiography protocol: use of 64-Section CT in low-to-moderate risk emergency department patients suspected of having acute coronary syndrome, *Radiology* 248:438–446, 2008.

Taourel P, Thuret R, Devaux-Hoquet M, et al: Computed tomography in the nontraumatic renal causes of acute flank pain, *Semin Ultrasound CT MR* 29:341–352, 2008.

Taylor AJ: *Atlas of cardiovascular computed tomography: an imaging companion to braunwald's heart disease,* 2010, Elsevier Health Sciences.

Tepel M, Aspelin P, Lameire N: Contrast-induced nephropathy: a clinical and evidence-based approach, *Circulation* 113:1799–1806, 2006.

Thomas BP, Strother MK, Donnelly EF, Worrell JA: CT virtual endoscopy in the evaluation of large airway disease: review, *AJR Am J Roentgenol* 192:S20S30, 2009.

Torres LS: *Basic medical techniques and patient care,* ed 4, Philadelphia, 1993, Lippincott Williams and Wilkins.

Tortorici MR, Apfel PJ: *Advanced radiographic and angiographic procedures,* Philadelphia, 1995, FA Davis.

Trotman-Dickenson B, Baumert B: Multidetector-row CT of the solitary pulmonary nodule, *Semin Roentgenol* 38:158–167, 2003.

Valentin J, International commission on radiation protection: managing patient dose in multi-detector computed tomography (MDCT): ICRP publication 102, *Ann ICRP* 37:1–79, 2007.

Vining DJ: Virtual colonoscopy, *Semin Ultrasound CT MR* 20:56–60, 1999.

von Schulthess GK, Steinert HC, Hany TF: Integrated PET/CT: current applications and future directions, *Radiology* 238:405–422, 2006.

Vu D, Lev MH: Noncontrast CT in acute stroke, *Semin Ultrasound CT MR* 26:380–386, 2005.

Wang CL, Cohan RH, Ellis JH, et al: Frequency, management, and outcome of extravasation of nonionic iodinated contrast medium in 69,657 intravenous injections, *Radiology* 180:707–710, 1991.

Wang ZJ, Coakley FV, Fu Y, et al: Renal cyst pseudoenhancement at multidetector CT: what are the effects of number of detectors and peak tube voltage, *Radiology* 248:910–916, 2008.

Webb WR, Brant WE, Major NM: *Fundamentals of body CT,* ed 4, Philadelphia, 2014, Elsevier.

Webb WR, Müller NL, Naidich DP: *High-resolution of the lung,* ed 5, Philadelphia, 2015, Lippincott Williams & Wilkins.

Wesolowski JR, Lev MH: CT: history, technology, and clinical aspects, *Semin Ultrasound CT MR* 26:376–379, 2005.

Wicke L: *Atlas of radiologic anatomy,* ed 5, Philadelphia, 1994, Lea & Febiger.

Wiest PW, Locken JA, Heintz PH, Mettler FA Jr: CT scanning: a major source of radiation exposure, *Semin Ultrasound CT MR* 23:402–410, 2002.

Wijetunga R, Doust B, Bigg-Wither G: The CT diagnosis of acute appendicitis, *Semin Ultrasound CT MR* 24:101–106, 2003.

Williamson EE, McKinney JM: Assessing the adequacy of peripherally inserted central catheters for power injection of intravenous contrast agents for CT, *J Comput Assist Tomogr* 25:932–937, 2001.

Willemink MJ, et al: Iterative reconstruction techniques for computed tomography Part 1: technical principles, *Eur Radiol* 23(6):1623–1631, 2013.

Willemink MJ, et al: Iterative reconstruction techniques for computed tomography part 2: initial results in dose reduction and image quality, *Eur Radiol* 23(6):1632–1642, 2013.

Wintersperger BJ, Nikolaou K, Becker CR: Multidetector-row CT angiography of the aorta and visceral arteries, *Semin Ultrasound CT MR* 25:25–40, 2004.

Wolbarst AB: *Physics of radiology*, Norwalk, CT, 1993, Appleton & Lange.

Wyatt SH, Fishman EK: Spiral CT of the pancreas, *Semin Ultrasound CT MR* 15:122–132, 1994.

Zacharias C, Alessio AM, Otto RK, et al: Pediatric CT: strategies to lower radiation dose, *AJR Am J Roentgenol* 200(5):950–956, 2013.

Zhang J, et al: The Importance of Patient Positioning When Using a Bowtie Filter in Computed Tomography Imaging, *Radiol Technol* 87(6):680–685, 2016.

Zimmermann E, Schnapauff D, Dewey M: Cardiac and coronary anatomy in computed tomography, *Semin Ultrasound CT MR* 29:176–181, 2008.

Zompatori M, Sverzellati N, Poletti V, et al: High-resolution CT in diagnosis of diffuse infiltrative lung disease, *Semin Ultrasound CT MR* 26:332–347, 2005.

A

Abdomen, 55–56
  axial image of, 60f–61f, 63f, 66f
  imaging procedures for, 7
  MIP image of, 65f
  MPR image of, 65f, 67f
  oral contrast agent for, 14
  special procedures for, 71–74
Abdominal aorta, 72, 72f
Abdominal-pelvic cavity, 55
Abscess, 30, 65
Absorbed dose, 24
Accessory spleens, 60
Acetabulum, 81
Acute stroke, 29, 35
Adrenal glands, 61–62
Adrenal "incidentaloma", 61
Adrenal masses, 61
Adults, acute reactions in, management of, 19b
Advanced single-slice rebinding (ASSR) algorithms, 105
Air, 14
Air kerma length product (P_{kl}), 25
Aliasing artifacts, 129
American College of Radiology (ACR) accreditation, 124
American Registry of Radiologic Technologists (ARRT)
  postprimary certification in computed tomography, 3
  study habits and, 4–5
  test-taking techniques and, 4–5
Analog-to-digital converter (ADC), 100
Anaphylactoid reaction, 19b
Angiocatheters, 15
Angiomyolipoma, of kidney, 63
Angular tube current modulation, 23
Ankle
  imaging planes for, 78–79
  MPR
    coronal, 79f
    sagittal, 79f
Anulus fibrosus, 74
Aorta, 53–55
Aortic aneurysm, 53–55
Aortic dissection, 53
Appendicitis, 68
Appendicolith, 68
Appendix, 68
  enlarged, 69f
ARRT. *see* American Registry of Radiologic Technologists
Arterial phase imaging, 71
Arteriovenous malformation, 30
Arthrography, CT, 82
Artifact, 42–43, 124. *see also* Beam hardening artifacts; Cone beam artifacts; Edge gradient artifacts; Equipment-induced artifacts; Hyperdense streaking artifact; Metallic artifacts; Motion artifacts; Out-of-field artifacts; Partial volume artifacts; Pulsation artifacts; Step artifacts; Streaking artifacts
Artifact recognition, 124–129

Artifact reduction, 124–129
Artifactual noise, 121
Aseptic technique, 16
ATCM. *see* Automatic tube current modulation
Attenuation, 21, 103, 125f
Attenuation correction, 85
Attenuation values, 103
Automated bolus-tracking software, 58
Automated tube voltage selection (auto kV), 23
Automatic tube current modulation (ATCM), 56, 90
Axial CT acquisition, 98, 101f
  helical CT acquisition *vs.*, 93f
Azimuth, 88

B

Barium contrast agent, 13
Barium sulfate, 13
Beam collimation, 120
  section width and, 98
Beam hardening artifacts, 28–31, 28f–30f, 91, 124, 124f
Beam pitch, 93
Beam reconstruction algorithm, 105
Bed index, 25
Benign neoplasms, of liver, 57
Benign prostate hyperplasia (BPH), 69
Biliary tract, 59
Biliary tree, 59
Binning, 98
Bismuth shielding, 24, 24f
Bits, 108
Blood-brain barrier, 33
Blood supply, to liver, 58
Blood urea nitrogen (BUN), 11
Body temperature, normal, 9
Body tissues
  Hounsfield values for, 106, 107t
  linear attenuation coefficients for, 107t
Bolus duration, in peripheral CT angiography, 83
Bolus injection, 17
Bone length study, 80
Bow-tie filters, 91
Bowel
  contrast agents for, 65–66
  preparation of, 73
BPH. *see* Benign prostate hyperplasia
Bradycardia, hypotension with, 19b
Brain, imaging in, 28–31
  axial images of, 28–31, 28f–30f
  CTA for, 34–35, 35f
    protocols for, 35
    spiral acquisition, 35
  CTV for, 35
Branches of celiac axis, 72
Breath-hold, 9, 71
Breathing instructions, 8
Bronchography, CT, 55

Page numbers followed by "*f*" indicate figures, "*t*" indicate tables, and "*b*" indicate boxes.